On All Frontiers
Four Centuries of Canadian Nursing

Editors

Christina Bates

Dianne Dodd

Nicole Rousseau

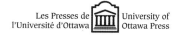
Les Presses de l'Université d'Ottawa — University of Ottawa Press

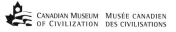
CANADIAN MUSEUM   MUSÉE CANADIEN
OF CIVILIZATION   DES CIVILISATIONS

This book has been published with a financial contribution from the Canadian Museum of Civilization Corporation.

The University of Ottawa Press gratefully acknowledges the support extended to its publishing programme by the Canada Council for the Arts and the University of Ottawa.

We also acknowledge with gratitude the support of the Government of Canada through its Book Publishing Industry Development Program for our publishing activities.

Library and Archives Canada Cataloguing in Publication

On all frontiers : four centuries of Canadian nursing / editors, Christina Bates, Dianne Dodd, Nicole Rousseau.

Co-published by: Canadian Museum of Civilization Corp.
Also issued in French under title: Sans frontières : quatre siècles de soins infirmiers canadiens.
Includes bibliographical references.
ISBN 0-7766-0591-7

1. Nursing–Canada–History. 2. Nurses–Canada–History.
I. Bates, Christina II. Dodd, Dianne E. (Dianne Elizabeth), 1955-
III. Rousseau, Nicole IV. Canadian Museum of Civilization.

RT6.A1O54 2005   610.73'0971   C2005-902398-8

Cover illustrations (top) by Joseph-Charles Franchère, *Dr. Hingston and the Operating Room* (Hôtel Dieu Hospital, Montreal, 1905), courtesy of the Collection of the Hospitalières de l'Hôtel-Dieu de Montréal; (bottom) *Northern Nursing* (1990s), reproduced from Health Canada website and Media Photo Gallery, Health Canada, (www.hc-sc.gc.ca), with permission from the Minister of Public Works and Government Services Canada, 2005.

Epigraph quoted from Isabel Huggan's *Belonging*, Alfred A. Knopf Canada, Toronto, 2003.

Copy editing: Trish O'Reilly
Cover design, interior design, and typesetting: Dan Sokolowski
English translation: Käthe Roth
Proofreading: Stephanie VanderMeulen

Published by the University of Ottawa Press, 2005
542 King Edward Avenue, Ottawa, Ontario K1N 6N5 Canada
press@uottawa.ca / www.uopress.uottawa.ca

© Canadian Museum of Civilization Corporation, 2005
100 Laurier Street, P.O. Box 3100, Station B, Gatineau, Quebec JX8 4H2 Canada
web@civilization.ca / www.civilization.ca

Printed and bound in Canada

Contents

I have the pearl buttons from [my mother's] nurse's uniform, and my sister has the navy blue wool cloak with the red lining. These are holy relics, for our mother made of her nursing years something out of which she instructed us about life — her value system, her sense of female identity and personal integrity inextricably tied to her profession.

Isabel Huggan, *Belonging*

Foreword

*O*n *All Frontiers* is a fitting title for a book that presents an in-depth and compelling look at the history of nursing in Canada at the beginning of the twenty-first century. From the earliest days of Canadian history four centuries ago, nurses have been an influence "on all frontiers" of society. As members of both secular and religious orders — from the very first wilderness settlements to the outposts of the westward push and beyond — nurses have made invaluable contributions to the building of this country.

Pioneers, educators, and leaders, Canadian nurses have accompanied us through birth, illness, injury, recovery, and death. They have led initiatives to improve the health of all Canadians and their communities. They have been witness to and participants in some of our society's greatest achievements — and some of its worst conflicts. Through it all, Canadian nurses have been innovators in the field of health care.

In this period of renewed focus on the transformation of Canada's health system, nurses are recognized as the most trusted health care professionals. They provide safe, competent, and ethical care to Canadians from coast to coast. They are on the front lines and at the heart of health care. The role of nurses in the delivery of health services is a critical one and their contribution to the research and development of public health policies is vital. Nurses are also pioneers on the virtual frontier, advancing technology and enhancing methods of communications through the Internet.

At a time when their voices are increasingly heard and respected, it is fitting that Canadian nurses devote energy to a book giving voice to the facts and stories that document their unique contribution to Canada's history. To this end, *On All Frontiers* is an important piece of work. Telling nurses' stories — collecting and sharing their history — is long overdue recognition of the key role nurses have played and continue to play in shaping this country.

Each chapter in this historical work offers a fascinating portrait of important events in time and place, telling stories as diverse as Canada itself. Stories of people meeting daunting challenges with courage and determination, seizing opportunities with innovation and imagination, and perhaps most importantly, bringing a sense of compassion and humanity to the work that defines the nursing profession.

Within these pages, you will meet people who have devoted their lives to nurturing Canada in its infancy, defending its best values in difficult times, and helping to rebuild in the aftermath of global conflict. People such as Regilee Ootova, an Inuit midwife; Kay Christie, a Canadian military nurse; and the Grey Nuns of St. Boniface. People with stories that are exceptional yet familiar to those in the nursing profession. The eye-opening accounts in this book will provide a new perspective not only on the traditional and evolving roles of nurses, but on the formation and development of a country. Among them is the history of the Canadian

Nurses Association, which celebrates its one-hundredth anniversary in 2008. And during this past century, Canadian nurses have been the instigators of great change — as well as having experienced it themselves.

For these reasons, *On All Frontiers* holds broad appeal. But it also holds a deeper and more intrinsic value. Telling the stories of nurses in the home, in the hospital, in the community, and on the frontier reflects the strength of character and spirit that drive the nursing profession. The stories show how, through leadership and unwavering vision, nurses have shaped their role in four domains: administration, research, education, and clinical practice. These remain the areas in which the impact of nurses' skills and dedication are most felt today.

In the past, Canadian nurses have faced danger in the hardships of settling a new land and in the hazards of a wartime theatre of operation. Today's dangers most often come from within the assumed safety of hospitals, clinics, and other practice environments. Nurses have witnessed the threat of new and emerging global diseases such as SARS. They experience stress due to increased productivity demands and reduced resources. They are more likely than prison guards or police officers to be attacked at work. Issues such as access, increased wait times, and a shortage of nurses are also front and centre in today's health system.

It is within this context that Canadian nurses continue to influence the agenda for transformative change in health care. They advocate for action to increase the supply of nurses. They work on initiatives to retain experienced nurses and mentor those who are new to the profession. They seek to integrate the nurse practitioner. Nurses are leaders in health promotion and prevention, continuously taking steps to improve the Canadian public health infrastructure. Advances in technology through initiatives in tele-health and tele-medicine are bringing new innovations to the workplace. The development of virtual libraries and the expansion of online resources will provide easier access to knowledge as well as learning opportunities to nurses across the country. Nursing research is growing and will continue to play an important role in building an evidence-based, decision-making climate within the Canadian health system.

As the health care providers with the greatest amount of patient contact, nurses are essential to ensuring that Canadians receive the best possible care. They are the patient's safety net. They watch. They listen. They act. Nurses apply critical thinking and best practices in the assessment and care of patients. When necessary — and it is increasingly necessary — they advocate on the patient's behalf, both inside and outside the care environment. In effect, nursing has become a political act. Considering the stories contained in this book, perhaps it always has been.

Spanning four centuries of Canadian nursing history, *On All Frontiers* proves that despite threats and risks, and despite the inherent challenges of the profession, the pioneering spirit of Canada's earliest nurses is alive and well in the twenty-first century. In the home, in the community, in the hospital, and on the frontiers of innovation in health care, nurses continue to make significant contributions to the well-being and safety of Canadians and society at large. In the national and global political arenas, Canadian nurses also make their voices heard, influencing international policies and practices.

The past helps us understand how to meet today's challenges as well as those of the future. In light of the stories of commitment and achievement that comprise the history of Canadian nursing, the future of nursing is hopeful. That is not to say the journey will be easy, but a heritage of resiliency, resourcefulness, courage, and determination will assist Canadian nurses in moving forward to advance the nursing profession and to provide quality nursing care for all.

Lucille Auffrey, RN, MN
Executive Director, Canadian Nurses Association

Acknowledgements

So many people have rallied round this book and its sister projects — the exhibition and the nursing collection — that it is difficult to name them all. We would particularly like to thank Lynn Kirkwood and Meryn Stuart from the exhibition advisory committee who suggested themes and authors for this book.

We would also like to thank the Canadian Nurses Association, the Canadian Nurses Foundation, the Historica Foundation, Associated Medical Services, Library and Archives Canada, the Canadian Museum of Civilization, and the Canadian War Museum for their support of this and other Canadian Nursing History Collection projects. Parks Canada was generous in providing Dianne Dodd with the time required to contribute to the editorial process. Our gratitude goes also to the Canadian Association for the History of Nursing for their support of the project, as well as their offer to publish in their newsletter the vignettes we were unable to put in this book.

For her extensive expertise and faith in this book, thanks to Deborah Brownrigg, Manager of Publishing at the Canadian Museum of Civilization, and to Publishing Coordinator Nancy Minogue for her 11th hour technical assistance with the images and production. We greatly appreciate Anne Youlden's photo editing. Thanks are also due to the museum's Khalil Ibrahim, Manager, Contracting and Administration, for his invaluable assistance.

At the University of Ottawa Press, we owe a debt to Director Ruth Bradley-St-Cyr, Production Manager Heather Ritchie, and the dedicated team that worked with them on this complicated, two-book project:

- Trish O'Reilly, English editor
- Käthe Roth, English translator
- Marie-Claude Rochon, French translator and editor
- Stephanie VanderMeulen, English proofreader
- Marc Desrochers, French proofreader
- Dan Sokolowski and team, design and typesetting

Together, they gently prodded us into shape with their numerous but always cheerful e-mails, and gave precious advice that helped us make this book accessible to a large audience while still meeting academic standards. As Ruth kept saying at the end of our long meetings, "Remember, this is going to be a great book."

Our sincere thanks also go to the many chapter authors who shared with us their research and/or personal experiences with nursing. To all the authors who responded to our call for vignettes, we thank you for enriching our volume with nursing stories. Special gratitude goes to the authors who went through the laborious process of finding and procuring illustrations, and to the archives, nursing organizations, and individuals who allowed us to use their historical photographs and documents.

Dianne has special thanks for Parks Canada colleagues Catherine Cournoyer, James De Jonge, and

Brigitte Violette, who heard her out about the "two soli-tudes" in nursing, and who helped to transform her early work on nurses' residences into a broader understanding of nurses across Canada. Dianne also thanks her reading group for their ideas and inspiration about the fascinating world of nuns and nursing, caps and habits.

Christina (Tina) received much inspiration and advice from Cynthia Toman at the University of Ottawa, and Felicity Pope, an expert in the history of medicine. Thanks to Marie Currie, interpretive specialist at the Canadian Museum of Civilization, who tutored Tina in "meaning-making." Tina has special thanks for the many pleasant and collegial hours spent with the Canadian Nursing History Collection working group: Andrew Rodger and Larry McNally, archivists with Library and Archives Canada, Cameron Pulsifer from the Canadian War Museum, Diana Mansell from the Canadian Association for the History of Nursing, and Janet Cater, formerly of the Canadian Nurses Foundation. Nicole is grateful to Johanne Daigle and Brigitte Violette for their helpful and encouraging comments on the chapter "Lay Nursing in Quebec" and for suggesting relevant references and archives.

We especially want to express our appreciation of our families and support networks for sustaining us through it all. No woman is an island, and we could not have succeeded without the support of family and friends. Dianne's thanks go to Michael, and her daughters Elizabeth, Kathleen, and Melanie for putting up with all those weekends when Mom was tied to the computer, working on "the book." Tina has her husband Phil to thank for his support through the good times and the "I'm fed up" times. Nicole is grateful to her friends as well as to so many volunteers and staff members of the Maison Michel-Sarrazin who often expressed their interest in "the Museum book."

Christina Bates
Dianne Dodd
Nicole Rousseau

Introduction

Christina Bates, Dianne Dodd, and Nicole Rousseau

*O*n *All Frontiers: Four Centuries of Canadian Nursing* introduces the rich and complex history of nursing from the beginning of Canadian history to the present. We hope to reach a broad audience of interested Canadians, but especially women, nurses, and other health care professionals. We invite all to learn about the practice of nursing, not only in the hospital, but on many frontiers: in the home, in the community, in remote outposts, on the battlefield, and in the innovation of health care practices to serve Canadians from coast to coast. This book represents the third stage of a unique joint venture to bring together and make accessible important nursing collections, initiated through a partnership among the Canadian Nurses Association, the Canadian Museum of Civilization, the Canadian War Museum, and Library and Archives Canada.

The Canadian Nursing History Collection

On All Frontiers is built upon the expanding body of research into nursing history that has been made possible by the pioneering efforts of nursing school alumnae associations; religious nursing orders; nursing history associations; federal, provincial, and municipal nursing organizations; and individual nurses to preserve their history through creating archival and artifact collections.

In particular, the Canadian Nurses Association (CNA) has, since its inception in 1908, produced and collected a substantial quantity of written material, photographs, and artifacts, documenting its own activities and those of other institutions involved in nursing in Canada and around the world. This special collection is now housed in three public history institutions.

In 1999, the CNA, faced with inadequate storage facilities and a change in mandate that eliminated the impetus for collecting, made the decision to dispose of its unwieldy collection. This caused considerable uproar among its constituents, and the CNA realized how important these archival and material things were to nurses' sense of their own identity, and put a great deal of effort into finding a suitable repository.

The CNA turned to the federal institutions, first sparking the interest of the Canadian Museum of Civilization (CMC), whose curator was interested in enhancing collections relating to women's history. The Canadian War Museum then came on board to assess the significant Nursing Sisters Association of Canada (NSAC) collection (originally compiled by the NSAC, this collection had been donated to the CNA and formed part of their holdings), and the National Archives of Canada (now Library and Archives

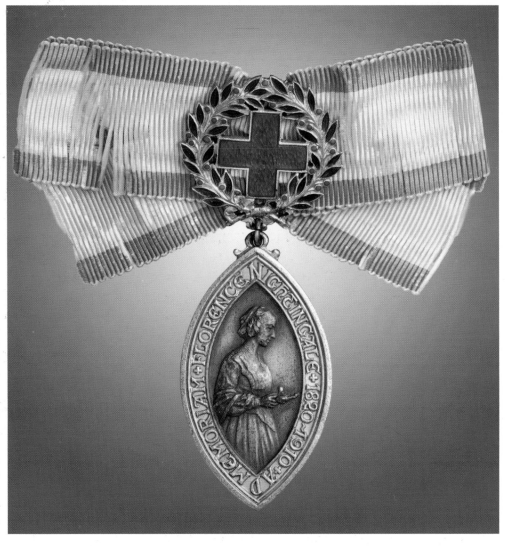

Figure 1
International Red Cross Florence Nightingale Commemorative Medal
1957
Photographer: Harry Foster
Canadian Museum of Civilization, 2000.111.102

This medal, presented to Helen McArthur, is the highest award for nursing given by the Red Cross.

Canada) became involved in the disposition of the extensive written, photographic, and audiovisual materials. Although parts of the collection would be entrusted to the institutions best able to look after them, the intellectual integrity of the collection as a whole had to be maintained. Thus a landmark partnership agreement among these three cultural institutions and the CNA was signed in June of 1999, creating the Canadian Nursing History Collection, as the combined holdings are now called. This collaborative approach will preserve and present a remarkable heritage, and will avoid the pitfalls that occur when varied collections are dispersed.

The archival material at the National Archives consists of 9000 photographs, 1600 audiovisual materials, and 35 metres of textual records representing the Canadian Nurses Association, the Nursing Sisters Association of Canada, and the Helen K Mussallem collection (all sub-collections of the CNA holdings). Approximately 950 documented artifacts related to civilian nursing were deposited at the Canadian Museum of Civilization, and 150 military nursing artifacts at the Canadian War Museum.[1]

The Nursing History Collection has been augmented by materials already in our holdings such as, for example, the medals belonging to Georgina Fane Pope, matron-in-charge of the nursing sisters during the South African War. Subsequent donations have enriched our collections such as minutes and cashbooks for four Victorian Order of Nurses (VON) branches at the National Archives, and 167 nurses' caps, dating from 1895 to 1983, at the CMC.

Portraying Heroes

Don Mayne, Toronto lawyer and artist

The SARS crisis in Toronto occurred two years after the infamous 9/11 terrorist attack on the World Trade Center. After that disaster, New York firefighters were celebrated as heroes worldwide. But after the SARS crisis, nurses received no international accolades. What was the difference?

Photographers focused on exhausted firefighters in New York. Photographers were prohibited from entering SARS units.

The sooty faces of firefighters displayed their char-acter. The faces of SARS nurses were hidden behind multiple masks.

Firefighters, at the end of their shift, were embraced by family, neighbours, and, indeed, the entire community. Nurses were shunned by a community fearing infection. Some nurses and their families were quarantined at home. Masked at home, they could not hug or even touch their families.

Firefighters were heroes. Nurses were nurses.

Nurses volunteered to work in SARS units knowing that their masks, gowns, and gloves might not fully protect them against the virus. One SARS nurse, who became infected, passed on the virus to her spouse and he died. She was on life support, and many nurses volunteered to care for her and other infected workers. This vulnerability shocks us. Nurses are not supposed to get sick. Nurses are not supposed to die.

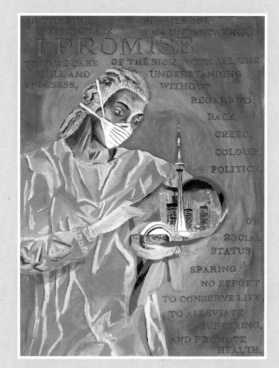

Figure 2
"I Promise"
Artist: Don Mayne
2003
Courtesy of Don Mayne

There are photographs showing a firefighter valiantly saving a firefighter. Where is the photograph show-ing a nurse caring for a sick nurse, who is caring for a sicker nurse — and so on....

This is the story behind the "I Promise" portrait. It depicts the strength of a nurse at the start of her night shift. With professional concern in her eyes and compassion in her touch she provides care for the life of the community. The words, visible in the colours of the sunset, are from the Pledge of the International Council of Nurses representing the goals of nurses worldwide.

Bringing the Collection to the Public

Providing students, researchers, and the general public with access to the collection was a priority. The first step was to transfer and organize the material. Each artifact was numbered and photographed, and material at the National Archives was described (this meant listening to endless hours of audio tapes), and guides to the contents prepared. In June 2004, a special portal called the Canadian Nursing History Collection Online was launched, providing access to the artifact collection.[2]

The second project is a major exhibition, "A Caring Profession: Centuries of Nursing in Canada/Une histoire de coeur : des siècles de soins infirmiers au Canada," which opened 16 June 2005 at the Canadian Museum of Civilization. Like this book, "A Caring Profession" explores nursing in various practice settings. The emphasis is on the human side of the story, which is conveyed through first person quotes, featured personalities from nursing history, nursing care artifacts, videos of nurses at work, and theatrical productions. This approach was based on a 2003 visitor survey conducted at the museum. It revealed that the general public holds nurses in high regard, as individuals full of "humanity, kindness and courage." It was difficult to elicit any negative comments about nurses, although the question, "do you think nurses have the right to strike?" brought out expressions of disapproval. Most people associated nursing with hospitals only, and nursing practice with "dirty work" exemplified by bedpans and diapers. The exhibition capitalizes on the regard visitors have for nurses by showing all the varied settings and challenges under which nurses worked and the direct impact nurses had on Canadians' quality of life. Visitors are introduced to the precision and knowledge required in nursing practice and procedures, as well as to difficult or controversial topics such as unionization and discrimination.

The third project of the Canadian Nursing History Collection Partnership is this book, which was launched at the opening of the exhibition. *On All Frontiers* brings together the results of over 50 years of research into a single volume, providing an overview of the state of nursing history at the beginning of the twenty-first century.

Our book is thematically organized by the diverse settings in which nurses practised: home, hospital, community, remote outposts, battlefields, and classrooms. Each theme is divided into chapters written by invited experts who have combined their own research with a synopsis of other related publications. The result is a broad, rather than deep, treatment of the themes, providing resources for further study and suggestions for further research. Peppered throughout the chapters are short vignettes related to a specific nurse, story, or event. Submitted through an open call for papers, the vignettes underscore and expand the contents of the chapters, adding a personal dimension.

Many paintings, photographs, cartoons, and artifact illustrations have been chosen to enrich the documentation of nursing history, and to encourage visual literacy. While most historians turn to the written record (newspapers, letters, census records, etc.) for evidence, visual and material sources can also inform our understanding of history, as they are profound evidence about beliefs and behaviours. Take, for example, the nurse's uniform: its introduction when a professional image was needed; its power in maintaining student nurses' allegiance to their hospital and school; and its rejection during the cultural revolution of the 1960s. Historians are beginning to tap these rich resources. Kathryn McPherson analyzed the 1926 Canadian Nurses War Memorial for visual clues to the role of nurses in shaping the national, and their own, identities. Dianne Dodd has found the design and decoration of nurses' residences projected an image of nursing meant to attract respectable young women into the profession.[3]

We hope that this book will reach both nursing historians and the general reader. Nursing history has largely been subject to a centripetal force: conducted for the deeper understanding of insiders in nursing organizations and in the academy. It is time for nursing history to reach out to the larger public. We trust that in these pages nurses, historians, and the general reader will gain up-to-date knowledge about the richness of Canada's nursing heritage.

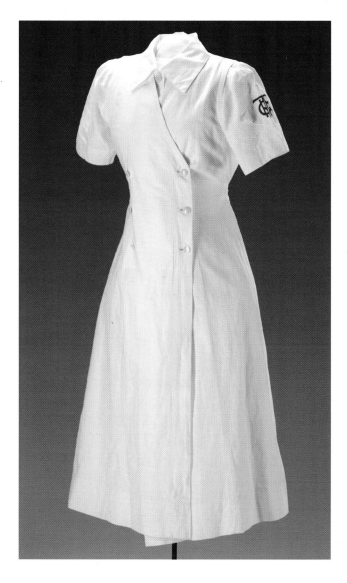

Figure 3
Uniform (dress and overall)
Toronto General Hospital
1949
Photographer: Doug Millar
Alumnae Association of the School of Nursing,
Toronto General Hospital Collection
Canadian Museum of Civilization, 2003.44.102

The Background: Nursing Historiography

The ambitious 1947 study *Three Centuries of Canadian Nursing*, written to commemorate the fiftieth anniversary of the VON, marks the last time a comprehensive history of Canadian nursing was published. That volume, covering New France to the contemporary period, admirably straddled the great divide between the late nineteenth century English, Nightingale nursing, and the much earlier Quebec, French-Catholic tradition.[4] Written in the liberal or "Whig" school, it focused on nursing leaders who established associations, released nursing education from the tyranny of the hospital apprenticeship system, and won the legal right to the title of Registered

Nurse.[5] Leaders' efforts to shape the humble work of the untrained nurse into a dignified, professional role, despite opposition from physicians and hospital administrators, were much exalted and seldom criticized. The historiography of nursing in French Canada focused on the religious vocation of their congregations' founders who build an impressive hospital system.[6]

Early histories of nursing focused on the other type of nursing sisters, those who cared for soldiers during armed conflict.[7] Indeed military nursing has received more recognition than most aspects of nursing history — even among mainstream historians. In chapters 10 and 11, Geneviève Allard and Cynthia Toman add to our knowledge of the bravery of military nurses with an analysis of the ambivalence of the military toward according nurses a permanent place in the Armed Forces or exposing them to risks they themselves were willing to assume.

In other published works, early nursing pioneers, a few of whom attained heroic status, became the subjects of biographies that did their share of myth-making: Jeanne Mance and Marguerite D'Youville, legendary for their pioneering nursing work as well as their religious and historic significance in Quebec, and Ethel Johns and Kathleen Russell in English-Protestant Canada.[8] In this vein also, many nurse-historians have contributed histories of nursing schools and alumnae associations.

Justifiably proud of their collective gains in a world stingy in granting women professional status, nurses have asserted that they have a past worth remembering. In 1987, Barbara Keddy and Margaret Allemang organized the Canadian Association for the History of Nursing, and in 1993, the Ontario Society for the History of Nursing created the Margaret M Allemang Centre for the History of Nursing. Other groups such as the Registered Nurses

Association of BC's History of Nursing Professional Practice Group have also joined this trend.

In the 1970s and 1980s professional historians also took an interest in nursing history. Under the umbrella of social history, they departed from the earlier approach to understanding the past through the eyes of leaders. The rank and file nurse in the wards, in private duty, and in public health came under the historian's microscope. Not surprisingly, historians began to wonder whether the term "professional" was appropriate to describe the gendered and subordinate work of nurses,[9] noting the failure of nurses to achieve a professional status comparable to that of the physician, who remained atop the health care hierarchy. Questioning whether nursing leadership's professionalization strategy was beneficial to nursing, others critically re-examined nurses' relationship with other female caregivers such as midwives and untrained nurses.

Interest in nursing history has also come from medical historians. Influenced by social history, they began to move away from the focus on celebrating great medical discoveries and scientists, to look more closely at some of the social factors that affected health. Some were perceptive enough to realize that nurses spent a great deal more time with patients than did doctors and recognized their role in the treatment successes.[10] Cynthia Toman is one of a number of historians now examining nursing practice.[11] In chapter 6 she analyzes the impact of technology on bedside nursing and the new status that operating increasingly sophisticated medical technology afforded nurses.

With a focus on male industrial workers, labour historians long shared the perception, cultivated by nursing leaders, that the nurse was a white collar professional. Led by Kathryn McPherson's innovative approach to nursing history, an approach that combined the insights of labour and women's history, labour historians began to see the nurse as a worker, studying unionization and nurses' work culture. Naturally, this led to a re-evaluation of professionalization. The post–Second World War demise of the private duty nurse, for example, is often cited as evidence that nurses, formerly private practitioners, were forced to accept employment as staff nurses in hospitals and thus underwent a process of de-skilling or proletarianization.[12] Unionization followed shortly afterward, cementing the nurse's status as worker. Chapter 3 of this volume, by Barbara Keddy and Dianne Dodd, examines the neglected area of private duty nursing in light of these arguments. And, in chapter 14, Sharon Richardson hints that the dichotomy between unionization and professionalization may be more apparent than real, showing that nurses negotiated perceived conflicts between the "ladylike" professional ideal and the new reality of collective bargaining.

In the first section of chapter 13, Diana Mansell takes issue with the labour historians' view. Outlining some of the conflicting definitions of professionalism that the debate has produced, she argues that, using criteria of professionalism that acknowledge differences between white collar women and the standard set by physicians, nurses did achieve professional stature. Her perspective underscores the importance of professional status to nurses, past and present. Closely tied to the professional debate are questions surrounding nursing education, and in chapter 12, Lynn Kirkwood examines the struggles of nursing leaders to move nursing education to the university, shedding light on the profound ambivalence demonstrated by physicians and university administrators toward accepting nurses as autonomous professionals worthy of a liberal arts education.

Whether nurses are workers or professionals or something in between, many historians share the view that nurses are relatively privileged. White, English- or French-speaking, and coming from the respectable classes until mid-century or later, nurses had superior educational status in relation to other workers and other women and achieved a level of recognition that afforded them a positive public image. It has long been acknowledged in the historiography that some nurses, particularly public health nurses, had considerable authority over others. In chapter 7 Marion Mackay shows that public health nurses, while conveying health messages that sometimes blurred the lines between health and cultural values, also provided pioneering services to needy populations.

Outpost nurses, examined in chapter 9 by Dianne Dodd, Jayne Elliott, and Nicole Rousseau, provided a

The Nurse's Cap: Symbol of a Profession

Christina Bates, Canadian Museum
of Civilization

Until the 1970s, the trained nurse was instantly recognized by her cap. The evolution of the nurse's cap reflects the history of hospital schools of nursing in Canada. The first nursing headdress in Canada was the nun's coif, worn by members of the religious orders that founded hospitals in Quebec and Montreal during the seventeenth century. In the British colonies, hospitals employed charwomen to provide rudimentary health care. Like all working women, they wore white caps to keep their hair neat and clean.

The first hospital nurse training program in Canada, based on the Florence Nightingale model, was established in 1874. Soon most hospitals opened nurse training schools, and created uniforms for their apprentice nurses to bring credit to the hospital and its students. A key ritual in the student's career was the "capping ceremony," in which a probationary nurse received her first cap. The next significant moment was gaining her black cap band upon graduation.

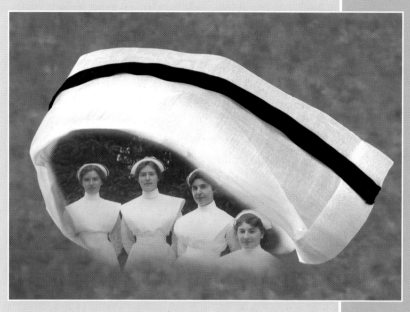

Figure 4
**Cap, Mary Bolton (second from left) and detail
of graduation photograph**
Cornwall (Ontario) General Hospital
1918
Photographer: Harry Foster
Gloria Barwell Kay Nurses Caps Collection
Canadian Museum of Civilization, 1999.267.29

Each hospital designed its own uniform and a lot of thought went into the image the hospital and nursing school wished to convey. Some of the caps resembled the nun's coif with its turned-back, winged brim, signifying the respected tradition of religious nursing and service to humanity. The nursing sister's veil, a type of coif, was the choice for Canadian nursing sisters who served in both world wars. Some hospitals chose the feminine mob cap, an oval of cloth gathered onto a band with a pleated frill. During the first few decades of the twentieth century, nurses' caps became highly stylized, perched on top of the head, with no functional value beyond the symbolic. Once nurse training entered the university, some hospitals capped their students with a mortarboard, albeit in starched white cotton.

When the hospital schools gave way to community colleges, allegiance to a particular hospital and school, along with the rituals of progress through its ranks, no longer dominated nursing education, and thus the cap lost much of its symbolic meaning. Capping ceremonies, and eventually the whole idea of a uniform to identify nurses, were abandoned. Some retired nurses and many patients lament its demise. However, the image of the starched white cap lingers in the public imagination and is still used to represent the profession in the media.

wide range of needed health services, including mid-wifery — services that went well beyond the confines of urban nursing practice. Their nursing stations and hospitals became community fixtures, and they lived and worked in isolated communities among their clients. Recent historiography stresses the role of these pioneering nurses in laying some of the foundations of the modern social welfare state. All nurses, in fact, played a role in this, an area that we hope will see further study in years to come.

Women's historians have stressed gender in the historiography of nursing, analyzing the tensions between female nurses and male doctors.[13] Initially, the history of women focused on extolling the historic achievements of a few feminist trailblazers, and in health care, these were the female doctors who opened the profession to women.[14] The question of why nurses, the numerically larger group, were so long overlooked is still relevant. Certainly there was and remains some reluctance on the part of feminist academics to embrace nursing — either because of the aura of "feminine virtue" surrounding its nurturing aspect and/or because of its subordinate status in relation to medicine. Fortunately, women's history is maturing, and historians are now looking at the quiet ways women expressed their agency, even in traditional areas. Nursing, one of the main professional categories for women in the late nineteenth and early twentieth century, is clearly of great significance. Indeed, as we alluded to earlier, the way professionalism plays itself out in a gendered workplace often uses nursing as a case study.[15]

Feminist historians have also critiqued the perception that women, by nature, are nurturers who should perform caregiving roles without asking for much by way of pay or recognition. These beliefs are deeply embedded in the historic baggage that all nurses carry. Thus any effort to organize, professionalize, or even unionize, serves to dispel these perceptions. Recently, women historians have examined the roots of nursing in unpaid domestic labour. Chapters 1 and 2 reflect this. In chapter 2 Cecilia Benoit and Dena Carroll explore the world of Aboriginal midwives, traditional lay/granny midwives and nurse-midwives. In chapter 1, Judith Young and Nicole Rousseau deal with skilled lay women who cared for

birthing women as well as the sick and dying in New France and pre-Confederation Canada. In this period before nursing became a profession, as was also the case in outpost nursing, nursing and midwifery could not be separated.

The Scope of Our Study: What is a Nurse?

No survey can claim to be completely comprehensive, and ours certainly is not. However, our strength lies in the wide geographic and chronological lens through which we view the history of nursing. We begin in New France and carry the reader more than 300 years into the present day, and cross this diverse country. More than this, we consciously use as inclusive an understanding of what it meant to be a nurse in Canada as is possible within the parameters of the available literature.

What is a nurse? This question is not straightforward. Veronica Strong-Boag has challenged historians of nursing to acknowledge that nursing history falls outside of the boundaries of the concept of a professional trained or registered nurse. She suggests that nursing history should include consideration of "women's longstanding responsibility for maintaining family and community health."[16] This inclusive approach allows the historian to highlight the wide-ranging impact of nurses. Like so many aspects of women's accomplishments, this contribution remains largely unrecognized. Many of the topics Strong-Boag cites as evidence of nursing's role in nation-building, such as Aboriginal health care and midwifery, the role of religious hospitallers, outpost nurses who settled new communities, and the many nurses who contributed to the modern social welfare state, are covered in our collection. We, too, want to stress the importance of nurses' work on a scale that is larger than the profession itself.

Still, not everyone is in agreement. Meryn Stuart and Kathryn McPherson have for example, cautioned against including all caregivers in the term "nurse." Too broad a definition of nursing might well prevent us from making needed distinctions both between historical periods and between different types of caregivers. While an informally trained lay woman caregiver working in Upper Canada might legitimately be called a nurse, can one say the same of a 1950s housewife who nurses a sick child in her own home? And, if all caregivers are nurses, how do we distinguish between the historical counterparts to the registered nurse and the practical nurse or between the nurse-midwife and the obstetrical nurse? Clearly we need more specific labels.[17]

Our goal is not to redefine nursing or to change the parameters of nursing history. We do take the spirit of Strong-Boag's challenge to heart by including a discussion of some of nursing's antecedents. We believe they are important because the women who did skilled nursing as part of their familial or community health care roles helped form the foundation on which the nursing profession was built. This is not to say that they did the same work, that we should call them all by the same name, or that their informal apprenticeship training was inferior or superior to that of the trained nurse. Rather, it is to say that the skills, traditional knowledge, and social perceptions surrounding pre-professional nursing have influenced the development of professional nursing. Whether for good or ill, one can see its influence in a professionalization strategy that had as its starting point a determination to banish the taint of domestic labour. We also see it in the nursing profession's alignment with physicians in persecuting lay midwives in order to attain a recognized role within modern health care, despite the fact that many nurses delivered babies in practice settings. And we see it in an educational campaign that devalued hospital apprenticeship training and asserted the nurse's right to formal education through the nation's universities and colleges.

It is of interest to note that historians of medicine trace their origins back as far as ancient Greece and Rome and do not claim modern medicine to be the beginning of medical history. Should nurses do no less? It would be ahistorical to date nursing from the emergence of the modern, professional period. Rather, acknowledging the long tradition of intelligently caring for the ill will allow historians of nursing to find names for — even enhance the legitimacy of — these other categories of caregiving. The strategy of devaluing lay nursing was a necessary step in the evolution of a new and insecure profession, but now, as nursing takes its rightful place in Canadian historiography, historians can enrich the scholarship by understanding nursing in the context of its full historic continuum.

Future Research: The Gaps in the Literature

The work of nurses in religious orders is much better documented and recorded than that of their less organized counterparts in other parts of Canada. In chapter 4, Brigitte Violette describes how the Augustines and other religious congregations built a network of Catholic hospitals across Canada. Some historians stress the positive role of these strong, business-like, competent women who did non-traditional work in a society that gave women few choices outside marriage and motherhood.[18] Still, this approach leaves some questions unanswered. What price did they pay for their relative autonomy? How did their efforts to gain heavenly salvation by doing good deeds affect their nursing work? Like public health nurses, did nuns use their power over others to indoctrinate them into the prevailing ideologies of the dominant elites?

In chapter 5, Kathryn McPherson outlines the development of the system of nurse training known as the "Nightingale system," as Violette did for French nursing; however, there are few comparisons of what happened when the two systems were mixed. We have tried to address this. In chapter 13, the authors critically re-examine the Nightingale myth in light of its divisive impact in Quebec, and in chapter 8, Pauline Paul looks at religious nursing in western Canada. Paul outlines the positive influence of the nuns who founded, developed, and maintained hospitals in all major cities of the West.

Some historians have suggested that similarities in nursing among all religious communities were indeed greater than the differences. While it is widely recognized that religion was central to Catholic nursing in Quebec and beyond, the literature has yet to fully explore religion in Protestant nursing. Even charity hospitals founded by secular women's groups often had religious overtones. Catholic influences in Protestant communities have not yet been fully explored.[19]

Religious nursing conjures up images of veils, habits, and crosses, and a similar Protestant phenommenon — caps, uniforms and pins. Few historians have looked at what function this clothing served.[20] Was it to identify nurses as special women, to identify them with a specific religious congregation or hospital, or was it to disguise the nurse's sexuality and protect her from the threat of harassment and abuse prevalent in a patriarchal society? Many nurses have suggested that their uniforms gave them status as well as a greater mobility than other women typically enjoyed. These are intriguing questions that await more systematic study in the future.

Who was allowed to nurse was not always a question of skill, but was, in fact, a projection of a society's values. It was no accident that nursing, until well into the twentieth century, was deliberately reserved for white, respectable, English- or French-speaking women. Although several historians have begun to study the question of what it meant to be a minority nurse and to tell the story of the pioneering nurses who gained entry into nursing schools for women of colour and Aboriginal nurses, definitive answers await further research.

Working together, nurse-historians and historians of women, of labour, and of medicine have gradually developed a sophisticated historiography of nursing, which we have tried to reflect in our book. We hope to bring the early focus on professionalism and nursing elites — a focus that suited a period of profession formation — together with new directions in the understanding of nursing history. Readers will also learn about unionization as the natural corollary of mid-twentieth century changes in nursing practice; the impact of technology on nursing practice; the predecessors to formalized, professional nursing; and the ways in which nurses have contributed to the building of the Canada we value, a Canada in which universal health care is accessible to all.

Lay Nursing from the New France Era to the End of the Nineteenth Century (1608–1891)

Judith Young and Nicole Rousseau

The work of religious caregivers throughout Canada's history has been well documented (and is, in fact, discussed in chapters 4 and 8 of this book); however, lay caregivers before the late nineteenth century have not received the same attention. Unlike religious communities, which have, for the most part, maintained abundant archives, lay caregivers left few traces of their work. To the paucity of archival material on lay nursing is added the difficulty in defining this category of work, since in French Canada the title "infirmière" came into use only in the first half of the twentieth century, while in English Canada the term "nurse" designated workers with a wide variety of skills long before nurses were officially trained and licensed. The celebrated midwives of New France, trained in French schools, and the self-taught "nurses," who essentially handed out medical prescriptions, had very different degrees of professional autonomy and social recognition. Within this wide range, two constants emerge: nursing workers were female caregivers, and their caregiving activities were most often associated with maternity. The work of Marie-Françoise Collière[1] is useful for distinguishing care activities that fall under nursing (care dispensed by women) and activities in other professions, particularly the medical profession (care dispensed by men). Collière includes in the first category practices whose goal is to maintain life; these practices were traditionally developed by midwives, wet nurses, and healers to deal with fertility, birth and development of the child, and the alleviation of physical suffering.

The training, the specific nature of the practices, and the working conditions of lay caregivers were very much shaped by their social and historical contexts; and the realities of French Canada (essentially Quebec) differed in many important respects from those of English Canada. We will, therefore, discuss French and English Canada separately. For Quebec, we will divide our discussion into three eras: New France (1608–1759); the effects of the Conquest (1760–90); and Lower Canada, which became the province of Quebec (1791–1891). For English Canada, we will also break our discussion down into three main time periods: early settlers and health care (1713–1840); "monthly" nurses and "sick nurses" (1840–75); and nurses in homes and hospitals (1875–91). Only those people for whom nursing was principal occupation, paid or not, are considered to be nurses for the purposes of this chapter.

Lay Nursing in Quebec

The Era of New France (1608–1759)

Because of the many difficulties involved with colonization, the first French colonists to settle the new

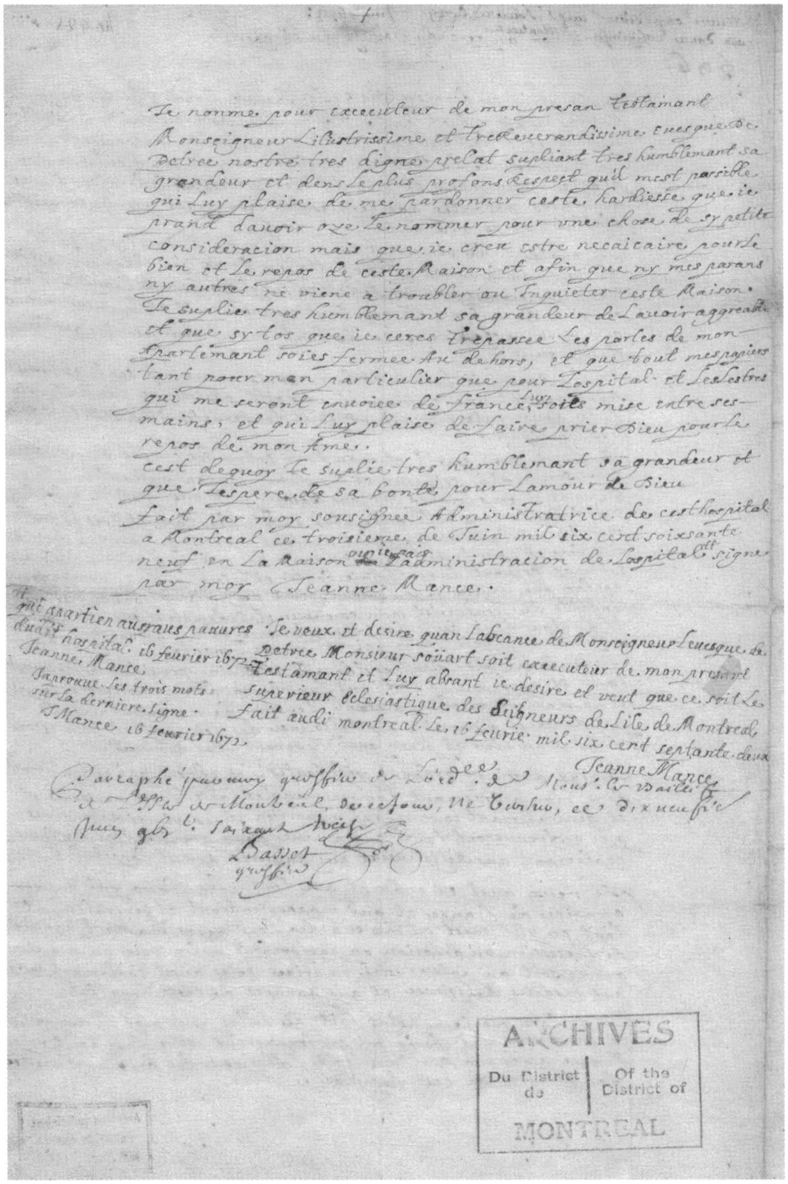
Je nomme pour executeur de mon presan testamant
Monseigneur Lillustrissime et treßreverandissime Euesque de
Petree nostre tres digne prelat supliant tres humblemant sa
grandeur et dens le plus profons respect quil mest possible
qui luy plaise de me pardonner ceste hardiesse que ie
prand dauoir oze le nommer pour vne chose de sy petite
consideracion mais que ie cree estre necaicaire pour le
bien et le repos de ceste Maison et afin que ny mes parans
ny autres ne viene a troubler ou Inquieter ceste Maison.
Je suplie tres humblemant sa grandeur de Lauoir aggreable
et que sy tos que ie seres trepassee les porles de mon
Parlemant soies fermee Au dehors, et que tout mes papiers
tant pour mon particulier que pour Lospital et les lettres
qui me seront enuoiee de france, soies mise entre ses
mains, et qui luy plaise de faire prier Dieu pour le
repos de mon Ame.
cest de quoy Je suplie tres humblemant sa grandeur et
que Jespere de sa bonté pour Lamour de Dieu
Fait par moy sousignee Administratrice de cest hospital
a Montreal ce troisieme de Juin mil six cent soixante
neuf en La maison de ladministracion de Lospital et signe
par moy Jeanne Mance.

Je veux et desire quen labcence de Monseigneur Leuesque de
Petree Monsieur Souart soit executeur de mon present
testamant et luy absant ie desire et veut que ce soit le
superieur ecclesiastique des Seigneurs de Lile de Montreal.
Fait audi montreal le 16 feurier mil six cent septante deux
Jeanne Mance

ARCHIVES
Du District de
Of the District of
MONTREAL

Figure 1
Jeanne Mance's Testament (detail)
1672
Archives nationales du Québec
Centre d'archives de Montréal,
CN601, S71, Greffe du notaire Bénigne Basset

territory were often risking their lives to do so. Although the settlement of Quebec was founded in 1608, it was not until 1617 that the first French family arrived: Louis Hébert and Marie Rollet (Hubou by her second marriage). In the first comprehensive history of Canadian nursing, Gibbon and Mathewson declare Marie Rollet to be the first "nurse" in Canada, since "...she spent such time as she could spare from her household duties in visiting sick patients recommended to her care by the Jesuit Fathers."[2] However, we cannot consider nursing to have been Rollet's main occupation: in reality, it was as assistant to her first husband, an apothecary, that Rollet's name entered the annals of women's history. Not until there was a more stable settlement did women begin arriving whose main occupation was the provision of care.

Among these early lay healers, Jeanne Mance is a particularly significant and memorable figure. Born in Langres, Champaign, in 1606 and died in Montreal in 1673, she has been the subject of many volumes.[3] Some historians consider her the "first lay nurse in America," while others see her, rather, as the co-founder of Montreal and the founder and administrator of the town's Hôtel Dieu.[4] Even for this heroine of Canadian history, however, there is a paucity of original documents available — especially regarding her training, the experience she acquired before her departure for Canada, and the precise nature of her work — and we are reduced to formulating hypotheses about these aspects of her life. We believe that she acquired her training in caregiving by helping to tend to the victims of the Thirty Years' War and the plague, two scourges that ravaged Langres in the 1630s. The official documents and accounts by her contemporaries attest that she knew how to read and write — a prerogative of the elite at the time — but there is no indication that she received formal training in nursing. Although there were well-known schools for midwives in France at the time, she does not seem to have attended one. It is plausible that she had access to one of the many republications of the book by Marie Maupeou (1590–1681), a collection written for charitable ladies who took care of the indigent sick.[5]

From 1642 (the year Montreal was founded) to 1653, Jeanne Mance was likely the only health care resource person in the colony, assisted by between one and four servants and at least two other women in the colony: the wife of Louis d'Ailleboust and Madame de la Bardillière. Although all the official documents designate Jeanne Mance as "administrator of the hospital of Montreal," there is reason to believe that she had other recognized skills. For instance, in 1645, the Société Notre-Dame sent her "medications for the ill [and] surgical instruments."[6] In this regard, it is important to consider the title that is given Jeanne Mance in the very first baptismal certificate made out in the colony — a baptism at which she was the godmother. This certificate, written in Latin, reveals that the baby, a girl, was born on 24 November 1648 and was baptized (without the usual rites), as she was close to death, by Jeanne, "*pappe chirurgo*," then was officially baptized by Father Dequen the same day.[7] Jeanne Mance may have been the midwife for this first birth, since she was the one who unofficially baptized the baby who was close to death; she was given, however, the title of "*chirurgo*" (surgeon). In the other baptismal certificates in which she figured as godmother, however, as well as in other official documents, she is always presented as "administrator of the hospital of Montreal." A single account relates her skills as a caregiver: On 6 May 1651, the settler Chiquot (or Cicot) barely escaped an attack by the Iroquois, but in the skirmish "they removed his scalp with a piece of skull. Through her care, Mlle Mance managed to heal him, and Chiquot lived almost another fourteen years."[8]

By 1672, the population of New France had more than doubled, reaching 6700. The state was beginning to take charge of certain services, such as occasional distribution of medications and other assistance to the poor, financial support for hospitals, and the care of the mentally handicapped and abandoned children. Midwives who came from France were also paid by the state.

Among the midwives, one stood out for her contribution as a herbalist: Catherine Jérémie, dit Lamontagne (1664–1744). In the fall of 1702, she and her second husband settled in Montreal, where she practised as a midwife and became known for gathering plants. Like the physicians Michel Sarrazin and Jean-François Gaultier, although to a lesser extent, she and amateur naturalists helped to spread knowledge of the medicinal properties of Canadian plants. She accompanied her shipments of "simples"[9] with notes indicating their properties and effects, and the intendant, Gilles Hocquart, remarked in 1740 that she "had long striven to discover the secrets of Indian medicine."[10]

The work of these pioneer caregivers fit within the relatively interventionist approach to health care by the French state compared to the more laissez-faire approach of the English state; therefore, the conquest of New France by England, which ended the French regime, had repercussions for all categories of health workers.

The Effects of the Conquest (1760–90)

Among the effects of the Conquest was the end of financial support by the state. Thus, after the surrender of Montreal, in 1760, the one employed midwife left the colony.

Aside from the cultural influence of the English on the training and practice of physicians and surgeons, there was a tightening of control over titles and practices that had an effect on female caregivers. In 1788, a statute granted a monopoly on practice to

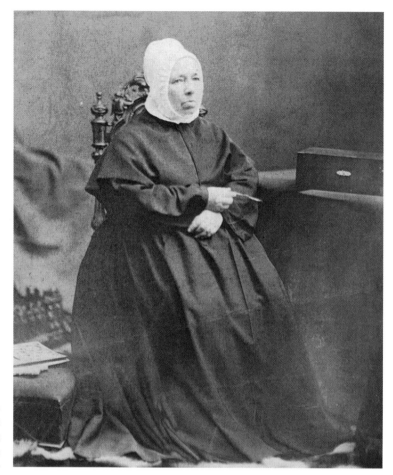

Figure 2
**Marie Métivier, founder of l'Hospice
Saint-Joseph de la Maternité de Québec**
Archives, Maison Généralice Bon Pasteur, Québec

the official medical corps.[11] Over the longer term, the Conquest was to have a disastrous effect on lay caregivers: the prospects of remuneration by the state faded and a new generation of caregivers could not be trained because the few qualified women had been trained in France. However, with the great epidemics of the early nineteenth century, the state was forced to invest in minimal health services. Thus, the government of Lower Canada, created in 1791, did hire a few women as nurses.

Lower Canada, Later the Province of Quebec (1791–1891)

Epidemics and Nursing

To deal with the epidemics that were brought from Europe, the Assembly of Lower Canada passed two statutes in 1832, one of which mandated the creation of a quarantine station at Grosse-Île, a small island in the St. Lawrence near Quebec City. Buildings were erected to shelter the ill, as well as houses for the doctors and nurses.[12]

How many nurses worked at Grosse-Île? The 1848 list of employees mentions the names of six women employed in this capacity.[13] It seems that most were of Irish origin, but Marianne O'Gallagher, in her 1987 book on Grosse-Île, states that in 1847, "Mrs Garneau and 'several nurses died after they left the island.'"[14] A Norwegian nurse, Margaretta Zelius, remained in her position from 1869 to 1879. All indications are that the nurses had no skills other than those acquired on the job, since these people, both men and women, went from one position to another according to the need. Christine Chartré, in her 2001 volume on the handling of epidemics at Grosse-Île, has found only one mention of the qualifications of these workers: a "professional," Helen Gorman, was hired in 1869 and worked in the hospitals of the station until 1879. The tasks of the nurses consisted of cleaning and changing patients' clothes when they

On All Frontiers

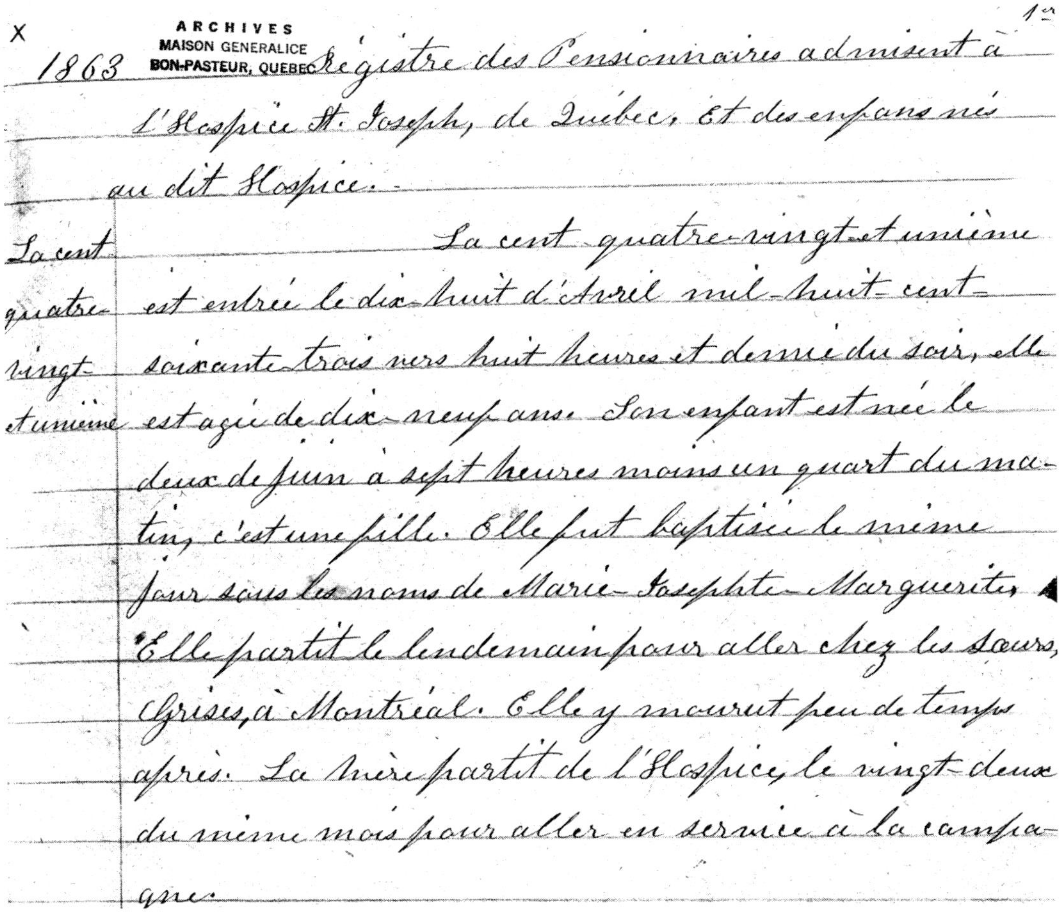

1863 *Régistre des Pensionnaires admisent à l'Hospice St. Joseph, de Québec, Et des enfans nés au dit Hospice.*

La cent quatre-vingt et unième

La cent quatre-vingt et unième est entrée le dix-huit d'Avril mil-huit-cent-soixante-trois vers huit heures et demie du soir, elle est agée de dix-neuf ans. Son enfant est née le deux de Juin à sept heures moins un quart du matin, c'est une fille. Elle fut baptisée le même jour sous les noms de Marie-Josephte-Marguerite. Elle partit le lendemain pour aller chez les sœurs Grises, à Montréal. Elle y mourut peu de temps après. La mère partit de l'Hospice le vingt-deux du même mois pour aller en service à la campagne.

Figure 3
Register of children baptised at l'Hospice Saint-Joseph de la Maternité de Québec 1863
Archives, Maison Généralice Bon Pasteur, Québec

were admitted, monitoring symptoms until the doctor stepped in, restraining delirious patients, changing patients' soiled bedding and bedshirts, distributing medications and meals, and cleaning the patients and the rooms.[15]

Nursing and Charitable Works

The quarantine measures and the resources deployed to house and care for thousands of ill immigrants quickly proved insufficient, and several thousand contaminated immigrants arrived in Quebec City and Montreal, where the existing hospitals were overloaded. It was at this time that the organizations founded in the early nineteenth century by charitable ladies began to reach beyond their initial mandate of assistance to the resident poor and care for the immigrants and the many orphans created by the epidemics.[16] Many of these women helped to ease suffering by using their privileged connections for charitable works, by donating money, or by managing charitable organizations, thus constituting a vast welfare network. Some were so committed that they delivered care directly as well as managing the charitable organizations.

It is not easy to separate the women whose work was situated in the domain of social services from those who worked as lay nurses, paid or not; here, we discuss only those who gave direct care (shelter, food, hygiene, care aiming to ease suffering and aid in recovery) to pregnant women, elderly and ill people, orphans and abandoned children, and the disabled. In this category, four women made a mark by starting up charities that later became permanent institutions.

In 1827, when she was 72 years old, Angélique Blondeau-Cotté (1755–1837) founded the Association des dames de charité with some 50 women of the Montreal upper class.[17] When Montreal was flooded with victims of the cholera epidemic of 1832, Mme Cotté and her companions rapidly organized, dividing up the city's neighbourhoods to provide assistance efficiently, in spite of the danger of contagion. The same year, the Association founded the Catholic Orphanage of Montreal, handed over to the Séminaire de Saint-Sulpice only in 1877.

Marie-Rosalie Cadron-Jetté, who began taking teenage mothers into her home after she was widowed and eventually founded a religious nursing order devoted to the maternity care of "penitents," is discussed at greater length in chapter 4.

Émilie Tavernier-Gamelin (1800–51), a wealthy member of Montreal high society, was widowed, without children, at 27 years of age; in 1827, she joined the Association des dames de charité, for which she made home visits, and in 1830 she opened a first refuge for aged, ill or infirm, and disadvantaged women.[18] On 18 September 1841, the Legislative Assembly recognized the legal existence of Mme Gamelin's refuge under the name Asile de Montréal pour les femmes âgées et infirmes; in December of that year, the Corporation de l'Asile de Montréal began construction of the Asile de la Providence. Two years later, Bishop Bourget decided to found a new religious community and appointed Mme Gamelin director of the new shelter that she had set up herself! He authorized her to act as superior of the new community, which she then joined at age 43, though she took her vows only on 29 March 1844, the day when the community attained canonical status. She survived the typhoid epidemic in 1838, and then the typhus epidemic in 1847, but she succumbed to cholera during the 1851 epidemic.

In 1852, Marie Métivier (1811–85) accepted the proposal of Father Auclair, curé of Notre-Dame-de-Québec, to found the Hospice Saint-Joseph. Unmarried, she was known as "matron," a title given to respected women, often responsible for an institution. She directed the hospice for 24 years without receiving a salary. It was administered by thirteen ladies' auxiliaries, and its mission was "...to receive pregnant girls, to have them give birth, to take care of them during their labour, and to place their children and them whenever possible."[19] Because the institution had a capacity of only 12 beds, it no longer met the demand by the time the Soeurs du Bon-Pasteur opened the Hospice de la Miséricorde de Québec; these nuns officially took over Métivier's hospice in 1876.

It is not surprising that so many women sought to fulfil themselves as volunteer caregivers, as physicians slowly but surely gained a monopoly in the health care field. Although laws passed in the seventeenth and eighteenth centuries were aimed mainly at men who claimed to be physicians or surgeons without having obtained a licence, those passed in the nineteenth century sought to exclude women from the medical field by reserving for physicians the profession of obstetrician, and in 1891, midwives disappeared from the censuses. A similar masculinization of professional health care, leaving women to labour in subservient roles or on the untrained and unrecognized margins, took place in English Canada.

Lay Nursing in English Canada

In times of illness and childbirth early colonists in English Canada had little choice but to rely on their own resources, and nursing care fell to the women of the family. Unlike the government of New France, which, to some extent at least, paid for hospitals and trained midwives, as well as assistance to the poor and care for the mentally handicapped and abandoned children, the British colonial government did not see fit to finance civilian health services, and it would be several decades before the Quebec nursing sisterhoods ventured into English Canada. Later, with population growth, a group of working class women emerged as hired nurses, most likely in response to a growing middle class expectation of domestic help. By the mid-nineteenth century in English Canada, it can be said that nursing had become a "trade" carried out by working class women (and a few men) of varying skills and respectability. Much of the remainder of this chapter will focus on these "untrained" nurses, a group frequently maligned in the history books. Who were they, and were they as bad as history has painted them? It is rare for working class women to leave personal records of their lives, but public records such as the census and city directories can provide information on early nurses, and as a result certain careers can be followed over a period of time.[20]

Mary Gapper O'Brien (1798–1876)

Jane Errington,
Royal Military College and Queen's University

In the world of Upper Canada in the first half of the nineteenth century, settlement was scattered, families were often isolated from each other, and it was up to the women to provide basic health care and "bind up the cares of others." Mary Gapper arrived in the colony in 1828–29, married Edward O'Brien two years later, and by 1838 had five children. She frequently recorded days of "nursing, cooking, nursing again, sewing, nursing, eating, sewing, nursing, talking, nursing, singing." As a responsible mother, Mary took care to make sure her family remained healthy and avoided situations that would have exposed her children to "fevers" or other "infectious disorders." But then, as now, nothing could stop her children from contracting colds, influenza, the measles, or other childhood diseases, and Mary spent considerable time serving as a nurse to her family. Indeed, many in the colony believed that an ill child could "be no better attended" than by its mother, whose love and attention and skills with home remedies were almost always the best "medicine" — better even, some asserted, than that offered by a doctor. When need demanded, Mary O'Brien also helped to nurse neighbours and friends and was herself attended by a local "granny" during each of her confinements. Although there were some midwives in Upper Canada who had formal training, were highly skilled, and received payment for their services, their numbers were few. Often an older woman who had a number of children of her own was pressed into service. A still unmarried Mary Gapper recounted how once she and her sister-in-law, Fanny, were called to attend "a poor Yorkshire woman who was apparently in immediate want of the assistance of a Granny." Neither Mary nor Fanny had any experience. They were the only help available, however, and — as neighbours and as women — they felt obliged to offer what support they could. Over the next decade, Mary attended at least five other women "whose time had come." Mary's confidence in her abilities as a nurse/midwife increased over the years. And as a woman, wife, mother, and neighbour she was one of the many keepers of the colony's health.

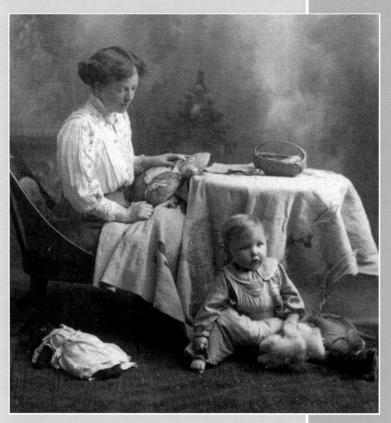

Figure 4
Mother and child
ca. 1900
Queen's University Archives, Grier Collection, 2326
Harriet Cartwright Dobbs File

Sources: Archives of Ontario, MS199, *The Journal of Mrs E G O'Brien*, 1828–1838; Archives of Ontario, MS78, Macaulauy Papers, letter of Ann Macaulay to her son, John, 23 July 1840.

In any account of early caregiving, nursing and midwifery are hard to separate. Some women combined nursing the sick with midwifery and with "monthly nursing" (care of mother and infant for four weeks after the birth). Thus any discussion of eighteenth and nineteenth century nurses must inevitably touch on midwifery. This account describes caregivers first during the early years of settlement, then at mid-nineteenth century, as numbers of hired nurses grew, and finally, late in the century, just before training programmes proliferated. Although the narrative centres on Halifax, St. John, and Toronto, the caregivers described can be seen as representative of lay nurses in English Canada at this time.

Early Settlers and Health Care 1713–1840

In 1713 the sparsely populated French colony of Acadia (Nova Scotia) was transferred to the British Crown but ongoing conflict with France, and later America, made the eighteenth century a time of great unrest in the colony. The port of Halifax was developed as a British garrison but colonization was slow. Following the American War of Independence a flood of immigrants, the so-called United Empire Loyalists, moved north and settled in Nova Scotia and along the St. Lawrence into Upper Canada (Ontario). The colonial government provided medical and hospital care for military personnel but little for civilians. Some officials were moved to help colonists and in 1755, for example, the Commander at Lunenburg, concerned over the number of infant deaths, requested that two midwives be appointed — although we do not know if his request was honoured. When faced with illness, settlers had to rely on their own resources and remedies. They also acquired medicinal knowledge from Canada's indigenous people.

The genteel but impoverished Catherine Parr Trail, who settled with her husband in 1830s Ontario, nursed her own large family and extended help to others. By the 1830s, doctors and midwives were likely available in the towns but travel to bush settlements was arduous and neighbourly help often the only recourse. Trail called herself a "regular old quack" but considered her knowledge came from "respectable sources." She used plant remedies such as balsam of wild cherry for bronchitis and favoured the time-honoured therapy of blistering for inflammations such as sore throats; a treatment, she considered, though "disagreable ... removed the inward evil."[21] Doctors, when available, attended in time of serious illness and were present for some confinements but, in the early nineteenth century, a midwife was more likely to aid women in childbirth.

Nurse/Midwives

For the less wealthy, midwives were more cost-effective than doctors as they stayed longer and helped with household chores. From the diary of Captain Johnson of Georgina, Ontario, we learn that in 1832 he paid $5 to a Mrs Elwes to attend the birth of his daughter, a sum that would have included care after the delivery.[22] Some midwives were known to be versatile. The diary of Martha Ballard, a late eighteenth-century New England midwife, revealed that she also made sick calls, dispensed herbs and pills, and laid out bodies for burial. In Upper Canada midwives were employed by benevolent societies organized to help the deserving poor. In York (Toronto), the Female Society for the Relief of Poor Women in Childbirth had, in its first year (1820), assisted seventeen women with "comfortable clothing of all kinds, a midwife, and Physician (if required)."[23]

Two midwives, Mrs Bennett and M McCaul, are recorded in the first Toronto directory (1833). Mrs Bennett may have been the first midwife in the town. In 1810, "Isabella Bennet, midwife from Glasgow" placed a sign on her house and later advertised a change of address in a York paper, the *Colonial Advocate*.[24] Her name can be found in directories up to 1846. M McCaul likely relocated to Brockville, Ontario, as a midwife named Mrs Margaret McCaul, advertising in the *Brockville Chronicle* of September 1835, considered that her "good reputation in Toronto" would make her popular with the local women. Midwives who were recent immigrants may have had some formal training. Many European cities had established lying-in hospitals and these institutions provided courses for midwives as well

The Kingston Female Benevolent Society: Caring for the Sick Poor in Early Nineteenth Century English Canada

Judith Young, Retired RN, MA History

In early nineteenth century Kingston, Ontario, the Female Benevolent Society provided the only hospital care available to the sick poor. Middle class women at the time played an important role in providing aid to less fortunate citizens. Spurred by the plight of destitute immigrants, the women of Kingston — and of Montreal and Toronto — organized to offer aid but hoped also to "stir the poor to industry." The Kingston ladies first set up a temporary hospital in 1818 to "avoid the expense of boarding the sick," but, as the years passed and the town failed to achieve a permanent hospital, it became a seasonal fixture. From November to May, in an abandoned military blockhouse, the women provided food, shelter, and nursing care to the indigent; others were "supplied with medicine in their lodgings." Local doctors contributed free services. Operation of the charity was given a boost in 1830 when male supporters managed to negotiate a small government grant. But, in 1836, disaster struck when the blockhouse housing the hospital burned down; it took several years

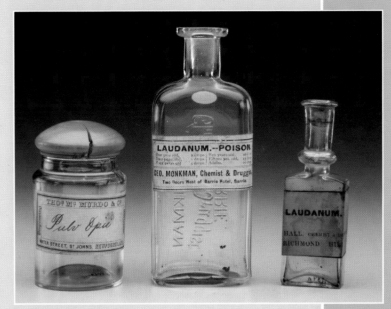

Figure 5
Opium and laudanum bottles
19th century
Photographer: Doug Millar
Canadian Museum of Civilization, D-16702
Gift of Mrs John Outram, D-14284, D-13639

to reopen the hospital, this time in an empty brewery warehouse. The town, meanwhile, had constructed a permanent hospital but lacked the funds to operate it (it proved useful as a House of Assembly during Kingston's brief tenure as capital). In 1845, still without funds, the town commissioners handed the hospital over to the Female Benevolent Society. By raising two hundred pounds, this enterprising group was able to equip two wards, hire a nurse/housekeeper and her daughter, and open the hospital. Society members visited daily to oversee operations. After four years and a terrifying typhus epidemic, the women gratefully handed over management to a Board of Trustees, but continued other charitable work. Through 30 years of immigration and epidemics, the women of Kingston had provided desperately needed hospital care for the sick and destitute of their community.

Source: Margaret Angus, *Kingston General Hospital: A Social and Institutional History Vol. 1* (Montreal & Kingston: McGill-Queen's University Press, 1973).

as medical students. Mrs Mahon, named in the 1843 Toronto directory, advertised her arrival from Dublin in the *Christian Guardian* and assured clients of her "real knowledge, experience and attention." It is difficult to know what kind of a living midwives made. Neither Bennett, McCaul, nor Mahon had husbands listed at their addresses so were likely widows eking out a living. Bennett, a longtime resident in an unsalubrious area of the city, was hardly prosperous but, like her colleagues, was educated and astute enough to advertise her services.

Early Hospital Nurses

We know little of nurses hired to work in early Canadian hospitals but it is apparent that hospital nursing was considered on a par with the lowliest servant work. Throughout the eighteenth and much of the nineteenth century public hospitals were a last resort for the indigent. Toronto, Halifax, and St. John were garrison towns so their first hospitals were for military or navy personnel with nursing care provided by orderlies. An early settlers hospital, erected in Halifax by the British government, was short-lived. Early public hospitals in Toronto, Halifax, and St. John had chequered histories. The Toronto General Hospital, though built in 1820 from public contributions, did not admit patients for nine years because it lacked operating funds. The hospital subsequently proved inadequate to meet growing needs.

Epidemics and Immigrants

At the best of times British colonial towns were poorly equipped to meet the social welfare needs of their citizens but in the 1830s and 1840s cholera and typhus epidemics, which came with an influx of sick, destitute immigrants, highlighted the inadequacies. Care during epidemics provides a sorry tale with boards of health ineffective, temporary hospitals pitiful, and nursing care abysmal. A surgeon appointed to administer the Toronto cholera hospital in 1832 complained that nurses were "unfit in every respect to assist him."[25] Lack of fitness may have indicated inadequate skill or poor personal qualities such as drunkenness. Given the extreme difficulty and

danger of caring for cholera patients in poorly equipped, hastily improvised surroundings, it is hardly surprising that the ill-prepared nurses were not up to the task.

Although the sheer numbers of immigrants arriving in English Canada were lower than in Quebec, all port cities had their share. A quarantine station on Partridge Island, St. John, was first established in 1832 and was later enlarged, though at peak times many were forced to sleep in the open air. In Toronto, sheds were erected close to the General Hospital and a citizen later recalled seeing great numbers of Irish immigrants "lying on beds or stretchers in rows of sheds, open at all sides";[26] nursing care was likely rudimentary. Lacking the presence of religious nursing orders, it was difficult to find nurses to staff hospitals, particularly during epidemics. The poor conditions of work meant that hospitals most likely could only recruit nurses from the lower echelons of society and the ranks of the desperately poor. By contrast, independent nurse/midwives, though also of the working class, can be seen as representing the "upper level" in a hierarchy of caregivers.

"Monthly" Nurses and "Sick Nurses" 1840–1875

Elizabeth Innes

One of the few early nineteenth century nurses to leave a diary was Elizabeth Innes of St. John, New Brunswick. Innes, born in St. John in 1785, was the daughter of a Scottish sergeant and a Quaker mother. A single woman, she remained living close to St. John in the parish of Portland. Much of her neatly written diary is taken up with local and family events and religious texts, but Innes tells us, "I have nursed in my time 168 women in their Confinement and 150 [in] Labour" thus indicating that she worked as both monthly nurse and midwife. She also cared for the sick and recorded her remedies for a "plaster for a weak joint" ("Rosin, Sulphur, Beeswax, Castile Soap and Lard boiled in half a pint of good spirits until thick enough for spreading") and for rheumatism ("Beeves' Galls, Camphor, Oil and Turpentine").[27] A photograph of Innes in old age reveals a dignified elderly lady in respectable attire.

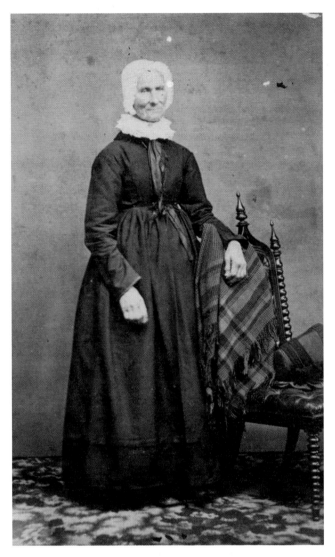

Figure 6
Elizabeth Innes
ca.1865
New Brunswick Museum, Saint John, NB, 7176

Plaster for a weak Joint

take 2 oz Rosin 1 tea spoonful flour of Sulpher
1 D° Beeswax 1 D° Hogs Lard 1 Castile Soap Boil all
together in half a pint of good Spirits till it is
a proper thickness for Spreading

Receipt for the Rheumatism

3 Beeves Galls half a pint Spirits turpentine 1 ounce of
Camphor Dissolved in a pint of Jamaica Spirits a pint
of neats foot Oil the whole mixed together and simmered
over a moderate fire till reduced to near a quart it must
be kept Stirring while on the fire

texts by the Lord Bishop of Nova Scotia

Genesis 2 Chapter 8 and 9 Verses
and the Lord God Planted a Garden east-ward in Eden
and there he put the man whome he had formed
and out of the ground made the Lord God to grow every
tree that is plesent to the sight and good for food,
the tree of life also in the midst of the garden and the
tree of Knowledge of good and evil

Acts 8 Chapter Verses 14 - 15 - 16, 17

14 now when the apostles which were at Jerusalem heard
that Samaria had received the word of god they sent
unto them Peter and John

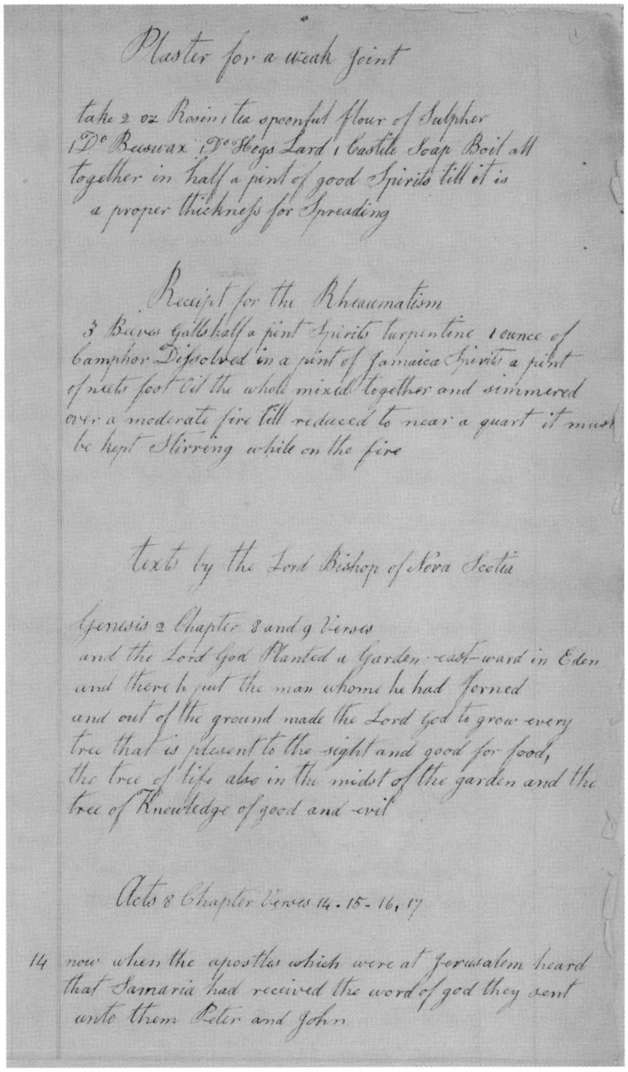

Figure 7
Page from Elizabeth Innes' diary
1840–1853
New Brunswick Museum, Saint John, NB, A273

Although we have limited information on Innes, as a literate, religiously-minded woman who aided the sick, her work was likely appreciated by local physicians. Hired nurses at mid-century struggled to carve out a role that was sometimes complementary to and sometimes independent of other practitioners. They were part of a divergent array of health care providers, which included regular physicians, druggists, midwives, and non-regular medical practitioners such as homeopaths. Physicians initially supported midwifery, but as doctors sought increasing control over obstetrical management, midwives suffered. It is not surprising that some midwives turned to monthly nursing.

The Monthly Nurse

Mrs Catherine Cole, a monthly nurse in 1860s Toronto, was a middle-aged widow. English-born, she had been practising for some years when she was enumerated, in 1871, caring for a new infant in the home of a barrister. The monthly nurse, also called "ladies' nurse" or "lady's nurse" was probably

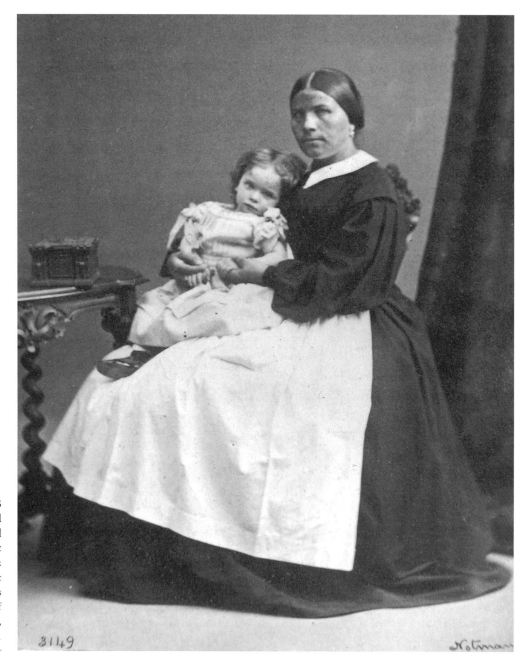

Figure 8
**R Masson's nurse and
child**
Montreal, Quebec
1862
Notman Photographic
Archives
McCord Museum of
Canadian History,
Montreal, 1-3149.1

the most frequently hired caregiver of the 1850s and 1860s. Catherine Parr Trail, unable to be present for her daughter Mary's second confinement, was pleased that she had found "a good nurse." From *Beeton's Book of Household Management* (1861), a popular English manual, we learn that a good monthly nurse should be "scrupulously clean and tidy in her person: honest, sober, ...possess a natural love for children, and have a strong nerve in case of emergencies."[28] The nurse was expected to be obser-

vant, to identify any illness, to be skilled in assisting with breastfeeding problems, and to carefully follow a doctor's orders. Women between 30 and 50 years were considered ideal, as they had both maturity and the necessary stamina to be on duty day and night.

In the early 1860s, Mrs Scott of Richmond Street West, Toronto, practised as a monthly nurse and as a midwife. An Irish-born widow, she lived in a one-storey frame house with her teenage children, Annie, a tailoress, and Ian, a printer. In Halifax the career of midwife/nurse Catherine Adams can be traced from 1871 for two subsequent decades. A 35-year-old widow in 1871, she had nine children at home ranging from three to sixteen years old. Adams was born in Nova Scotia of English or Irish background and was literate. Twenty years later three children remained at home including the two youngest sons, a merchant and printer respectively. Lacking a male breadwinner, Scott and Adams relied on the wages of their children to supplement their own income while ensuring that they learned a respectable trade.

The "Sick" Nurse

The term "sick nurse," though not widely used, does appear in the records and helps to differentiate nineteenth century nursing work. Beeton emphasized ventilation, cleanliness, diet, the importance of keen observations, and proper conduct in the sick room, instructions taken directly from Florence Nightingale's popular *Notes on Nursing.* Nightingale advised against "reckless physicking" and Beeton urged nurses to forget their own remedies and follow the advice of physicians. Contemporary physicians expected nurses to provide assistance with procedures such as bloodletting, to give medications and diets as ordered, and to carry out treatments (poultices, douches). Describing an "unusual" postpartum case, a physician in the *Canadian Lancet* relied on the attending nurse to observe keenly, to administer medication every four hours, and give enemas and warm poultices, as well as strengthening nourishment. For this patient, "the presence of anyone but her nurse gave her emotions of unease."[29] Another physician discussed the use of "hot water injections in uterine disease": this treatment "best done by an intelligent nurse." As there were no nurse training programs in Canada at the time of these case studies, physicians were relying on the skills of an experienced but untrained nurse.

As the population and wealth of cities grew, it is apparent that a demand was created for private nursing. By the 1860s, monthly nurses appeared more prominently in the records than midwives. It is possible that some women masked their midwifery practice behind the title of nurse. In Ontario, this seems more likely after 1865, when midwives could be prosecuted for practising without a licence. Some may have just preferred the steadier and more lucrative work of monthly nursing.

Nurses in Homes and Hospitals 1875–1890

Industrialization and Population Expansion

The final decades of the nineteenth century were a time of great change as cities industrialized and populations grew. In Toronto, with its large population growth, the number of private nurses grew significantly. This increase was less dramatic in St. John and Halifax, where industrialization proceded at a slower rate, and in Winnipeg the population did not appear sufficient to support private nurses until a later time. The growth of private nursing, it seems, depended on the existence of a prosperous middle class. Physicians supported the private nurse and, in 1883, the Toronto Medical Society set up a "Directory for Nurses" which must, at this time, have had mainly untrained nurses on its books. Along with the growth in private nursing, most cities, by the 1870s, had public hospitals. Hospital expansion occurred both in eastern Canada and in the developing West. An array of nurses, of varying reputation, continued to provide hospital care.

Hospital Nurses in the 1870s and 1880s

In 1871 Halifax and St. John each had a general hospital, which continued the military tradition of employing male nurses. The St. John hospital staff consisted of a matron and two nurses, William Grant, aged 32, born in New Brunswick of "African" parentage, and Susan Smith, a 22-year-old widow. A later Halifax census recorded four male nurses living with their wives and families and designated "hospital nurses." Toronto General had, in 1871, a matron and five female nurses, ranging in age from 18 to 46 years. For accounts of these early nurses we must rely on Charles Clarke, Medical Superintendent, and Mary Agnes Snively, who became Lady Superintendent in 1884. Of staff in the 1870s, Clarke later recalled that two or three were experienced; the rest "raw and uncultured ... (but) good enough girls." Eliza, an older woman, kept the patients in order at night but was not considered a good nurse.[30] Snively described the untrained nurses as mostly illiterate and some intemperate. Her comments on literacy are not exactly born out by census information, since from 1871, all nurses at the General were recorded as literate. The charge of intemperance more likely holds, as excessive use of alcohol was common at all levels of Victorian society. Living conditions at Toronto General were rough. Nurses slept on straw beds on the wards and had meals in the basement. Pay was $9 per month, though if an employee gave up the daily beer allowance, wages were increased to $10.

Margaret Davis, one of 16 nurses at Toronto General in 1881, is one of the few it is possible to describe in more detail. A middle-aged widow, she continued to work at the hospital after the nursing school was introduced in 1881 and was seen as a link between the "old-time" nurse and the "new." In a short obituary in 1905 in the newly published journal *The Canadian Nurse*, Davis was described as lacking professional instruction but able to do "good work" according to her abilities: a person who possessed "good common sense, loyalty and discipline."[31]

Early nurses at Toronto's Hospital for Sick Children (HSC) were respectable, working class women. Although suitable staff was not always easy to find, the Ladies Committee, which founded the hospital in 1875, would never have tolerated disreputable women. Solicitous of the welfare of their staff, the Lady Managers provided decent accommodation, and certain valued workers were allowed to keep older, dependant children with them. The nurses bathed, fed, and dressed the children, took them for airings in Queen's Park, treated wounds and sores, and taught bedtime prayers.

In contrast to the situation at HSC, temporary isolation hospitals still, on occasion, "recruited" from the dregs of society. In 1870s Halifax, Margaret Howard was pressed into service to "nurse" patients in a Halifax smallpox hospital. Habitually in court for drunkeness and fighting, Howard's nursing service was a condition of her early release from gaol. Women such as Davis of Toronto General and

Howard in Halifax illustrate the best and the worst of the untrained hospital nurse.

Private Nurses in the 1870s and 1880s

One overwhelming fact about nineteenth century private nurses was that the majority were widows. Apart from their working class status, widowhood stands out as the single most defining characteristic of private nurses and of midwives up to the training school era. Rosanna Baillie, a monthly nurse, was at the time of the 1871 Toronto census in the home of a physician and his wife caring for their new baby. We do not know when Baillie was widowed, but she was still wage earning in 1891. Annie Bell of St. John was a 58-year-old widow in 1881. She was still working as a "sick" nurse ten years later, living with two single daughters, a dressmaker and a fur store machinist. Eliza Schwartz, a nurse in 1880s Halifax, was unusual in that she was unable to read and write. She was still working at age 66. The census only occasionally recorded a private nurse who was unable to read or write, a fact that challenges the way they are often presented in history.

Conclusion

It seems quite obvious that in French Canada before the nineteenth century, lay caregivers could legitimately provide their services as midwives, a vocation that was not limited to tending to childbearing alone, as shown, for instance, by the case of Catherine Jérémie. After the Conquest, we must jump to the nineteenth century to find lay caregivers whose contribution can be specifically described. Aside from the work of the "nurses" of Grosse-Île, the vast majority of these women provided their care free of charge within charitable organizations that eventually became religious institutions. Laywomen made a considerable contribution to health care in the nineteenth century, since, in addition to the direct care that they dispensed to the needy, some also founded and managed care institutions funded by public charity. Three of the four founders discussed in this chapter, Blondeau-Cotté, Cadron-Jetté, and Tavernier-

Gamelin, fit this description. They became engaged in and laid the foundations for their charities after they were widowed, and all three benefited from the financial support of the Montreal bourgeoisie. Angélique Blondeau-Cotté never took religious vows, while the other two did so only late in life (Mme Jetté when she was 54!), probably more to ensure the continuity of their work than through a desire to blossom within a religious community.[32]

Untrained lay nurses in English Canada, though undoubtedly of the working class, were of diverse characters and levels of skill, ranging from highly respectable, intelligent practitioners to those who were ignorant and disreputable. In the words of British historian Anne Summers, many were "neither unskilled nor unkind, just unrefined."[33] During the nineteenth century, as family care gave way to hired care, increasing numbers of working class women, usually middle-aged or older widows, earned their living as private nurses. It is unlikely that without a degree of respectability these women would have been accepted into middle class homes and, judging by the trades of their children, many came from the upper echelons of the working class. While very early hospital nurses gained a poor reputation, once hospitals became better organized, they appeared to attract women who were more competent and respectable. The decline of midwifery can be traced through public records, but there is evidence that some midwives "re-invented" themselves as nurses. Whether they still practised midwifery but under the guise of nursing can only be conjectured. When training schools were established, young trainees quickly supplanted existing hospital nurses. This did not happen in private work where many old-time nurses remained working well into the twentieth century.

CHAPTER 2

Canadian Midwifery: Blending Traditional and Modern Practices

Cecilia Benoit and Dena Carroll

The history of midwives is virtually absent from standard medical historical texts and nursing records, yet Canadian midwives have survived in various forms, despite difficult circumstances, internal divisions over education and practice, and ongoing struggle to achieve autonomy and recognition as health professionals on par with physicians and nurses. For Aboriginal midwives, the history of midwifery has been further affected by colonialization, criticism of traditional healers, and the imposition of Western medicine. A genuine retelling of the history of midwifery in our country is overdue.

In this chapter we examine Aboriginal midwives, traditional lay/granny midwives and finally nurse-midwives, ending with a postscript on the present day status of midwifery. We draw upon a diversity of sources to highlight common themes that mark the history of midwifery. Despite the continuum of midwifery types, differing in regard to their recruitment, training, place of work, access to technology and economic rewards for services rendered, all midwives perform common activities during pregnancy and childbirth, and provide not only emergency, but social and emotional care, for birthing women. Given the challenges to their autonomy that all midwives have faced, past and present, from other professionals as well as their clients, there has also been a great range in public perceptions surrounding their occupa-

tion. It is now common knowledge that pregnancy and childbirth are as much a social and cultural process as they are biomedical and thus require sensitivity by health providers to women's personal needs.

Aboriginal Midwives

The history of Aboriginal midwives predates European settlement in Canada; its survival has ebbed and flowed, but its traditions have been revived in parts of Canada in the last decade.

Despite few historical accounts of early traditional midwives in pre-contact societies, there is reference to Aboriginal women (and sometimes men) who occupied privileged positions in their communities, providing maternity and general health care. Due to the sacred nature of childbirth and dependence on oral history stories about midwifery and childbirth were seldom recorded.[1]

Young girls were chosen at an early age to be apprentices, though few actually occupied the role of midwife until later in life, attending the births of their female relatives in order to build a solid basis of local knowledge and rituals. They were sometimes taught to recognize the "birth energy" — a special communication between the labouring woman and her baby. Skills included the preparation and administration of herbal medicines, acquiring knowledge of

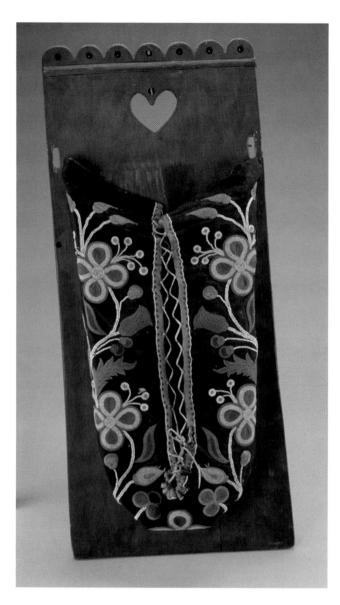

human anatomy, and the cultural and spiritual knowledge related to childbirth.

Recent linguistic research suggests the term *midwife* focused on the roles and responsibilities of providing care for women in need, and lifelong commitment to their children and families. The Nuu-chah-nulth people, located on the West Coast of BC, translate the term midwife as "she can do everything," the Coast Salish of Vancouver Island, BC, describe the role as "to watch/to care," and the Chilcotin people of the province define it as "women's helper." Anthropologist Franz Boas described the complex social organization of pregnancy and childbirth in Aboriginal societies, noting that often one or more trained midwives stayed with the woman during labour.[2] Traditional stories and dances, such as the Atlak'am masks and legends of the G*exsem of the Kwakiutl people, illustrate the spiritual and cultural connection between midwife, mother, and child.

Aboriginal women elders (also referred to as "grannies or aunties") assisted with births. Katsi Cook Bareiro, Akwesasne midwife, director of the Lewirokwas (Pulling the Baby Out of the Earth) midwifery program and former midwifery instructor at Six Nations Birthing Centre at Grand River, Ontario, emphasizes how roles were passed down from generation to generation. Katsi notes that her midwife relatives required no sanction from an outside medical, legal, or political authority, nor were they required to have a formal midwifery certification. Considered "keepers of the culture," due to their rich personal experience of childbirth and other aspects of female life, their role was to help pass down moral and ethical values through generations.[3]

Using a holistic approach to childbirth, considerable time and attention was given to the needs, concerns, and obligations of the birthing woman, an approach that still exists today. Pregnant women were required to follow specific regulations, rituals, and obligations, pay careful attention to their activities, and avoid certain social networks and foods, in order to ward off danger to their baby. The midwife was closely involved with the newborn's family circle during the four-week postpartum "healing period," and midwifery care was often extended throughout the child and mother's life cycle. Small communities and the close proximity of the people facilitated this type of care.

The midwife also oversaw a variety of preparations for labour and delivery and the welcoming of the new baby into the community. Among the Cree, tasks included gathering wood, making and beading the *tikinagan*, preparing the "birthing hands" through cleansing and blessing, honouring the placenta, using

Regilee Ootova, Inuit Midwife, Mittimatalik (Pond Inlet)

Cecilia Benoit, University of Victoria (BC) and Dena Carroll, Aboriginal researcher

Regilee Ootova exemplifies how traditional midwifery knowledge has survived over the ages and continues to be useful in modern times. Regilee entered into the midwifery profession after consulting with her grandmother, who was a traditional midwife, as well as with her maternal uncle's wife from Ikpiarjuk (Arctic Bay) about Inuit traditional birthing ways. Regilee obtained formal apprenticeship with relatives and started practising midwifery in a concerted way at age 30. Her paternal Aunt Aksi also assisted her in being a midwife several times for home births, including that of her daughter (Regilee's cousin). Working as a traditional Inuk midwife, she developed an appreciation of the high level of skill needed to assist Inuit births within local communities. She talks about the close relationships she developed with women and how critical monitoring abilities helped to encourage short labours. In 1989, she wrote a paper identifying the need to bring birth back to Inuit women's homes and communities and presented it to the Northwest Territories legislative assembly. She has learned much about the traditional procedures, and recognizes and points out that labour is not an illness. Years ago, she says, Inuit knowledge guided childbirth, and women delivered babies after hiking all day. Labour was not a big deal and it did not cause anxiety or concern for them.

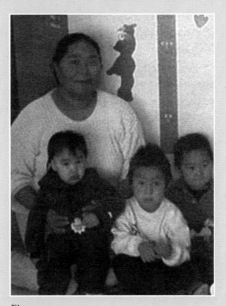

Figure 2
Regilee Ootova
ca. 2000
With permission of Regilee Ootova
Inuktitut 88 (2000)

Source: J Kusugarmit,"President's Message: Inuit Midwifery," *Inuktitut Magazine 88* (2000): 7–10.

traditional medicines to aid birth, preparing the rabbit skins, gathering moss, and preparing special foods. For Inuit women, childbirth preparations also included making the *amautiq*, the traditional clothing for transporting the baby in the new mother's pocket located in the back of her parka. Other practices included care of the afterbirth. One elder described how the "the afterbirth was commonly placed in a clean, white cloth and tied in a tree in order for it to dry naturally. This symbolized keeping the stomach clean. A boy's cord was cut and dried and put under deer or moose tracks. If [the cord] was a girl's, it was put under a berry tree." Sometimes cords were clamped on newborns' backs so that others would never lose sight of them, or kept in a drawer in a white cloth, or hidden under the house so that the infant, when it was older, would not run away. In other groups, navel amulets were used to encase children's navel cords and hung from their cradle-boards or their clothing to protect them from bad spirits. Related cultural practices included naming the baby and his/her relationship to nature and refraining from intervening in the natural process of growth by not cutting the baby's hair.[4]

Colonial laws and policies, the introduction of alcohol and the imposition of "white man's medicine" led to the demise of Aboriginal midwifery, which negatively affected the health of Aboriginal peoples. Individual physicians were often attached to government appointed Aboriginal agents who usually had no formal medical training. Many Aboriginal midwives and other healers found themselves threatened, punished, and/or ignored by both missionaries and non-Aboriginal government officials. One exception was a Tsimshian midwife from Vancouver Island, Mary Wiha, who died in 1917 at the age of 87. The notice of her death in a local paper suggests that she continued to hold a vital place in her community even after the arrival of settler populations. Other Aboriginal midwives, however, were labelled as charlatans and their birthing practices dismissed as outdated and harmful. The transmission of crucial traditional knowledge from elder to youth or from midwife to apprentice was discouraged. By 1922, mobile nurse-visitor services complemented the work of medical officers and the federal government

eventually established nursing stations in rural and northern Aboriginal communities where pre- and postnatal care was provided by station nurses, often nurse-midwives. While allowing Aboriginal women to at least give birth in their local communities, most nurse-midwives were trained within a Western biomedical model of care, and these outsiders often failed to provide effective care.[5]

By the 1970s, the federal government had closed down most nursing stations, and Aboriginal women were pressured to travel long distances to give birth in urban hospitals. Some resisted being evacuated and continued to give birth in their own communities, attended by elder midwives and/or members of their family and community. Women who left their communities to give birth were attended by English-speaking nurses and physicians who knew little about Aboriginal language and traditions, and they often experienced serious disruptions of their family life. These developments also eroded the central role of Aboriginal midwives and fewer women had access to the midwife's traditional practices and to lay medicines. A Stony Creek Band elder sums up the impact of these outside forces on their once intact culture: "[B]etween 1920 and 1993 we have seen a big change in our population. Years ago there were no drugs and we used herbs. The traditional art of midwifery was learned from mother and grandmother."[6]

The tide finally began to shift in favour of Aboriginal people and cultural revival in the 1970s and 1980s, leading to a national movement to create locally-based education, social, and health programs in Aboriginal communities across Canada. The innovative health representative program, for example, played a key role in assisting Aboriginal women to have their babies in their own communities.[7] Local maternity/birthing centres have been established. Quebec was the first, setting up the Puvirnituq Maternity Centre, which was opened in the mid-1980s as a pilot birthing centre for Inuit "trainees." It has allowed Inuit women to give birth among their own people with Inuit birth attendants who can communicate in Inuktitut. It also provides an apprenticeship model of training for Inuit women. In 2000, Inuit midwives cared for approximately 70 to 80 Inuit women. To have maternity workers to speak to them in their

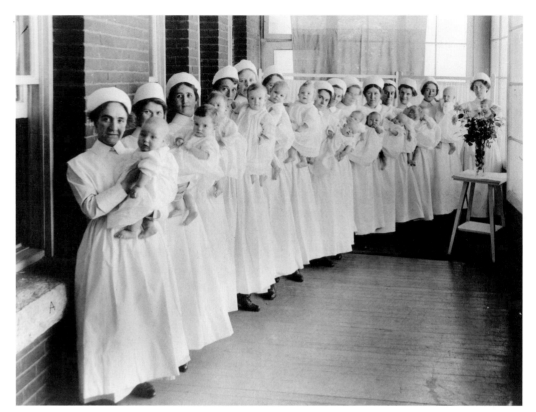

Figure 3
Student nurses holding babies
Grace Hospital,
Winnipeg, Manitoba
1914
Manitoba Archives
Foote Collection, 1522

native tongue and to be able to give birth on their traditional land without facing legal action is a major step forward. Unfortunately, recent provincial legislation in Quebec recognizes only the five existing trained Nunavik Inuit midwives, restricts their membership to the Nunavik territories, and denies membership in the Quebec Order of Midwives to any other Aboriginal midwives. Aboriginal midwives in Quebec are campaigning to change this ruling.

Other Aboriginal birthing initiatives include the birthing and training centre in southern Ontario known as the Tsi Non:we Ionnakeratstha (the place they were born) Onaigrahsta' (a birthing place) Six Nations Maternal and Child Centre, located on Six Nations Reserve in Hagersville. This unique birthing centre incorporates traditional practices with modern midwifery services, and offers a three-year training program for Aboriginal midwives. Although the Six Nations midwives do not currently have formal hospital privileges, they hold formal certification as "Aboriginal midwives" and work closely with physicians. In 2002, there were two full-fledged community midwives on staff and two Aboriginal midwife apprentices overseeing nearly 200 births. Other

recent developments include the Lewirokwas Midwifery Program, located in Akwesasne, a Mohawk reserve that straddles Quebec, Ontario, and New York State. This group is campaigning to obtain an exemption for Aboriginal midwives in the Quebec midwifery legislation and to bring midwifery back into the hands of the community. Finally, mention should be made of the Rankin Inlet Birth Centre, which, while not yet sanctioned under provincial legislation, nevertheless provides vital, culturally unique services to local women.

In summary, recent legislation has provided opportunities to revitalize traditional Aboriginal birthing methods and enable the development of birthing centre programs, both through exemption from and inclusion within existing legislation. However, only a small number of Aboriginal certified midwives work today in Canada. Equally sobering is the fact that there are few elders remaining to transmit the cultural knowledge around childbirth and traditional parenting to help Western-trained midwives blend traditional and modern day maternity care practices. On the positive side, Aboriginal midwives are gaining greater public attention, are being recognized for their unique professional practices, and have begun to organize on a national level.

Traditional Lay/Granny Midwives

Immigrant groups settling in present day Canada date back to the 1700s. Over time, settlers began to develop systems of maternity care that were a combination of customs and traditions learned in their country of origin as well as the Native practices found in their new homeland. The traditional lay midwives who cared for settler women during pregnancy and childbirth were mostly older local women who had little or no formal education, yet demonstrated strong skills and were well integrated into their ethnically-diverse settler communities. One of the first references to lay midwifery appears in a deed published by a Mr Massicotte, "which reveals that the women of Ville-Marie [Montreal], in solemn conclave assembled, on February 12th, 1713, elected a midwife Catherine Guertin for the community."[8]

Much like their Aboriginal counterparts, lay midwives in settler communities followed local protocols regarding their proper roles, duties, and responsibilities; they also faced legal impediments to practise in later centuries. Physicians began to influence health legislation as early as 1795 in "Upper Canada" (present day Ontario), with the introduction of the first *Medical Act* which essentially made it illegal to practise midwifery without an official licence. Due to the impracticality of such a ruling, the small degree-holding segment of the medical profession, mainly located in the few urban centres, was left vulnerable to public criticism and the Act was repealed in 1806. From 1806 to 1866, traditional lay midwifery remained immune from the licensing laws of the Ontario Medical Board. However, by 1866, permission that had been awarded by the provincial government to unlicensed female midwives was withdrawn, and midwifery practice was henceforth restricted exclusively to physicians. Given that no female physicians were licensed in Ontario until the 1880s and few women worked in this capacity for many decades to come, licensed male physicians enjoyed an official monopoly over childbirth and other "medically-designated" health events. In larger urban areas of Ontario,

competition between physicians and midwives as to who had authority for home births continued for several decades after Confederation. Although "doctor births" were eventually to become the norm, midwives continued to attend women in rural and remote areas of the province, as well as among the urban poor who could not afford physician attendance fees for some time after.

Outside Ontario, midwives in other settler communities remained active long after their Ontario counterparts had been displaced. In Quebec, as early as 1788, formally-trained midwives (examined by a health board to determine their proficiency), were granted the right to practise alongside male physicians. Meanwhile, in the countryside, traditional lay midwives (*sage-femmes*) continued to remain unregulated, controlled by local clergy and by birthing women themselves. In 1879, the Quebec College of Physicians and Surgeons, following events in Ontario, extended control over traditional lay midwifery. Nevertheless, for the next half century, Quebec midwives in rural areas were permitted to practise, provided that their competence was physician certified. Such was the case as well in New Brunswick and Saskatchewan, where as late as 1924 at least 50 percent of births were not attended by medical doctors.

Things looked hopeful for midwives in central Canada in the 1930s, when prominent Canadian health reformers started advocating for "health teams," comprised of midwives, physicians, and public health nurses working out of community clinics, a model that had been implemented in some European countries, including Sweden. However, medical and nursing associations, worried that competition from midwives might reduce work for their own members, lobbied against these recommendations. Ultimately, the hospital-based physician–obstetrical nurse team replaced the community midwife as primary attendant during childbirth, initially among the urban middle classes and eventually reaching other sectors of society. The obstetrical nurse became known as the "doctor's handmaiden" and was expected to show "wifely obedience to the doctor, motherly self-devotion to the patient and a form of mistress/servant discipline to those below."[9] The commonly adopted perspective promoted by the

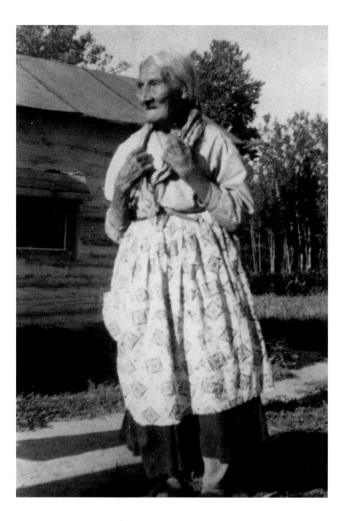

Figure 4
**Mrs Adam Callihou, Metis midwife
Hazelmere, Alberta**
1955
Glenbow Archives, Calgary, Alberta, NA-1271-1

simply did not arrive on time, and those at hand did what they could to make sure all was okay. Social historian Nancy Langford researched childbirth on the Canadian Prairies from 1880 to 1930 and noted that homestead birthing women hoped to find experienced midwives. Some women were forced to rely on inexperienced neighbours who did not always want to be a midwife but became one through necessity. Mrs Elizabeth Akitt of Edmonton, Alberta, who was attended by a doctor and a nurse with midwifery training, indicated that "I know what lots of women have gone through by not having a doctor. Sometimes, there was just a neighbour; no midwife." In recalling the beginning of labour, a first generation settler in Alberta noted that "some good friends were with us; one of them wasn't exactly a midwife, but people used to call her that." According to her grand-daughter, Karen Kobb (a British-trained midwife currently practising independent midwifery in St. John's, Newfoundland) Eileen Lillian Cleary of Beaver Harbour, Halifax County, Nova Scotia, helped deliver seven of her nieces and nephews in the late 1940s and early 1950s out of both necessity and generosity. She also helped seven other local women birth their babies.[11]

Lay midwifery survived well into the twentieth century in Newfoundland and Labrador; the province, in fact, has arguably the best records of this form of health care for child-bearing women in the country. Midwives from Canada's most easterly province were often given the epithet of "granny" or "auntie," signalling the wisdom and practical skill that comes with age and experience, as well as denoting the respect that these women often held within their outpost and rural communities. Like their Aboriginal counterparts, many of these Newfoundland and Labrador traditional midwives learned their craft from female relatives or senior midwives as well as via personal experience (most had given birth themselves, often many times over); they thus learned

medical and nursing professions was that "the art of midwifery belongs to prehistoric times; the science of obstetrics is the latest recognition of all ancient sciences."[10] However, historical continuity can also be observed with these developments. Women continued to aid one another during pregnancy and in childbirth. Though obstetrical nurses were formerly subordinate to doctors and denied the technical training required to be effective autonomous birthing care providers, in practice many continued to serve as women's primary attendants at birth, on occasion even with the attending physician's acquiescence.

The midwife story is even more complex when we look at settler communities where access to trained health professionals was limited. Often stories arise about male relatives who were forced to "fetch" the midwife, if time and weather permitted, while the woman laboured alone or perhaps with a neighbour standing by. In many cases, the birth attendant

by observation and simply by doing the work. According to one granny midwife from the west coast of the island, "I first learned to doctor the women and others in the village from my dear mother. I learned to give a newborn a steeped brew from weeds—caraway seeds perhaps [and to be] always present during birth, consoling and guiding the expectant mother." These traditional midwives were often called upon to provide an array of nursing services to local families, most of whom had no access to professional health care: "I had to do the other things besides bringing along babies 'cause there was no nurse there for a long time. So I had to do that work too. When anybody got sick, they'd call." Similarly, accordingly to midwife Aunt Gertie Legge from Heart's Delight in eastern Newfoundland, "we understood sickness and set bones and everything, and even did animals." Clara Tarrant, a granny midwife from St. Laurence, Newfoundland, who practised until the arrival of nurse-midwives and the cottage hospital in her town in 1953, described her experience this way: "I got into a situation when I just had to [do midwifery] and there was nobody but myself. I had been at a birth and had seen deliveries and I had children. Seeing is believing but feeling is the naked truth."[12]

As on the island of Newfoundland, until well into the twentieth century, most Labrador families resided in small fishing villages or rural farming communities separated from each other by considerable distances. Access to the services of local midwives was crucial to survival. Bertha Anderson or "Aunt Bertha," as she was affectionately known in her home community of Makkovik, Labrador, was one such local midwife; she travelled "no matter how great the storm," by dog team, boat, or overland "to answer a call of mercy."[13] Susan Andersen (1914–2000), another local Labrador lay midwife, is recorded as having delivered 50 babies in her lifetime, many of them at the "White Elephant," a multi-purpose building located in Makkovik where women from nearby fishing villages went to deliver their babies.

While variation existed in skill level and dedication to task, what stands out about these examples of traditional lay midwives from the Prairies and eastern coastal communities is their willingness to provide care for needy birthing women, often with little or no remuneration for services rendered. Aunt Ri from L'ance au Loup on the Labrador coast recalled that "I received one five dollars once, and that was for a month's work in Pinware. Usually it was one dollar, sometimes nothing at all." While traditional lay midwives were rarely paid in cash for their work, they frequently received gifts in kind (root vegetables, milk or fresh butter, wild meat). One of them from the west coast of Newfoundland said, "when they didn't give me money, they'd give vegetables and things like that. It was all money in a way, my dear." Sophia Anstey from Saskatchewan, who practised midwifery over much of the first half of the twentieth century, was rarely paid for her work but sometimes was awarded a hot meal. This was the case even though many of these midwives were themselves widowed and without other economic means to support themselves and their families. One Newfoundland midwife described one of her peers: "[S]he was a poor old granny, a very poor woman. She charged $5 but some people couldn't afford even that. I used to give her my old clothes."[14]

Just as their experience, skill level, and payment for services rendered varied, so did the contents of their "maternity bags" and the tools to which they had access. Mme Hubert from rural Quebec carried "the burnt rag for the cord; the great scissors to cut the tongue-tie; the large teaspoon of thick castor oil to 'cut the phlegm' in the baby's throat." Granny midwife of Newfoundland Gertrude Thomas had been given by a local doctor a "big book with all sorts of medical things in it" and a "maternity bag," which contained medical and personal items she collected herself over her midwifery career: clean towels, olive oil, soap, scissors, needle and thread, vinegar and baking soda, hot water bottle, Vaseline, safety pins, diapers and baby gown, and "medicinal drops" for the baby's eyes. Aunt Lou Dove from Chanceport, Newfoundland, recalled that her mother, also a traditional lay midwife, referred to her maternity bag as a "personal suitcase."[15]

While lay midwives in urban areas of central Canada were experiencing serious challenges from the neighbouring professions of medicine and nursing as early as the late 1800s and by mid-twentieth century had all but disappeared, lay midwives in rural

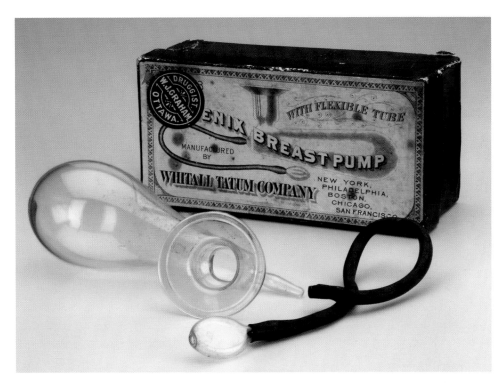

Figure 5
Breast pump
early 20th century
Photographer: Doug Millar
Canadian Museum of
Civilization, D-1583.
Gift of Mrs John Outram

areas and those practising among the numerous ethnic groups residing in the inner city and in settlements to the east and west continued to work as midwives for some time. Sometimes it was because there was no one else to help out. Other times lay midwives were simply preferred by rural women and those from different ethnic backgrounds over professional nurses or physicians more attuned to urban, white, middle class women. Periodically these professional providers came in direct competition with community lay midwives, while at other times the two groups worked together, on occasion along with a third type of midwife found in Canada's historical record: nurse-midwives.

Nurse-Midwives

Nurse-midwives were the only type of midwife legally allowed to practise in Canada throughout most of the twentieth century until the mid-1990s, and even so they were not free from government restrictions. Mainly trained overseas and holding two foreign education certificates (nursing and midwifery), nurse-midwives in the Canadian context were by and large able to provide primary care to only those pregnant women located in non-urban and northern Aboriginal

communities where trained physicians and nurses were in short supply or non-existent.

Records of nurse-midwives in Canada date back to at least the 1920s and 1930s with the establishment of nursing outposts by the Red Cross in Ontario and the efforts of the United Farm Women and United Farmers of Alberta and the National Council of Women to lobby their government to supply midwives to under-serviced communities. Elizabeth Hutchinson, nurse-midwife from Durham County, England, emigrated to New Waterford, Nova Scotia, with her husband around 1919–1920. Her nurse-midwifery training placed her on par with the local doctor and so he let her handle the deliveries unless there was a complication. Midwife Hutchinson maintained that she was trained to turn a baby in utero and knew how to perform instrument deliveries. Not all nurse-midwives were so lucky. In Vancouver during the 1930s, most Japanese immigrant mothers were attended by trained nurse-midwives from Japan who, however, had no licence to practise in BC.[16]

Local institutions also responded to the needs of pregnant women and established formal midwifery training programs. In Newfoundland in 1920, a group of women from St. John's and other parts of the

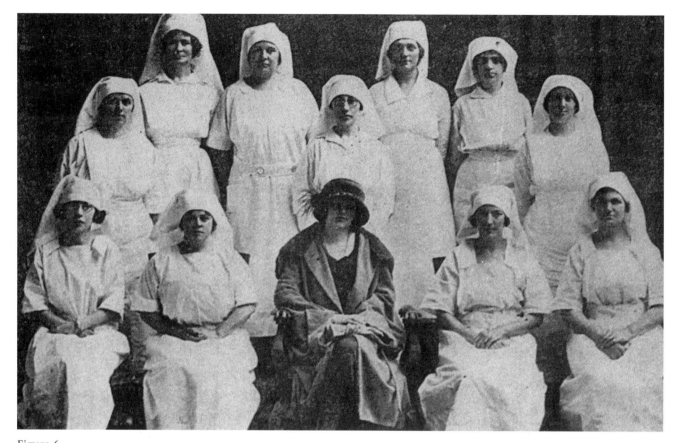

Figure 6
A graduating class of midwives from the Midwives Club
St. John's, Newfoundland
1924
Newfoundland Quarterly, Autumn, 1924; Harry Cuff Publications

Island, received formal training in midwifery and nursing skills and became the first graduates of the "Midwives' Club." One Newfoundlander who made the trip to St. John's for formal training explains: "When I was young my grandmother was a good granny midwife. There were two or three others. But when I came out [to St. John's], they were getting too old to do any work. I always liked helping people but I never done any midwifery before I trained.... Father Thomas asked me to go to school in St. John's. They wanted to get someone young, not an old person."

Another of her peers put it this way: "I was 32. I packed my bags and went to St. John's.... After it was over, I got a license. I was a licensed practicing midwife." Like the granny midwives before them, these newly trained nurse-midwives had a very demanding role. Olive Bishop, from Pass Island off the South

Coast of Newfoundland in Hermitage Bay handled an array of normal births as well as abnormal ones, including twins and breeches.[17]

As outlined in chapter 9, between 1925 and 1934, the Newfoundland Outport Nursing and Industrial Association (NONIA) recruited nurse-midwives, mainly from the British Isles, to work in the outports. Nurse-midwife Myra Grimsley Bennett came from Britain to Newfoundland in the early 1920s to practise her skills and eventually married a local man in Daniel's Harbour on the northwest coast. By 1938, 143 outposts and villages had access to trained midwives in 23 districts. By the late 1940s, a Cottage Hospital Plan (CHP) had been established, based on eighteen community hospitals, with referral of serious medical concerns to three regional hospitals. In the capital city of St. John's a base hospital operated by the Department of Health was also established. Fourteen additional small community facilities and a larger regional hospital were established in the north of the province under the auspices of the religious-based International Grenfell Association, subsequently also placed under government direction. Cottage hospitals were comparatively small, 30- to 50-bed institutions employing a work team comprised of one or a few staff physicians, a number of nurses and nurse-midwives, and a small support staff. As Margaret Maloney, a retired cottage hospital nurse-midwife from Burgeo, southwestern Newfoundland, recalled: "to the women of Burgeo, coming into the cottage hospital to have a baby was like eating a piece of pie, you know…. And people were having an average of five or six children, so you got to know the mothers."[18]

Other nurse-midwives, recruited from the British Isles, New Zealand, and Australia, were employed by the philanthropic International Grenfell Association (later renamed Grenfell Regional Health Services) located in the western regions of Newfound-land and parts of Labrador. The Association relied heavily on the expertise of immigrant nurse-midwives to care for birthing women in these sparsely populated, and medically under-serviced regions; although some midwives were Canadian-born midwives and received their training in Britain.[19] One of the immigrant nurse-midwives recalls her experience working on the maternity ward in the hospital in Goose Bay, Labrador in the late 1980s:

> I was in Goose Bay [southern Labrador], yeah. It was busy. We worked as midwives in as much as you don't anywhere else in Canada within a hospital system. Like we did the deliveries and gave the care. …[W]e had a [British] obstetrician who had been brought up in a system with midwives so he was really good. …[E]ven the GPs we had up there, if they were on call and everything was straightforward, quite often they'd say, "Well go ahead."[20]

In 1944, in Edmonton, Alberta, the first of its kind nurse-midwifery training program "Advanced Practical Obstetrics Course for District Nurses" was established. Another educational program was developed for nurse practitioners in 1967 in Halifax,

Nova Scotia, and a similar program, boldly titled "Nurse-Midwifery," was launched in 1978 in St. Johns, Newfoundland. The establishment of these latter two programs reflected the development of nurse-midwifery practice opportunities in rural and remote Canada.

By the late 1950s and early 1960s, Health and Welfare Canada established networks of nursing stations and cottage hospitals across the North and expanded nurse-midwifery services. Many who came were British-trained nurse-midwives who worked in the North for only short bouts, sometimes returning home or immigrating and settling down in urban areas, perhaps working as obstetrical nurses. Other nurse-midwives stayed in the Canadian North for extended periods. One example was the British-born nurse-midwife Lesley Knight, who worked in Gjoa Haven, Northwest Territories, in the mid-1970s and later practised nursing and midwifery in Pond Inlet on Baffin Island and in Inuvik. Lesley was especially liked by the local people for her attempt to integrate traditional midwives into the maternity care system, often despite opposition from medical authorities.[21] Such was also the case for both Glad Reardon, an Australian nurse-midwife who worked extensively among First Nations people across northern Canada, and Kathleen Mary "Jo" Lutley, who spent a quarter of a century working as a nurse-midwife in the Canadian North.[22]

Pat Kaufert and John O'Neil point out the positive contribution of nurse-midwives among Inuit women in the Keewatin region of northern Manitoba:

> [The midwife] was a positive figure when at the centre of the stories women told about their experiences of childbirth in the nursing stations, but midwives were also recalled as representatives of government, as authority figures. Despite this ambivalence, women complained bitterly about the disappearance of the midwife, seeing her as the key to the returning of birth to the community setting.[23]

Indeed, nurse-midwives' knowledge of pregnancy and childbirth sometimes proved useful in separating birthing women at genuine medical risk from those who could deliver their babies in their own home communities. One Scottish-trained midwife, Pearl

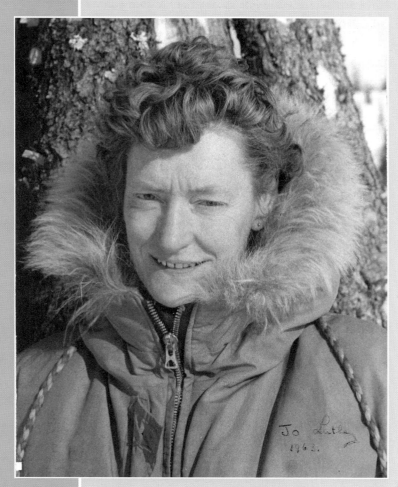

Figure 7
Kathleen Mary "Jo" Lutley
1962
Courtesy of Jo Lutley and Cecilia Benoit

Jo Lutley

**Cecilia Benoit, University of Victoria (BC) and
Dena Carroll, Aboriginal researcher**

British-born Kathleen Mary "Jo" Lutley spent a total of 26 years in health service work in Canada's North, working for long stints in Labrador, northern Quebec, and Manitoba, attending to birthing women in teepees, nursing stations, and airplanes. The Royal College of Midwives in Britain awarded her midwifery and nursing certificates in 1953. Part of her training involved attending women in labour and catching their babies in the hospital setting as well as "on the district." Jo chose to work her practicum in the London working class district known as the East End. She says that it was here she got "toughened up" and was "put in good stead" for her work in Canada's North. Jo worked in dwellings in the East End where "mice were running around" and she had to send her husband away with some of her own money to buy mousetraps! Jo was given a soapstone sculpture for helping an Inuit woman whose baby "was born in a coil" (with the umbilical cord around its neck).

Source: Personal communication with Kathleen Mary "Jo" Lutley, May–June 2000.

Herbert, recalls her initiation into a Northern Ontario Native community:

> The woman had only contractions when they called for me. She had several babies before and I had seen her at the nursing station. So when I arrived at her home I said: "Well, where do you want to have the baby?" I knew that they had cleaned a [seal] skin especially for her to have the baby on it. So I asked, "You got some skin?" "Oh yes, I got plenty of sealskin, clean and wiped." So I asked, "Where do you want to be, on the bed?" She said, "Well, no, I want to be on the floor." They used the floor to press against, you see. One of the other women sat behind her to give support. ... So, anyway, I ended up delivering the baby. Everything I did was all commented upon. I didn't know the dialect enough to really understand it all. But what I did was approved 'cause after that I got called for just about all deliveries.[24]

Despite these positive outcomes, Health and Welfare Canada policy in the late 1970s and early 1980s forced all pregnant women residing in isolated and remote areas of Canada to travel to large urban hospitals, sometimes several weeks prior to their delivery date. This policy reduced opportunities for nurse-midwives to practise and tighter immigration policies meant few nurse-midwives were available to practise autonomously.

On a different front, a group of nurse-midwives in 1973 presented a statement to their provincial association in Ontario outlining how they might be integrated into the mainstream maternity care system in Canada. A catalyst for these early efforts was the attendance of British-trained midwife May Toth at the International Confederation of Midwives conference in Washington, DC, the year prior. As most of the members of what became known as the Ontario Nurse-Midwives Association (ONMA) were British trained, the preferred model of care was the British independent midwifery model. Concerns about political expediency led them to pursue a less contentious American nurse-midwifery model where attendance at birth was limited to institutional settings. Nurse-midwives in British Columbia, Alberta, Saskatchewan, Northwest Territories, and the Yukon also adopted the Ontario statement and established the Western Nurse-Midwives Association. Subsequently, a Canadian National Committee on nurse-midwives emerged to promote nurse-midwifery nationally.[25]

These efforts were supported by the larger nursing profession through the Canadian Nurses' Association (CNA), which contrasted the approach adopted in the early decades of the twentieth century. In 1974 the CNA recommended that a nurse-midwife be recognized as "the health professional best equipped to meet the growing needs for counselling services and for greater continuity of care within this area of the health system."[26] In Ontario, the Registered Nurses Association of Ontario (RNAO) supported the development of nurse-midwifery as a complementary element in the provincial maternity care system. The RNAO's statement followed the ONMA's efforts but also the recommendation of the government appointed Committee on the Healing Arts (1970) to integrate nurse-midwifery into the health care system as a strategy to address the physician shortage and foster cost-effective maternity care. The RNAO subsequently proposed negotiations with the College of Nurses of Ontario, provincial medical organizations, and the Ontario government to draft enabling legislation. These negotiations, however, never came to fruition, due in large part to the opposition of the medical profession and public submission to medical authority. The end result was that Canada would remain for some time to come the only advanced industrial country with no provision for legalized midwifery.

Postscript

While nurse-midwives made little headway at gaining recognition in mainstream Canada, the resurgence of feminism eventually led to a version of traditional lay midwifery in a small number of rural and urban pockets of the country. In BC, "independent lay midwives" struggled to gain training by forming their own underground school for a short while; others acquired their craft through apprenticeship. Some held midwifery and/or nursing credentials or academic degrees attained from institutions in other countries or locally while others had no advanced training at all.

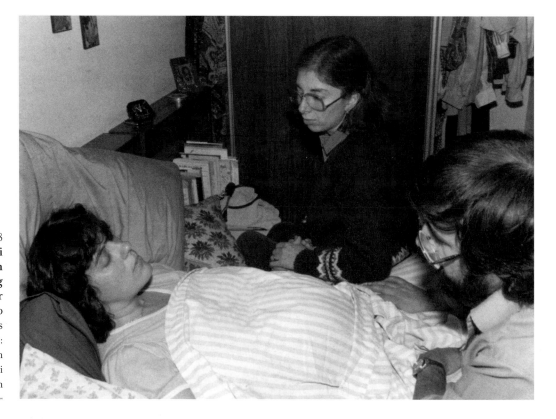

Figure 8
**Midwife Bobbi
Soderstrom
attending
birthing mother**
Ottawa, Ontario
1980s
Photographer:
Bonnie Johnson
Courtesy of Bobbi
Soderstrom

Estimates indicate that by the early 1990s there were about 100 independent lay midwives across Canada with a full-case load — that is, attending 40 or so births a year. About the same number were estimated to be attending five or fewer births per year. Due to the legislative ban, many independent lay midwives faced risks of being prosecuted for practising medicine without a licence. Despite this, small groups continued to operate underground, sometimes using secret codes during telephone conversations in fear that their phones were tapped by the authorities. Others influenced by US training schools sought to upgrade their skills south of the Canadian border and attain some form of professional certification.

In the early 1990s, some provincial governments became increasingly concerned about legal cases against unregulated midwives, brought on by physicians opposing illegally attended home births or clients unhappy with the aftermath of a midwifery-attended birth. Simultaneously, some midwives, concerned about their legal risks, pushed for regulation of midwifery under a professional association. The time was right as provinces were seeking to reorgan-

ize their health care services, and were facing considerable pressure from international and local groups to regulate midwifery. As noted above, Canada was the only industrialized country not to recognize midwifery as a profession distinct from nurse-midwifery.

In the last half decade, midwifery leaders in Ontario, Quebec, and British Columbia have established university training for midwives distinct from educational programs for nurses and physicians. Manitoba is currently in the planning stages of a baccalaureate midwifery program at the University of Manitoba and apprenticeship programs approved by the College of Midwives of Manitoba. Both of these educational routes would equip the future midwife with the core competencies required for practice in the province. Certification programs have also been established in Ontario, British Columbia, Alberta, Quebec, and Manitoba; however, public funding is not yet available in Alberta. A *Midwives Act* has been passed in Saskatchewan, but is not yet proclaimed. Legislation is proposed in some other provinces and territories.

The practice of today's midwives has changed considerably compared to earlier periods. Certified midwives are trained to use obstetrical instruments, prescribe pharmaceutical aids, as well as homeopathic remedies and natural aids, and are permitted to attend births in hospital settings and birthing centres and/or women's homes, depending on provincial legislation. A professional college oversees the midwifery profession, and certified midwives must maintain a specific caseload each year and carry medical malpractice insurance similar to physicians.

Summary and Conclusion

The above historical overview shows that midwives of different types have been active in Canada from before the arrival of European settlers up to the current time, providing crucial services to enhance the health and well-being of women and babies. In this way, midwives in Canada parallel nurses who, virtually all women as well, responded to the call for help during sickness by members of their local communities.

Individual midwives have for the most part been courageous healers, willing to attend birthing women when no nurse or doctor was at hand and tend to the sick or victims of accident or injury, despite difficult working conditions and little or no economic reward. It is because of this, perhaps, that Canadian midwives in earlier times held relatively high status in their local communities, although this did not extend to formal recognition of their profession until less than a decade ago.

The dominant model of midwifery being endorsed in many Canadian provinces today is the end result of a centuries-old history of women caring for other women during pregnancy, childbirth, and the postpartum period, influenced by pre-colonial Aboriginal societies and waves of immigrant women from Britain, the US, and other countries. While most lay midwives in urban English Canada and in French Canada were no longer practising by the turn of the twentieth century, their counterparts in Aboriginal communities and among the country's numerous ethnic groups living in the inner city and in rural settlements to the east and west continued to provide care into the post–World War II period. In all of this, the neighbouring professions of nursing and medicine have played major roles; indeed, in the case of nurse-midwives, the professional body overseeing their work was nursing not midwifery, which was not then recognized.

There have been a variety of overlapping and often competing discourses among midwives themselves regarding their education, place of work, and use of technology. Most recently, an autonomous form of midwifery has become legitimized in parts of Canada, and certified midwives have finally secured a stable niche in the modern health care system alongside their nursing sisters. Yet, as with nursing itself, we can be fairly sure that the midwifery profession will continue to evolve, as it has in the past, to meet the changing needs and concerns of birthing women and their families and communities across Canada.

CHAPTER 3

The Trained Nurse: Private Duty and VON Home Nursing (Late 1800s to 1940s)

Barbara Keddy and Dianne Dodd

This chapter examines the much neglected area of nursing in the home, principally the private duty nursing that the vast majority of graduate nurses performed prior to the Second World War, as well as the bedside nursing of organizations such as the Victorian order of Nurses (VON). While employment as private duty nurses was plentiful in the first two decades of the twentieth century, it declined in the interwar years, markedly so during the Depression, leaving many nurses under-employed and often unable to collect their fees. Following changes in the health care system, particularly the increase in hospitalization for birthing, surgery, and other medical care, as well as the implementation of medical insurance, most private duty nurses became hospital employees.

The field of private duty nursing suffers from relative neglect within nursing history due to its association with the domestic sphere and a lack of documentary evidence. However, historians are beginning to sketch its outlines. No doubt its private nature held attractions for many graduate nurses who worked, in essence, as entrepreneurs, receiving fees for their services much as physicians did. Often their work was fulfilling and they enjoyed a certain measure of autonomy that the supervised hospital or public health nurse did not. However, they worked in a gendered job market, where patients and doctors alike linked nursing with "feminine" traits such as compassion and caring, and it was soon clear that nursing would achieve only partial recognition as a profession. Working conditions were not always ideal, the pay was low, and job security non-existent. As health care shifted from the home to the hospital, many nurses found the security of full-time hospital employment preferable and began to look to unionization as a way to protect their interests. Now it seems that the nursing profession has come full circle and much nursing care is being transferred to the home.

What Is a Nurse?

The concept of nurse and nursing has always been somewhat ambiguous. Prior to the late nineteenth century in Canada, a nurse was a woman who gave care in the home, usually to members of her own family who were ill, or giving birth. This private care could also extend to the preparation of the dead for burial, and was viewed as a domestic skill that most women possessed. In an era before sophisticated medical treatments, these nurturing traits qualified women to watch the patient, keep the patient and sickroom clean, change dressings, provide comfort and food, and perhaps administer some herbal medicines. Hospitals in this period were centres for the custodial care of the very poor and offered few

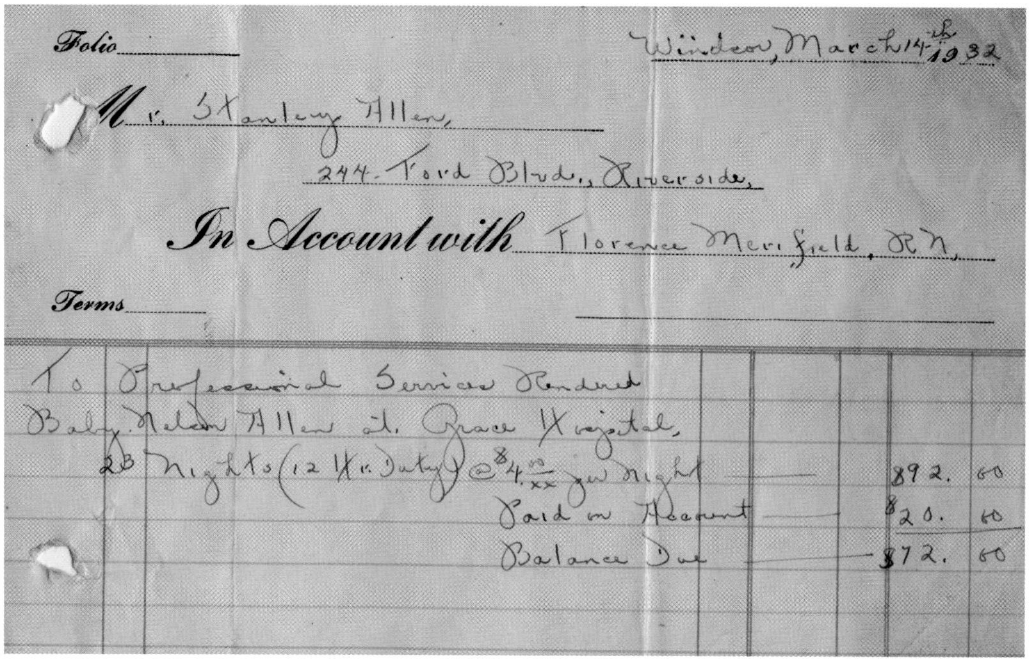
Folio
Windsor, March 14th 1932
Mr. Stanley Allen,
244 Ford Blvd., Riverside,
In Account with Florence Merifield, R.N.
Terms
To Professional Services Rendered
Baby Nelson Allen at Grace Hospital,
23 Nights (12 Hr. Duty) @ $4.00 per night $92.00
Paid on Account $20.00
Balance Due $72.00

Figure 1
Bill for Florence Merifield, RN, post-natal private-duty nursing services
Grace Hospital, Windsor, Ontario
1932
Canadian Museum of Civilization Archives
Gift of Lynn Kirkwood

Nurse Merifield charged $4 per night to care for a newborn baby and his mother.

resources to cure their patients. Thus domestic nursing was the norm and seldom was the nurse paid for her services. Indeed many, notably those belonging to religious orders, provided nursing services for altruistic or religious reasons.

The emergence of the "trained" nurse followed dramatic changes such as surgery, new diagnostic tools, and other medical techniques successfully undertaken in the hospital setting. Here, paying patients expected to be treated and cured. As hospitals evolved, it became evident that a skilled, literate, and qualified nursing workforce was needed to replace the working class women, often former hospital patients, who had previously provided nursing care.

By the end of the nineteenth century, new hospital-based schools of nursing, influenced by the Nightingale tradition and religious hospitallers, were systematically training nurses. Student nurses worked as apprentices in exchange for their training, doing most of the hospital nursing. Supervised by a few graduate nurses, the students worked strenuously, 12 to 14 hours a day, were paid a meagre allowance of $8–10 per month and were exposed to dangerous contagious diseases on wards. Indeed many historians describe them as exploited, oppressed, and usually exhausted.[1] Still, nurses learned the skills they needed to care for sick patients using modern techniques.

As graduates of these schools came onto the labour market, they helped change the concept of the nurse from that of a domestic worker, who could be any woman with nurturing skills, to a trained "professional." At this time, nursing leaders were working to dissociate the profession of nursing from the untrained domestic labour that passed for nursing in former times. The North American nurse began to claim social legitimacy and prestige as one of the few occupations considered appropriate for women. Indeed nurses remained somewhat privileged vis-à-vis other women workers. They were chosen from the respectable classes and from English- or French-speaking Canadian women. The nursing schools made it very difficult for ethnic, Aboriginal, or women of colour to gain admittance until the mid-twentieth century in Canada. Although the now familiar term, RN, or "registered nurse" did not become widespread until the 1940s, these early nurses called themselves "trained," or "graduate" nurses in order to distinguish themselves from the untrained women who also hired themselves out as nurses.

A Neglected Majority

The graduates of the early nursing schools, estimated at only about 300 at the turn of the century, quickly grew to a workforce of over 20 000 by the beginning of the First World War. Most of this first generation of trained nurses worked as private duty nurses, largely in other people's homes. Prior to the Second World War, 43 percent of nurses worked in private duty, while 26 percent were employed in institutions and 20 percent in public health.[2]

Yet, despite these numbers, most of the literature examining nursing history deals with the small minority of nurses who worked in hospitals or in public health. Why this neglect of private duty nurses? In part this silence can be explained by the lack of documentary sources on nurses who worked in the domestic realm, but also by the hierarchy of values within nursing. Publicly- or even privately-funded hospitals, religious communities, and publicly accountable agencies like the VON kept records. Private duty nurses generally did not. While indirect sources are available, such as nurses' journals and reports in which private duty nursing was discussed, the nurses themselves seldom had a voice. There are few biographies, letters, or diaries documenting the day-to-day lives of these nurses. In contrast to this silent majority, are the well recorded voices of the profession's elite: nursing superintendents in hospitals who founded alumnae and professional associations fought to have nurses' residences built, and to improve educational standards. Also enjoying a very positive image were public health or district nurses who required advanced training and were selected for such qualities as tact and leadership ability. They were often held up as models for other nurses to emulate. Another group that overlapped somewhat with public health nurses were outpost nurses, heroic pioneers celebrated in literature and their communities, where they cared for isolated populations in newly settled territories.

By contrast, private duty nurses, like ordinary women raising their children, domestic servants making their living, or workers toiling in factories, represent the less glamorous, day-to-day bedside nursing. Often their work bordered on domestic labour, and discussions concerning private duty nursing often focused on the obstacles its domestic associations posed to the long-standing goal of professionalization. The history of the VON demonstrates this bias.

Secondary sources focus on the organization's public health work, the controversies surrounding its origins, and its battles with physicians and nurses over practical midwifery for poor and isolated populations. By contrast, there is a relative dearth of information available on the home nursing care that constitutes the backbone of its work. The voices of the women who worked for the VON are seldom heard. Yearly VON records are mainly accounts of funding and numbers of cases attended to by the nurses. We know relatively little about what nurses thought of their challenges, struggles, rewards, and contributions.

Recently, there has been a resurgence of interest in rank and file nurses, and some historians and nurses have conducted oral interviews which reach back to the period after 1920. However, we still know little about private duty nurses in the first two decades, and much of that comes from the voices of the nursing leadership, who had their own perception of the private duty market.[3]

The Early Years of Private Duty Nursing

Initially private duty nursing was a relatively well paying job for women, given the limited options that "respectable" women had in the marketplace. Besides teaching, there were few options for a young woman who wanted to enjoy the status that came with the notion of being "trained." Little wonder many took pride in their uniform, a symbol of their stature and independence. Indeed many were attracted to nursing out of a sense of adventure. Interviews indicate that most nurses believed that their uniforms allowed them to travel more freely than could other women. It did not always work, however. Kathryn McPherson cites one example of a young nurse who was being harassed by a man while going home on a city bus. On disembarking she shouted out to him, "If you can't respect me, you might have respected the uniform."[4]

Among the early group of nurses who graduated from the first hospital schools, private duty employment was relatively easy to find, as the nursing profession was in a state of expansion.

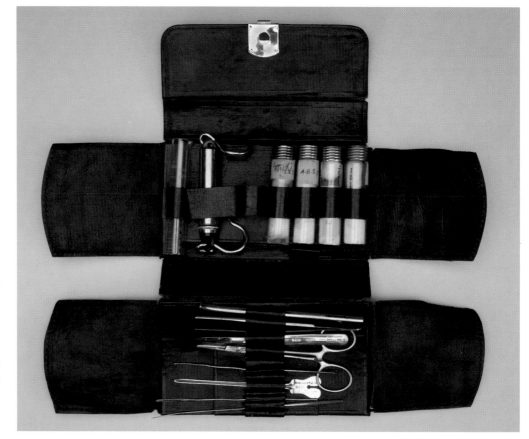

Figure 2
**Instrument kit, used by
Ruth Vivian Hart,
graduate Royal
Victoria Hospital
School of Nursing,**
Montreal, Quebec
1916
Photographer:
Doug Millar
Canadian Nurses
Association Collection
Canadian Museum of
Civilization, 2000.111. 492

*A kit containing
instruments,
medications,
thermometer and
scale was essential
to the private
duty nurse.*

Most private duty nurses lived with patients in their own homes on a daily basis for varying lengths of time, depending on the need. In 1934 an RN could expect to receive $5 per day for a 12-hour shift, $4 per day for an 8-hour shift, and $6 a day for a 24-hour shift, varying somewhat from province to province. Nurses were paid directly by the patient's family and in some cases their wages were covered by private insurance policies. Private duty nurses could also be found in hospitals, where they provided the well-to-do with around the clock nursing care and were referred to as "specials." Although working in the hospital, they received their fee, much like the doctor did, from the patient. By the wartime period, private duty nursing in homes had significantly declined and hospital employment had increased correspondingly.

Historians have speculated about whether student nurses preferred to work on their own in patients' homes or did so out of necessity. Strong-Boag, for example, has pointed out that private duty nurses had the benefit of being their own bosses in the home, and if times were good they could choose their own places of employment. Following their student experiences, in which they were closely supervised and regimented, many nurses may have found the relative freedom refreshing. McPherson, who interviewed private duty nurses, found that "the perils inherent in the unregulated private health care market were more than compensated for by the autonomy, variety, mobility and equality they enjoyed." Still, for many there was little choice, as there were only a few jobs available in hospitals and public health agencies. Most hung out their shingle as private duty nurses.[5]

Although less restrictive than the hospital environment, such work was still not independent. A nurse needed a good relationship with a physician or several physicians, as she was often dependent on them for patient referrals. There were central registries, at hospitals, sometimes in doctor's offices or sponsored through nurses' alumnae associations, where patients could find the names of trained nurses

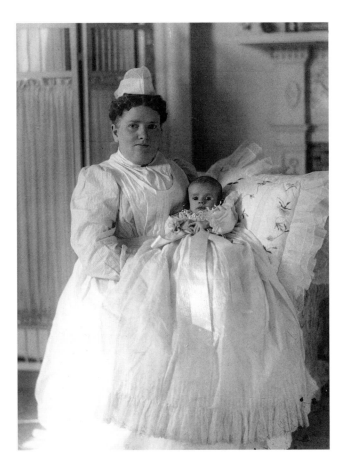

Figure 3
Mrs Allan's nurse and baby
Montreal, Quebec
1898
Notman Photographic Archives
McCord Museum of Canadian History, II-127160

the chronically ill, for accident or burn victims, for children affected by childhood diseases, for young adults or children with tuberculosis, for newborn babies and their mothers, and for the elderly. Certain types of work seem to have been preferred over others. For example, assignments in country districts, 24-hour work (as opposed to working 8- or 12-hour shifts), and cases involving contagious disease were least popular, while maternity cases were often welcomed. George Weir found in his 1930s study that private duty nurses in the Prairies, hardest hit by the Depression, were more likely to accept the hated 24-hour jobs and to perform household duties than those better situated. One would expect that nurses developed considerable expertise over time. Nurses certainly needed the skills they learned in hospital schools, even if the conditions they encountered in homes were vastly different than those in the highly regimented hospital setting.[7]

Early graduate nurses faced competition from those who advertised themselves as nurses, but were not bona fide graduate or trained nurses. While the distinction was clear to the trained nurse, the public often did not see the difference. Many nurses wore their caps and uniforms as visual proof of what they considered to be their superior training and nursing skill, in an effort to demonstrate the benefits to the public of the trained nurse.

Related to the issue of competition from untrained nurses was the pressure to blur the distinctions between nursing and domestic work. In private duty the nurse was often responsible for preparing meals and that could be extended, "into more substantive household chores." Much depended on the resources and goodwill of the patient and family. While special duty nurses in hospitals were generally hired by those who were relatively well off, nursing in the home was quite different. In the few homes where there were paid housekeepers, the nurse's work

to live in with them. The market was competitive, in spite of the fact that the nursing jobs were arduous.[6]

What kind of work did private duty nurses do? Certainly bedside nursing was quite different then than it is today. Many minor surgeries, births, long term care of the sick and other types of medical care that we would now associate with the hospital took place at home. Prior to the development of sulfonamides, penicillin, and other antibiotics and vaccines, nurses employed labour intensive measures to combat infections that could easily take the life of a new mother or child. Recovery was often slow. Maternal and infant death rates were high, and contagious diseases such as tuberculosis, smallpox, measles, and scarlet fever were common. Graduate nurses became experienced at dealing with these life-threatening diseases, yet they often faced the death of a patient from infections resulting from accidents to puerperal fever to pneumonia. And, of course, they could contract disease themselves and had to be vigilant to protect their own health.

Private duty work was varied. Nurses cared for

was easier. However, like a governess, the private duty nurse could get caught between being accepted on equal footing with family members and their need to assert some authority over domestic staff. But in many homes, private duty nurses were seen as "Jill of all trades" and were expected to carry out the tasks of a housekeeper, parent, companion, cook, maid, servant, and nanny. Duties were often of a personal and domestic nature, rendering the trained nurse in the home a subservient quasi-family member, under the authority and direction of the physician as well as the patient and family members who paid her, "solving their servant problem." While it could be said that nurses in hospitals in the 1920s and 1930s were also expected to perform many of these same domestic tasks, they were done in the regimented setting of a public institution, with fellow students. The domestic duties of the trained nurse in the home were performed in isolation, in another person's home, and were often more intense. Sometimes nurses were able to sleep only when the patient slept. And they could work for long stretches without days off, making a social life difficult. As well, the facilities and resources to do their work adequately varied enormously from one home to the next.[8]

It was indeed a role enmeshed within peculiar domestic relationships. A private duty nurse might feel she was at the mercy of an individual patient, and/or the patient's family. As illness can be a time of tremendous stress, private duty nurses had to avoid involvement in family conflicts. Although few nurses are willing to discuss this, they may occasionally have been subjected to sexual or physical abuse by patients, their families, or even the doctor, whose orders the nurse was expected to follow. While a private duty nurse had the option of quitting the job to avoid a difficult situation, she did not have the institutional support to protect her that she might have had working in a hospital. Such problems required a certain amount of resolve and confidence to deal with and we might surmise that nurses developed good business sense, people skills, and leadership qualities as well as enhancing their nursing skills.

Working in a home could have its benefits, however. Changing jobs regularly gave the nurse a variety of health conditions to deal with, added experience,

and day-to-day autonomy. And a close relationship with the patient and his/her family could be rewarding. Nurse Rebecca Bancroft cared for one man in his home who had a ruptured appendix and subsequently had three operations because of delayed treatment. He had been relatively wealthy during the first days of being in his home but later was unable to pay her as well as he had originally. Yet, she insisted on staying with him until his complete recovery. She felt that the experience of learning about his trade as an interesting antique dealer was compensation enough. No doubt she felt satisfied in seeing him through to recovery and in shouldering responsibility for his care.[9]

Amid all the discussions about what constituted a nurse, the VON was established in 1897. Not surprisingly this high profile agency was careful to select the most poised women to be trained as VON nurses, and then established training schools to give them a further six months of training in public health or district nursing, the first such schools in Canada. In the work of public health, VON nurses needed to be ambassadors for healthy living and a credit to the new nursing profession all in one. When it was formed, the VON had hoped to tackle the desperate need for outpost nurses, or better yet, midwives, in isolated parts of the country. Sadly, that turned out to be prohibitively expensive, and professional rivalries also stood in the way of effective action. However, by early century, the VON was becoming a quiet, effective force in performing much day-to-day bedside nursing work among the urban poor, including working class and ethnic populations. Nurses, usually young single women, generally lived in settlement-like residences in cities, often located in working class areas in order to be close to their patients. They wore their own distinctive uniform, visiting families who could not afford to pay for a private duty nurse. They did much of the same work, except that they did not live in: monitoring new mothers and babies and in some cases delivering them when the family didn't want or couldn't afford to hire a physician; caring for children afflicted by childhood illnesses; administering first aid and changing dressings; attending to the elderly and chronically ill; and working among neglected

Appearance and Technique: VON Nursing Manuals

Christina Bates, Canadian Museum of Civilization

During the period from the 1920s to the 1950s, when the home nursing service of the Victorian Order of Nurses (VON) flourished, the organization put out nursing manuals every few years. These gave detailed instructions on personal appearance and strict procedures to be followed by all their nurses. Like public health nurses, their demeanor had to be lady-like, with not a trace of sexuality: "The nurse who goes into the school and homes of the poor dressed in a low-neck silk waist, fashionable skirt, silk stockings and high-heeled boots will only antagonize.... Any nurse on duty should be dressed neatly and smartly but plainly," wrote Lina Rogers Struthers, Toronto's first school nurse.

The process of crossing the threshold into a patient's home was carefully regulated in the manuals — to avoid contamination and perhaps also to illustrate to the patient and to the family that the VON nurse was refined, even fastidious: "Coat and hat should be placed on a wooden chair drawn away from the wall, the coat folded with lining inside, cuffs may be placed inside the hat." The outfitting and use of the VON bag, the essential accoutrement of home nursing, was methodically outlined in the section "Bag Technique":

> ...the nurse rolls her sleeves well above her elbows...opens her bag and removes paper napkin, paper towel and bottle of green soap. The paper napkin is spread on the table which has been protected by a newspaper and the green soap and towel are placed thereon.... She washes her hands thoroughly.... [She] returns to her bag and takes from it her apron which she puts on.... The bag is then closed and if for any reason it must be re-opened the nurse should thoroughly cleanse her hands.

The combination of personal grooming and strict procedure served to give the VON nurse authority in homes where there was a perceived resistance, since the success of her ministrations was dependent upon the families' co-operation.

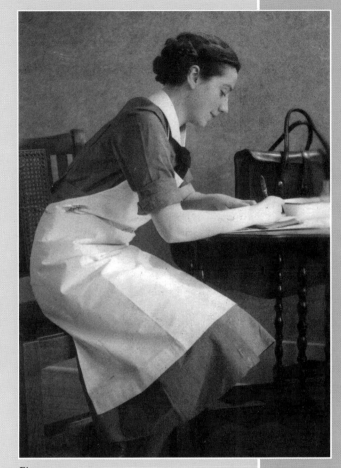

Figure 4
VON nurse in studio portrait
1920s
Courtesy of VON Canada

All is neat and tidy in this posed portrait of a Victorian Order nurse.

Sources: Lina Rogers Struthers, *The School Nurse* (New York: Putnam's Sons, 1917); *Victorian Order of Nurses for Canada, Nursing Manual, 1940.*

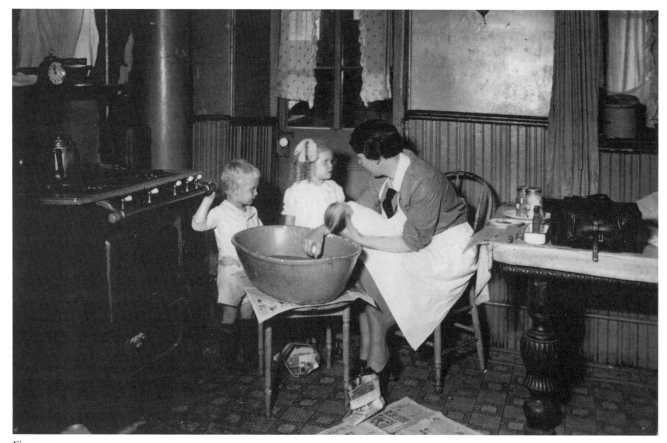

Figure 5
VON nurse on home visit
Winnipeg, Manitoba
1920s
Courtesy of VON Canada

tuberculosis sufferers. While VON nursing work compared with private duty nursing, the former had the advantage of greater institutional support, companionship of colleagues, better pay, and more steady employment. Also the VON nurse was usually the social superior of the patient and could exert some authority, while those roles were often reversed for private duty nurses.

The VON hoped that by offering much-needed bedside nursing to these families, they could also impart some public health messages at the same time. While attending a newborn baby and her mother, for example, a nurse might also educate the mother about new techniques in childcare, prenatal care, and prevention of disease in her family. Indeed VON nurses served as proof that bedside and public health nursing could not be entirely separated. This leaves us to

wonder just how much work the private duty nurse also did to convey the same health messages.

The Interwar Years: The Crisis in Private Duty Nursing

Beginning in the late 1920s and accelerating in the 1930s, an era of unemployment and scarcity of jobs began for private duty nurses. This was caused not only by the economic instability of the Depression, but by hospital training schools turning out too many nursing graduates, and the shift from home to hospital care. Student nurses still provided the lion's share of the nursing workforce for hospitals, which were reluctant to give up this source of labour. At the same time, surgery was becoming a safer procedure, as hospitals improved their hygiene and sanitation and bought new technological tools for treatment and

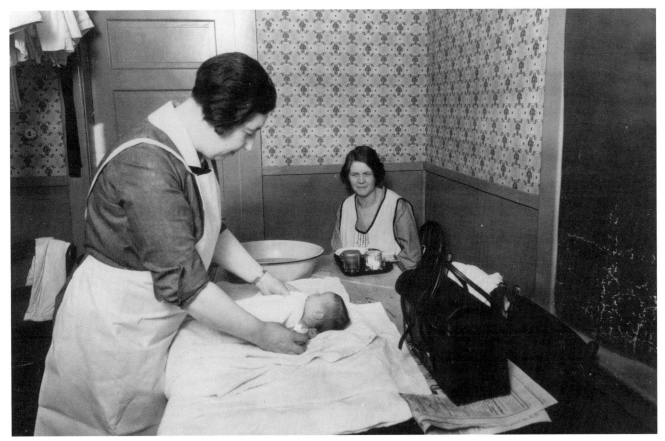

Figure 6
VON nurse
Calgary, Alberta
1929
Glenbow Archives, Calgary, Alberta, NA-3445-17

diagnosis. As paying patients went to hospitals for their care, the long-standing stigma of hospitals as filthy, dangerous places was changing. Special duty nursing in hospitals was on the increase and nursing superintendents often tried to get hospital work for their unemployed graduates.

Just as the Depression hit and more and more families could not pay for health care, a surplus of private duty nurses came onto the job market. The result was hardship for many. Historian Mary Kinnear found that pay for private duty nurses in Manitoba ranged from $4 a day to $6 depending upon the hours of care expected. And there were few such jobs available, as student nurses were still used as a source of cheap labour in hospitals, and public health employers, in financial straits themselves, were hiring few new employees. Private duty nurses encountered

more and more families who could not afford to pay for their nursing care. Attempting to eke out a living, many were only able to find work in private homes for substandard pay. "We were very, very happy to have a nursing job, mostly. There was so much unemployment. In fact, I can recall nurses offering to work for their room and board," said one nurse who worked in Nova Scotia during the 1920s and 1930s. Others resorted to family support. As one nurse said: "We waited to do special duty nursing, it was all you could do, and, you see, we were getting into the Depression then. I lost thirty dollars saved, that was a fortune, the little bank closed up like a clam so fast, I just never got over that thirty dollars. I came home in December, it was either that or starve to death."[11] Some nurses responded to the crisis by taking jobs that were outside the profession, such as sales clerks or waitresses, and others emigrated to the United States, where their skills were welcomed.

As an entrepreneur, the private duty nurse had always had to deal with both job insecurity and delinquent accounts, problems that doctors also faced with increasing severity during the Depression. There could be weeks or even months between assignments. Kinnear cites a Manitoba nurse who preferred private duty nursing to hospital nursing but recognized that "one might not get a case for a month." Susan Reverby uses language such as "shame," "despair," "disgrace," and "wanting work, not charity," to describe the angst of the American private duty nurse, always awaiting the call for the next nursing position in another home. As intervals between jobs grew longer, so did the problem of patients who did not pay. One private duty nurse recalled: "Oh, of course you took the job. You didn't ask them for money. Maybe they would give you a bag of potatoes. One woman gave me a jug of soft soap."[12]

Yet the same nurse was unwilling to shirk any of her perceived responsibilities. She reported:

My brother had a market and he had lots of meat and potatoes and the people that called needed me and I went. The only time my brother and I had any words at all was one time I was out somewhere, I worked a great deal, and someone came for me to go out to the river. A woman was very sick out there, and my brother didn't call me to go and I said "Walter, don't you ever as long as you live, while I live here, ever do that to me again.[13]

Clearly the charitable origins of nursing did not die easily. "He said he thought that there was too much work for me and he knew that they didn't have any money. I said 'don't ever let that happen again,' and he never did. He never interfered again." Clearly nurses faced complex decisions, sometimes pitting economic survival against patient care. While on the one hand the private duty nurse needed money, she was also dedicated to the lives of those to whom she was providing care, or even potentially providing care. The extent to which nurses worked on a charitable basis is difficult to estimate.[14]

Historians note that private duty nurses often found themselves in precarious financial straits, whereas those who managed to get hospital or public health positions were at least guaranteed constant employment. Although public health nurses were grateful to have greater job security, pay, and benefits, they too were affected by the Depression. They faced greater need in the homes of the families they visited. For example, the VON caseload increased, despite the fact that many patients who could once pay for services no longer could. Families on relief or close to it were in crisis, and this led to greater illness. Visits to homes became longer, as nurses sometimes spent as much time counselling and trying to arrange for such basic social services as food, clothing, and fuel for destitute families as they did in providing actual nursing services. Hospitals, also strapped for funds, began to release patients earlier. The VON was left to pick up the slack.

On the other hand, there were still rich patients and the experience of caring for them could be quite different. One nurse looked after a relative for eight or nine months as a nurse companion. She recalls that there were no set wages, but that they paid her what they thought was fair and that they were quite generous. The woman she cared for did have a slight heart condition but was in otherwise good physical health, although she was senile:[15]

I had to stay with her every minute really. Her son and daughter-in-law, they had been tied with her and the daughter-in-law wasn't too well and her doctor had decided she should have some time off. During that time they went to England and I was left in charge of her with a maid but I didn't leave her. When I heard her moving in the morning I got up and she got up very early. I had no time off with her. I put her to bed at night. But they had a chauffeur — and she would go for a ride each afternoon.

Economic duress reinforced existing inequalities in the work situation of private duty nurses. Physicians could wield a great deal of power over nursing jobs — but more so in times of hardship when nurses had fewer options. While some hospitals would recommend nurses for positions in the community, doctors would often call the nurse directly, particularly if he — given that they were almost exclusively male at this time — had a favourite.

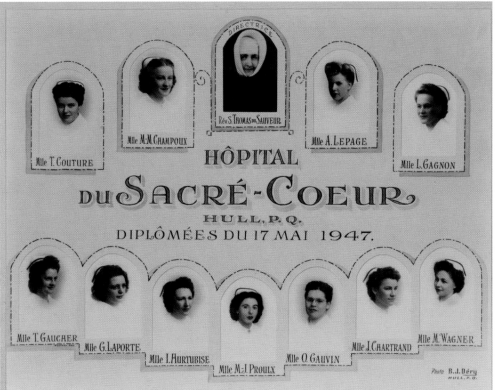

Figure 7
Gertrude Laporte's graduation photograph
l'Hôpital du Sacre Cœur
Hull, Quebec
1947
Photographer: Harry Foster
Canadian Museum of
Civilization, 988.1.34
Gift of Charles Morin

Laporte is bottom, second from left.

Oral histories reveal how intricate the relationship was between nurses and doctors, and its impact on nurses' economic situations. Writing about the American experience, Reverby discussed how physicians preferred "young," "pretty," and "vigorous" nurses because they "would evince a better cure." While there is little concrete Canadian evidence to suggest that doctors preferred "prettier" nurses, they did indeed have favourites whom they took along with them. For example, Sister Alice Clare Salterio spoke of hopping on a train in Nova Scotia with a doctor where he removed tonsils for five children in one family in a little village about 100 kilometres from Halifax. The doctor then left her there in charge of the children, which she described as a frightening experience.[16]

Evidence from oral history points to the degree of trust physicians had in private duty nurses, and that they recognized the strain on the nurse's income. Flora MacDonald, from Cape Breton, Nova Scotia, was nursing a patient in a coma who was not going to survive. She spoke of calling the doctor whom she described as an excellent surgeon. "I said, 'Doctor Green, I'm afraid we are going to lose our patient.' And here I am with the family listening to me, and

he said, 'That's your hard luck,' meaning, you know, that it was Depression and there were very few jobs."[17]

Private duty nurses often took obstetrical cases particularly in less settled areas, and like public health and outpost nurses, sometimes delivered the babies. One nurse remembers being sent to a confinement case by the doctor's wife, because the doctor was away dealing with an eclamptic woman and no one else was available. So she undertook the journey, carrying her brown bag. She knew that she was expected to deliver the baby and told the mother "I will do my best for you." She described the house as being very plain but also very tidy and clean, although she noted, "I didn't let on to her, but I was quite uneasy, but however, a lovely baby girl." She clearly knew what to do with the placenta and how to tie the cord and when all was finished, she was delighted to sit down to a dinner prepared for her by the woman's sister who was also near her delivery date.[18]

By the 1930s, private duty nurses working in the home were showing increasing dissatisfaction with uncertain job opportunities, poor pay, domestic

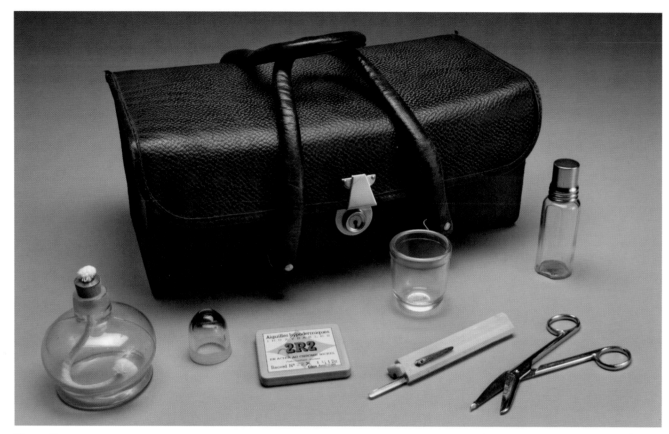

Figure 8
Gertrude Laporte's nursing bag
Photographer: Doug Millar
Canadian Museum of Civilization, 988.1.1-40. Gift of Charles Morin

Nurse Laporte's large private duty bag contained over 50 items, from an alcohol burner for sterilization of needles to a St. Christopher medallion.

responsibilities, and the lack of freedom to enjoy a social life. Lacking many options, Mabel McMullen, a private duty nurse in St. Stephen, New Brunswick, asked the Association in New Brunswick in a paper read at their annual meeting to open up discussion on ways to "ease the present situation among private duty nurses." She thought that they should consider "increased fees and shorter hours of service." She stated: "Personally I do not consider our fees exorbitant, and I would suggest that they remain as they are. The unemployment situation at present would not warrant an increase, and we could not work for less and earn a decent living." In 1936 an editorial in *The Canadian Nurse* addressed the problems facing the private duty nurse: "The double problem of providing continuous nursing care and domestic assis-

tance in the home will never be solved until its real implications are frankly faced by all concerned. It is physically impossible for a nurse to perform heavy household tasks and, at the same time, to give adequate nursing care to a sick patient."[19]

Nursing organizations did address these concerns, although it appears they did so with their own preoccupations in mind. The Private Duty Section in the Canadian Nurses Association (CNA) looked at the question of hours, pay, and other inequalities, making such suggestions as group nursing, a system whereby nurses could substitute for each other. Some also looked to general staff nursing in hospitals. In 1937 Jean Church, Chairman, Private Duty Section, CNA wrote: "Hours of recreation depend on the available assistance from members of the household in looking after the patient." In 1935–36, the Private Duty Section of the Registered Nurses Association of British Columbia, meeting in Vancouver at the CNA Biennial Convention, focused primarily on the establishment of the 8-hour duty, although they also discussed money issues, recommending that nurses be paid an additional 50¢ for each hour over eight hours up to 12 hours.[20]

Of all these suggestions, however, it was only the proposed reduction in the student population that received any serious attention by the CNA throughout the 1930s. This strategy was also reflected in George Weir's nationwide study into issues within nursing. He found that private duty nurses were underpaid, underemployed, and living with uncertainty. The average annual income for private duty nurses in 1929–30 was only $1022 compared with $1385 for institutional staff, and $1574 for public health. He addressed the issue of oversupply, recommending that nurse training be moved from the hospital training schools to the universities, and that hospitals hire more general duty nurses to provide their nursing services, rather than relying on student labour.[21]

While nurses' associations met, and Dr Weir conducted his study, private nurses continued to work in homes where they were not given anything like the advantages being proposed. Such discussion proved futile as the era of the private duty nurse came to an end in mid-century. In 1943 the CNA estimated that over 14 000 of its members were employed by hospitals and public health agencies, while only 6000 were in private health services. Canadians saw increased hospitalization, more specialized medicine, more hospital births, more general duty nurses in hospitals, and eventually better insurance coverage for hospital and medical care.[22]

Although the private duty nurse was something of an entrepreneur, working on a fee-for-service basis, nurses failed to negotiate as attractive a "professional" deal in the new health care environment as physicians were able to do. They obtained a fee-for-service arrangement with governments in health and hospital insurance plans that provided them with greater economic certainty while retaining their professional autonomy. However, most nurses, although they could use the title Registered Nurse in most provinces by 1940, became the employees of hospitals. Their professional stature remained conditioned by their gender as did their subordinate status vis-à-vis physicians.

However, as the longevity of the VON has demonstrated, the need for professional care in the home did not disappear. Indeed one of the strengths of this organization remains its ability to take its cues from patients in their homes and to fill the many gaps left vacant by other health care players. The VON evolved from a nursing service focused on public health, tuberculosis, and maternity care to home care directed at the elderly and chronically ill.

There are more questions than answers in this overview of private duty nursing history. How did private duty nurses see their "entrepreneurial" status? Were they practical businesswomen with strong leadership skills in health care, or the exploited underdogs of nursing? What were their lives really like, and did they manage to maintain social lives? Did the private duty nurse accept her leaders' orthodoxies concerning professionalism and reject the domestic, charitable and/or religious side of nursing? And to what extent did and/or could private duty and VON nurses negotiate with a distant, sometimes unwieldy health care system and bring their patient's needs to the health care table? Did they serve as a foot soldier in bringing public health messages back to patients?

Back to the Future

From the vantage point of the late nineteenth century, who could have foreseen the dramatic changes in nursing that would occur in the 1980s and 1990s? After the relative prosperity of the 1940s, 50s and 60s, once again nurses cannot find full-time jobs. Who could have predicted that the term "nurse" could conjure up images of the bachelor, master, and doctorally prepared nurse, Advanced Practice Nurse (APN), Registered Nurse (RN), Nurse Practitioner (NP), Licensed Practical Nurse (LPN), Certified Nursing Assistant (CNA), Personal Care Worker (PCW), Registered Practical Nurse (RPN), Home Care Worker, Patient Attendant, and the myriad of other health care providers who provide nursing care of one sort or another? Even more significant, how could one have envisioned that there would be a shift back to home care as a result of health care cutbacks? Now nursing is often left to the unprepared family member — usually a woman — without training or recognition for such work, just as it was in the days before the nurse training schools opened. Suddenly we are seeing another nursing shortage accompanied by shorter hospital stays for patients who are acutely ill, with nursing care of both the young and elderly taking place in the home. If the history of nursing reflects the high value that Canadian society places upon an individual's health and well-being — enough to ensure that the person is cared for by a trained, educated nurse — have we made a backward move in recent years?

Healing the Body and Saving the Soul: Nursing Sisters and the First Catholic Hospitals in Quebec (1639–1880)

Brigitte Violette

The genesis of a large part of the hospital network in Quebec and, indeed, across Canada cannot be separated from the history of female religious orders.[1] For more than three centuries, over 50 religious orders were associated with development of the Catholic hospital network across Canada and the delivery of care to patients inspired by an age-old caregiving philosophy.[2] Behind the foundation of these establishments were conceptions of the human being, health, and illness based on Christian faith. From this conception flowed modes of intervention in which the nursing sisters played a paramount role. The funding and management of the institutions, and the organization of care within them, were based on practices in which charity was deemed essential.[3]

In this chapter, I will attempt to show how the traditional conception of the hospital enabled nursing sisters to play a central role in organizing and delivering health care within the Quebec hospital system for two centuries. In the mid-nineteenth century, however, a shift took place in which the medical establishment was constituted as the sole repository of medical science and guardian of health; this changed mentality caused an upheaval in the hospital sector and imposed new ways of doing things. The consequent rise of the medical profession within hospital organizations was to lead to the medicalization of hospitals and the gradual imposition of the biomedical model of care. This new model led to a subjugation of the nuns that, in the end, would cause them to lose control of their centuries-old institutions in favour of state-run medicine.

The literature includes works on the history of hospitals, as well as publications on specific aspects of health or public health and monographs devoted to certain religious orders. However, research has not yet advanced to the point where we have an overall view of the development of the hospital system and an account of the role assumed by the many religious orders that were associated with it.[4] In fact, the history of religious orders working in the health care field in Quebec[5] and across Canada remains to be written. Because of the embryonic state of the research in this area, this chapter is based on documentation that highlights the work of the Augustinian Nuns of Mercy and the Religious Hospitallers of St. Joseph. The chronological framework extends from the foundation of the Hôtel-Dieu de Québec, the first hospital in North America north of Mexico, in 1639, to the opening of Notre-Dame Hospital in Montreal in 1880; the latter, owned by a lay corporation, was managed by a board of directors from which nuns were excluded, a first in the Catholic hospital network.[6]

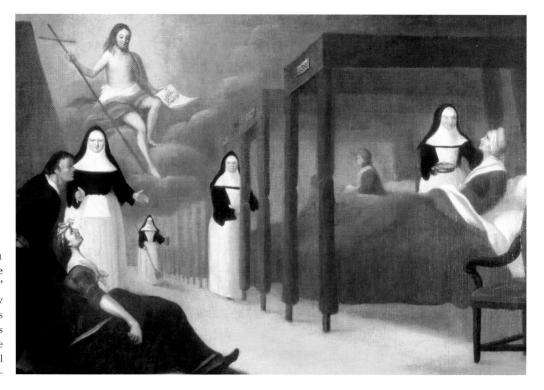

Figure 1
"Ex-voto of the Women's Ward"
18th century
Collection des
Hospitalières
de Saint-Joseph de
l'Hôtel-Dieu de Montréal

Establishment of a Centuries-Old Tradition and the Nuns' Place in the Hospital System: 1639–1840

The presence of religious orders in the hospital sector can be understood only through the traditional function of the hospital in Christianity. Arising from the need to do charitable works, most hospitals hosted, indiscriminately, pilgrims, travellers, the indigent, ill and infirm people, old people, orphans, widows and widowers, and others, as an embodiment of "the direct image of the Crucified, whose sufferings conferred upon them a redemptive value of cooperation."[7] Thus, the hospital was a religious space in terms of both its origins and its purpose. It was configured essentially in the perspective of salvation — salvation of the weak and suffering people whom it took in, but also of those who worked there, since charity had a redemptive value for those who practised it. The nuns thus embodied the words of Christ: "I was hungry and ye gave me to eat; I was thirsty and ye gave me drink; I was a stranger and ye took me in; naked, and ye clothed me; I was sick, and ye visited me... inasmuch as ye did it unto one of these my brethren, even these least, ye did it unto me."[8] It was in these

words that the foundation of works of mercy — the Hotels-Dieu and general hospitals — by the religious nursing orders resided.

In the late seventeenth century, the towns of Quebec, Trois-Rivières, and Montreal already had a Hotel-Dieu, and the two largest towns, Quebec and Montreal, also had a general hospital. "Usually founded and managed by the [Catholic] church and supported by the state, these institutions remained essentially French. Their architecture, operations, and ideology resulted from a long hospital tradition. The regulations and constitutions of the French religious communities also served as a framework for their activity in the colony."[9] In principle, the general hospitals were distinguished from the Hotels-Dieu by the fact that they were intended to be mainly residential shelters for the poor, the old, orphans, prostitutes, and the infirm; they also provided work for the indigent and asylum for the insane. But in practice, the general hospitals were sometimes devoted to patient care, particularly of soldiers.

The Hotels-Dieu clearly did not have the role of social detention and occupation (asylum, shelter, and workhouse) that the general hospitals had until the early nineteenth century. From the start, they were

Table 1

Health Institutions in Quebec and Female Religious Orders Associated with Them (1639–1880)

Hôtel-Dieu du Précieux-Sang, Quebec City (1639)	Augustinian Nuns of the Mercy of Jesus
Hôtel-Dieu de Montréal (1642)	Hospitallers of St. Joseph, starting in 1659
Hôtel-Dieu de Trois-Rivières (1697)	Ursulines of Trois-Rivières
Hôpital Général de Québec (1693)	Augustinian Nuns of the General Hospital
Montreal General Hospital (1737)	Grey Nuns of Montreal, starting in 1747
Hôtel-Dieu de Saint-Hyacinthe (1840)	Sisters of Charity of Saint-Hyacinthe
Hospital of Mercy, Montreal (1845)	Misericordia Sisters
Hôpital Saint-Camille, Montreal (1849)	Sisters of Providence
Hôpital Saint-Eusèbe, Joliette (1855)	Sisters of Providence
General Hospital of Sorel (1862)	Sisters of Charity of Saint-Hyacinthe
St. Joseph Hospital, Trois-Rivières (1864)	Sisters of Providence
St. John Hospital, Saint-Jean d'Iberville (1868)	Grey Nuns of Montreal
Hôtel-Dieu du Sacré-Cœur de Québec (1873)	Augustinian Nuns of Hôtel-Dieu du Sacré-Cœur
Sacred Heart Hospital, Montreal (1874)	Sisters of Providence
Hospital of Mercy, Quebec City (1874)	Sisters of the Good Shepherd of Quebec City
Notre-Dame Hospital, Montreal (1880)	Grey Nuns of Montreal

devoted to patient care. Medical care was provided by physicians or surgeons usually appointed by the state. They were organized according to the French model, but were distinguished from their contemporaries in France because they housed patients from all social classes rather than only the disadvantaged. Although they were, in essence, charitable institutions, they were not out of step with the medical wisdom of their time. Their rudimentary technical and surgical equipment conformed to the current scientific knowledge of the seventeenth and eighteenth centuries. Physicians were a daily presence among the patients. In this sense, they were also places of healing. In the nineteenth century, many physicians (including those who were to give medical care in the Hotels-Dieu) went to Europe — London or Paris — for training and brought back, with their intellectual baggage, technical innovations. Thus, "...contrary to what some historiography presumes and notwithstanding the importance of the religious and charitable functions assumed by the Hôtels-Dieu, these institutions always played an important medical role with the population.... It was in fact to care and treatment...that the hospitallers of these institutions devoted themselves in large part."[10]

This said, in the late nineteenth century, some Hotels-Dieu, notably those in rural regions, often assumed functions that fell, in principle, to the general hospitals; they, too, devoted much of their space to housing orphans and old people.

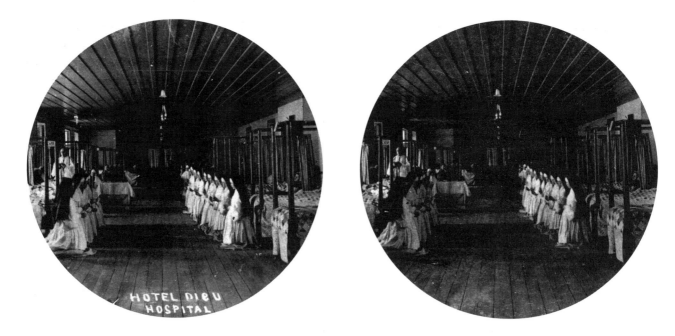

Figure 2
Last Rites, Hôtel-Dieu
1877
Photographer: Louis Prudent Vallée
Collection des Augustines de l'Hôtel-Dieu de Québec

Healing the Body and Saving the Soul: The Care Philosophy of the Nursing Sisters

Although in the seventeenth century the Hotels-Dieu were medicalized institutions devoted to care of the ill, it is important to understand that the general perspective that gave meaning to the work of the nuns and the life of the institution was still the hereafter. Although there was a manifest desire to heal the body, it was of paramount importance to save the soul. This meant that the spiritual dimension of the nuns' activity prevailed over the temporal dimension; they were out to win souls through hospital care.

Similarly, their caregiving was based on a conception of illness and medicine in which God, more than anyone else, dictated the process of healing:

> In the millennia that preceded the advent of "scientific" medicine (nineteenth century), it probably seemed inconceivable, if not heretical, to dissociate human action from divine intervention, both in the course of disease and in healing.

This was because the human animal was not yet considered...to be a biological mechanism, furnished or not with a religious spirit, as we represent it today in a materialist approach to nature. Man was, above all, perceived as a whole (microcosm) in constant relation with the forces of the cosmos (macrocosm). Any rupture between these two worlds caused illness. In fact, disease — that is, any assault, other than an accidental one (fracture, snakebite, etc.), on the human biological balance — was considered to be the result of heavenly intervention.[11]

These precepts guided the action of the religious nursing orders and were at the origin of a caregiving ritual that had already been in use for centuries in Europe. Prayer was an integral part of the caregiving regime; prayers were recited several times a day and the hospitallers encouraged patients to take the sacraments (confession, communion, extreme unction). They conducted spiritual readings in the public wards; they performed blessings with holy water, crucifixes, statuettes, and pious images; and they named wards after saints. A whole series of rituals and signs accompanied the discourses on suffering, sacrifice, and surrender to Providence.

The concern with salvation of the soul was also conveyed in the hospital's architecture. At Hôtel-Dieu de Québec, for example, the women's ward was simple and plain and gave onto a generously lighted and richly decorated chapel; by its plainness, the ward symbolized time on earth, the vale of tears, while the chapel prefigured paradise, the ultimate stage of life, an end to hope for and to attain. The beds were aligned on either side of the ward, with the heads to the walls, the feet toward the central aisle. This arrangement was still in existence in 1877, as shown on stereograms made at the time. Since the men's ward did not give directly on the chapel, an altar was erected, which also served the officers' ward. The three paintings that were hung above this altar evoked divine mercy and the mystery of redemption.

Organization of Caregiving in the Hotels-Dieu

Organization of care in the Hotels-Dieu was not haphazard. Notwithstanding the general considerations demonstrating the nuns' caregiving philosophy, their constitutions explicitly set out the division of labour and the tasks delegated to each level of the hospital hierarchy. For instance, once a year, the mother superior of the order gathered together the nuns and assigned the tasks that would be assumed by each. The various tasks were divided into "offices," each under the direction of a nun called an officer. A nun who became an officer after training in the pharmacy managed a ward (this would be the equivalent of "head nurse"). Until the late nineteenth century, the officers working in the wards of Hôtel-Dieu de Québec and those responsible for private patients dispensed only general care: reception of patients, washing, beds, meals, general cleanliness, assistance to the dying, and so on. Medical care was given by physicians. The converse nuns (lower in rank than the officers), assigned to maintenance of the wards and equipment (basins, spittoons, etc.) by the hospitallers, completed the caregiving hierarchy.

The most senior hospitaller — later called the head hospitaller — was the de facto superintendent of the hospital; she was responsible for management, organization, and general administration of the institution with regard to hospitalization of patients. She was the key person in the health care organization. All issues relating to the hospital, whether they were professional or scientific, fell under her authority. Doctors had authority over medical decisions only, and carried out their work under the administrative supervision of the head hospitaller. Under orders from the superior of the religious community, she admitted patients after — according to the regulations — the doctor or surgeon had examined them and certified in writing that they had no contagious or incurable disease. Then, the head hospitaller assigned the patients to her companion officers. She made sure that the doctor was punctual in his visits and went with him on his rounds, made sure that his prescriptions were filled, and kept up to date on the status of convalescing patients. She granted hospital leaves, but she could not release patients without notice or without the permission of the superior. Finally, she made sure that the chaplain visited the patients every day, that they made their confessions and received their communion, and that no one died without having received the final sacraments. Through her management style, her organizational abilities, and her sense of human relations, the head hospitaller stamped the entire hospital with her personality. Her companions had to obey her on all matters related to patient care, and her authority also extended to lay employees of the hospital.

According to a time-honoured tradition, the philosophy of patient care was transmitted from master to apprentice, from generation to generation. The first hospitallers in New France received their training in Europe. The Augustinian Nuns of Mercy learned the art of caregiving from their sisters at Hôtel-Dieu de Dieppe, while the Hospitallers of St. Joseph completed their apprenticeship at Hôtel-Dieu de la Flèche.[12] Some of these pioneers had studied pharmacology. At the time, caregivers had to have skills based mainly on medication, hygiene, and wound dressings. Caregiving techniques, knowledge about making and administering medications,

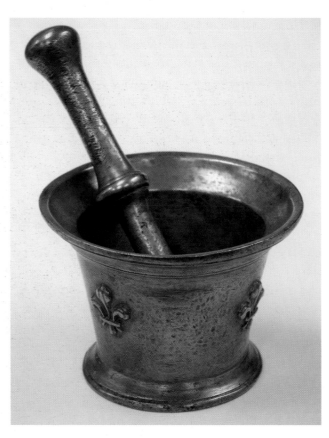

Figure 3
Bronze mortar and pestle
Collection des Hospitalières de Saint-Joseph de l'Hôtel-Dieu
de Montréal

and treatment methods were learned essentially
by observation.

Training was acquired in stages, first at the bedside of patients, and then by an apprenticeship with
the pharmacist, who had "scientific" knowledge.
Guided by the ward officers, postulants and novices
learned first to provide basic services: serving meals,
making beds, settling patients in and making them
comfortable. They then began to learn about nursing
treatments. In the last part of their apprenticeship, all
caregivers had a training period at the hospital pharmacy. This step conferred a certain uniformity on the
training: "A true focus of training, a centre where the
art and science of nursing care converged, the pharmacy served as a school before such schools existed,
and the officer and pharmacist as teachers."[13] Once
they had solid caregiving experience and training in
the pharmacy, the nuns became, in their turn, hospi-

tallers. All choir sisters[14] — at least, those in the large
religious nursing orders — followed this mode of
apprenticeship in the profession.

In spite of this empirical education system, most
historians maintain that the skills of hospitallers were
completely on a par with medical knowledge at the
time. Historian François Rousseau believes that the
opening of the new Hôtel-Dieu de Québec in 1825
and the organization of real medical services probably had a concomitant effect on the care dispensed
by the nuns. According to Rousseau, biographies of
the Augustinian Nuns mention their often exceptional skills, notably in pharmacology. As some physicians admitted, "If one considers the state of medicine
in the seventeenth and eighteenth centuries, and in
the first part of the nineteenth century, one is forced
to conclude that the nuns did much more, thanks to
their care, to cure the ill than did the surgeons, with
their repeated copious bleedings, sweats, drastic
purges, enemas, and counter-irritants."[15]

The Apothecary, or the Knowledgeable Nun

Until the late nineteenth century, the apothecary (or
pharmacy) was the nerve centre of the entire system
of health care distribution in Quebec hospitals. To
know the diagnosis of each patient admitted to the
institution, the apothecary had to accompany the doctor or surgeon on his daily rounds to note his opinion, inquire about the remedies and diets that he
prescribed, and follow up on treatment. At Hôtel-Dieu
de Montréal, until 1900, she was also responsible for
organizing the laboratory and the operating room,
and she assisted the surgeon.

Because the "scientific" part of the caregiving
organization was her office, it was to the apothecary
that the responsibility for "cures" belonged; she was
seen as the expert — the knowledgeable nun or *soeur
savante* — by her companions and was in charge of
their training. She saw to all dressings, treatments,
remedies, temperature notations, and vital signs in
the wards and private rooms. All remedies, instruments, and apparatuses needed for treatments were
kept in the pharmacy and returned there after use.
The postulant apothecary learned to apply rubs, phe-
nol sprays, poultices with linseed flour and mustard

Marie-Angélique Viger, known as Saint-Martin (1770–1832)

Brigitte Violette, Parks Canada

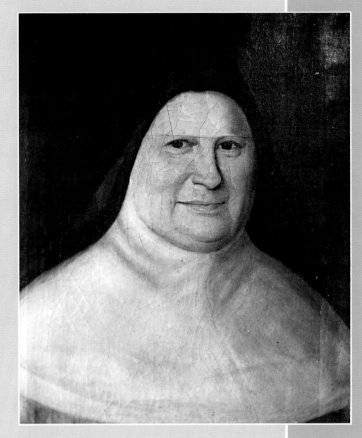

Figure 4
Marie-Angélique Viger
Collection of the Augustines of the Hôtel Dieu
de Québec

The daughter of Louis Viger and Marie-Agnès Papineau, Marie-Angélique Viger received part of her education from the Ursuline nuns of Trois-Rivières. She was said to have "a lively and penetrating mind, which [took in] everything ... quickly becoming the equal of her teachers." She entered the Hôtel-Dieu de Québec on 16 June 1788 and took the name Sister Saint-Martin. The community placed much hope in her. Soon after she took her vows, on 21 December 1789, she became the apothecary, "an office for which she had a distinguished talent, and a boundless charity." Over the years, this apothecary healed many patients suffering from cankers.

In the opinion of Mother Saint-Pierre, superior of the community (1831–34), Viger also excelled in surgery. She related a case in which "the Doctor of the Hospital not having succeeded in a first" amputation on a patient, Sister Saint-Martin took the initiative of making a second attempt, which was successful. According to this account, the surgery involved a resection of bones protruding from the stump.

A multi-talented woman, Viger was a trustee of the community for 11 years. She played an important role in the planning and implementation of the hospital's reconstruction (1816–25). Thanks to the influence of members of her family who were elected to the House of Assembly, the congregation was able to obtain government grants. Viger had already had an opportunity to show her know-how in designing plans for the construction of the church and the chancel a few years earlier, and had been lambasted by the bishop of Quebec City, Bishop Plessis, for her "brusqueness and independence."

Marie-Angélique Viger, dite de Saint-Martin, died on 28 June 1832 of an apoplectic fit after three days of illness during the cholera epidemic.

Sources: Archives of the monastery of the Hôtel-Dieu de Québec, 124th Circular Letter of Marie Angélique Viger of Saint Martin (T 12, C 510, no. 2); François Rousseau, *La croix et le scalpel : histoire des Augustines et de l'Hôtel-Dieu de Québec*, vol. 1: 1639–1892 (Quebec, Éditions du Septentrion, 1989), 193–4, 249, 343.

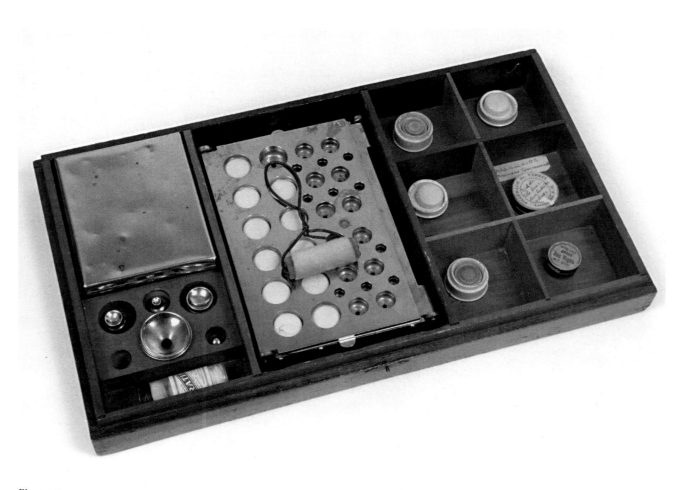

Figure 5
Pharmaceutical kit for making pills
Collection des Augustines de l'Hôtel-Dieu de Québec

(mustard plasters), and to wash and clean bottles, pans, and other instruments used to make remedies.

In this context, the apothecary was therefore called upon to occupy the top of the hierarchy since, of all the nuns, she had the most responsibility for caregiving itself. The regulations at the Hôtel-Dieu de Québec and the Hôtel-Dieu de Montréal were unequivocal in this regard. The holder of this position had to see to the supply and operation of the apothecary, regularly check the quality of the products, and, of course, make the medications every three months, including compositions, syrups, preserves, distilled water, *miel violet*, and other preparations. In addition, she had to make sure that no product became spoiled and that the contents of each container were clearly marked. Once or twice a year, she made an inventory of the products needed to make the medications. On the other hand, the superior determined the quantities to be produced. The apothecary was usually assisted by another nun, but she might have to use a lay employee. Under the French Régime, simple or composite medications were the same as those used in French hospitals, and most were imported from France, notably from Dieppe in the case of the Hôtel-Dieu de Québec. To these were added the medicinal plants that might be grown in a corner of the garden.

Alongside traditional products arose a pharmacopoeia that integrated local products, metal-based medications, and very new medicines such as cinchona and ipecacuanha. In short, the apothecaries had to stay up to date, and they were not reluctant to use new treatments; their pharmacy was well supplied with bottles, bowls, jars, and other containers for herbs, powders, unguents, lotions, potions, and other substances. The utensils and instruments used by the apothecary went from copper kettles to mortars of different sizes; bottles, flasks, and stills for distilling water and essences; ovens; cast-iron and marble mortars — in short, everything they needed to prepare medications. As needed, they could consult a number of books in which different preparations and their uses were explained. The apothecaries of the Hôtel-Dieu de Québec had a well-established reputation and taught other orders to make remedies.

The Growth of Female Religious Orders and Expansion of the Hospital Network: 1840–1880

New Actors in the Health Care Field

In 1838, there were 322 nuns in Quebec, all functions combined. The Anglo-Protestant authorities were more tolerant of female religious orders (than of male orders) because of their "utilitarian" function. Between 1840 and 1850, female orders had the best opportunity ever to prove their usefulness. Population growth, stimulated by successive waves of immigration, exerted considerable pressure on the church's charitable works. Cholera and typhus epidemics, the growing number of abandoned children, and the precarious situation of single mothers were among the motivations for recruiting religious orders in Europe or for creating new ones.

The proliferation of religious orders in the second half of the nineteenth century — and, more particularly, of female orders — was striking, especially because each diocese tended to possess a good network of religious orders and charitable institutions. Following an appeal by the parish priest of Saint-Hyacinthe, the Grey Nuns of Montreal founded the Hôtel-Dieu de Saint-Hyacinthe in 1840.[16] Their house was independent of the one in Montreal. This same order had taken on management of an orphanage in Quebec City in 1849 and became known as the Sisters of Charity of Quebec City. They also opened a dispensary and visited patients at home. In the same period, the Hospitallers of Joseph, who had been working

at the Hôtel-Dieu de Montréal since 1659, responded to a number of appeals from outside of Quebec.

Among these new actors in the health care field, some were asked to manage institutions with specialized vocations (such as hospitals for people with contagious diseases — usually temporary — sanitaria, children's hospitals, dispensaries, etc.), which were added to the landscape of the hospital network. The increasing numbers of nuns also resulted in a diversification of their activities. The most innovative order was no doubt the one organized by the widow Rosalie Cadron-Jetté and a group of midwives. Created in 1848, the Institute of the Misericordia Sisters provided assistance to single mothers during childbirth and afterward. They took charge of the Maternité Sainte-Pélagie (1845) maternity ward, which later became Hospital of Mercy, a general hospital. In their early years of practice, the Misericordia Sisters attended the births of an average of 200 poor women at home and almost 80 "penitents" in the maternity ward.

The Rise of the Medical Establishment: Toward a New Conception of the Hospital

In the second half of the nineteenth century, the hospital network began a new phase of development, and the landscape of the health care system underwent major transformations. If the nuns' sphere of action seemed at first glance to be expanding, all the actors in the health care field now had to deal with an increasingly powerful factor: medical science was advancing[17] and medicine, an ancient profession, was becoming organized; its prestige was rising, and its power was increasing.

The changes in power relations began with the professionalization of the medical establishment in Quebec, which became official in 1847 with the creation of the College of Physicians and Surgeons of Lower Canada.[18] Concerned with improving and standardizing the theoretical training of practitioners, the College advocated a theoretical and clinical education to be provided by private schools; the long-established tradition of apprenticeship with an experienced physician was discredited, and a few years later faculties of medicine were established.[19] Very early, physician-professors sought access to the major religious orders' large hospitals in order to profit

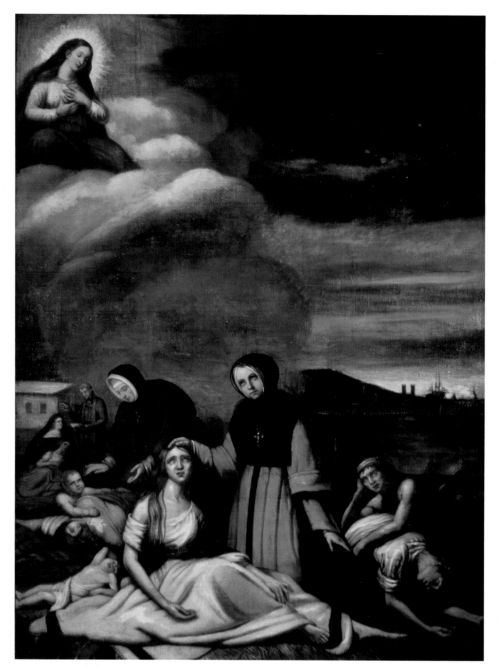

Figure 6
"Typhus"
Artist: Théophile Hamel
1849
Photographer: Bernard Dubois
Musée Marguerite-Bourgeoys,
Montreal

Montreal was hard-hit by the epidemics, which ravaged the population during the nineteenth century. Here, a Sister of Providence and a Grey Nun nurse Irish immigrants struck with typhoid fever.

from the advantages, both clinical and surgical, that such institutions were able to offer. These affiliations had a decisive impact on the future of the hospitals and the medicine practised in them and, consequently, on the work of the hospitallers.[20]

Gradually, the physical changes made to hospitals (for example, subdivision of the wards, expansions, new buildings, introduction of new equipment, etc.) led to changes in vocation; these arrangements were oriented to respond to the needs of hospital medicine. The new requirements of the science led to the modernization of infrastructure, the purchase of increasingly costly equipment, and a rise in the numbers of caregiving personnel. As the services offered by the new charitable institutions (the orphanages, sanatoria, and temporary hospitals discussed at the beginning of this chapter) were differentiated, the Hotels-Dieu began to be devoted exclusively to the care of the ill. Similarly, the term "general hospital" now corresponded to hospital institutions that, like English-Canadian general hospitals, offered a variety of medical services to the population as a whole.

These transformations in the hospital sector did not always occur without pain and friction. The requirements of the medical establishment, confronted with the skills of the hospitallers, inevitably affected relations between the congregationist management of the Catholic hospitals and its attending physicians assembled within medical bureaus.[21] Similarly, initiatives such as the one by Marie-Angélique Viger (1770–1832), apothecary of the Hôtel-Dieu de Québec, who undertook to perform a second amputation on a patient — which was successful — after the hospital physician failed on the first attempt, would no longer be tolerated.

In spite of the increased power of physicians, some researchers have shown that the religious orders that owned hospitals still managed to exercise some control over medical practice within their institutions. Concerned with maintaining control over operations at Hôtel-Dieu de Montréal, the Religious Hospitallers of St. Joseph imposed a rather restrictive and rigid schedule of clinical rounds, and professors were admitted into the wards only one at a time and for a period of three months. The Augustinian Nuns of the Hôtel-Dieu de Québec also set out a profusion of rules that provided supervision for students. They were worried that the presence of young people with varying degrees of self-discipline would disturb their caregiving ritual. The order was not resistant to innovation, but had reservations about anything that might affect the "regularity" of its routine and charitable work.[22] The growing medicalization of the hospital therefore posed a number of challenges, but the Augustinian Nuns did not intend to cede their management prerogatives.

Because the Augustinian Nuns and the Religious Hospitallers of St. Joseph managed to impose relatively severe restrictions on the physician-professors, should we conclude that these two large orders enjoyed greater autonomy in the management of their institutions — that they were treated with greater deference than were the new communities, which

had no solidly anchored hospital traditions? Or was it, rather, that these orders did not present a competitive threat for the medical establishment, so that it was less inclined to contest their authority within the hospital environment? Given the current state of historiography, it is difficult, if not impossible, to answer these questions with certainty, but it seems that they warrant being asked. The subsequent experience of the Misericordia Sisters seems to be revealing in this regard, as we shall see.

Because they became the only actors in the health care sector who could define their own sphere of activity, the physicians were able to take advantage of their power to circumscribe and constrict that of other practitioners. "Thanks to these assets, the College of Physicians engaged in a battle against certain competitors during the second half of the [nineteenth] century."[23] A group of monopolistic manoeuvres were initiated against those whom the College deemed charlatans (healers and bonesetters) and against midwives. After 1850, medical journals were bursting with complaints regarding the latter. They were blamed for their ignorance, for the fact that they were consulted for services other than those linked to pregnancy and childbirth, and above all, for the fact that their customary practice deprived physicians of appreciable profit. The complaints directed against midwifery in general were aimed mainly at the Misericordia Sisters.

In 1849, the eight founders, including Cadron-Jetté (Sister of the Nativity), were given their midwife certificates.[24] "Their professional competence, consolidated by an Ecclesiastical pastoral letter and an apostolic non-profit community engagement, particularly threatened young physicians [seeking new clients]."[25] Increasingly harassed by physicians and their students,[26] the bishop of Montreal, Ignace Bourget, held the fourth vow[27] of the Misericordia Sisters up to question in 1853. Cadron-Jetté, very aware of the "casual manner" with which some students treated the penitents, opposed this position. According to the testimony of the first superior, their presence was proving difficult on more than one level. Complaining to Canon J-O Paré, ecclesiastic superior of the community, Mother Sainte-Jeanne-de-Chantal (first superior) wrote, on 24 February 1861,

Marie-Rosalie Cadron-Jetté, Sister of the Nativity (1794–1864)

Brigitte Violette, Parks Canada

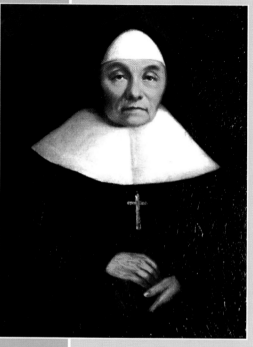

Figure 7
Rosalie Cadron-Jetté
Artist: Sister Marie Perras
1860s
Misericordia Sisters, Montreal

Marie-Rosalie Cadron was born in Lavaltrie on 27 January 1794 to a farmer father and a midwife mother, and she married Jean-Marie Jetté in 1811. They had 11 children, five of whom died at a young age. She was widowed in 1832, and in 1840 she began to take teenaged mothers into her home. In 1845, Bishop Ignace Bourget formulated a plan to assist teenaged mothers who had been rejected by their families and scorned by society. Instead of entrusting this mission to an existing religious community, he hoped to create a new one "free of traditions or previous hampering ties."

Despite the opposition of her children, who feared the reaction of Montreal society, Mme Jetté accepted Bourget's proposal, and on 1 May 1845, she and a "penitent" moved into a small house donated by a rich benefactor of Bishop Bourget's charitable works.

On 16 January 1848, Mme Jetté, then 54 years old, and seven collaborators, took nun's vows. The Institute of the Misericordia Sisters, created by l'Église de Montréal, received the ecclesiastical mandate to "live the mercy of Jesus the Saviour with girls and women in a situation of maternity out of wedlock and their children, and with the mothers of families who are having a difficult time with their maternity." Up to that time, no religious community in Canada had received a similar mission.

Mme Cadron-Jetté, now a Sister of the Nativity, refused to be considered for the position of superior of her community. Humility was certainly one motive for this move, but it seems that she had recognized in Josephte Malo-Galipeau (Sister Sainte-Jeanne-de-Chantal) a talent for managing the community's temporal affairs. In addition, her own predilection was for being a caregiver — taking in penitents, caring for newborns in the maternity room, caring for ill people in their homes (until 1862), visiting prisons, and other similar activities.

When she died on 5 April 1864 the community was composed of 33 professed religious, 11 novices and postulants, and 25 magdalens and other women attached to the Institute of the Misericordia Sisters. The community founded by Mme Jetté had taken in 2300 teenaged mothers over the years. It continued its work until 1973 at Hôpital de la Miséricorde and was active in three other Canadian provinces.

Sources: *Béatification et canonisation de la Servante de Dieu, Rosalie Cadron-Jetté, en religion Mère de la Nativité (1794-1864), fondatrice de l'Institut des Sœurs de Miséricorde de Montréal: positio sur les vertus et la renommé de sainteté*, vol. 1, Rome, Congregation for Beatification, 1994; Andrée Désilets, "Cadron, Marie-Rosalie, dite de la Nativité (Jetté)," in *Dictionary of Canadian Biography*, vol. 9, 1861–1870 (Toronto and Quebec City: University of Toronto Press and Université Laval, 1976), 111–2.

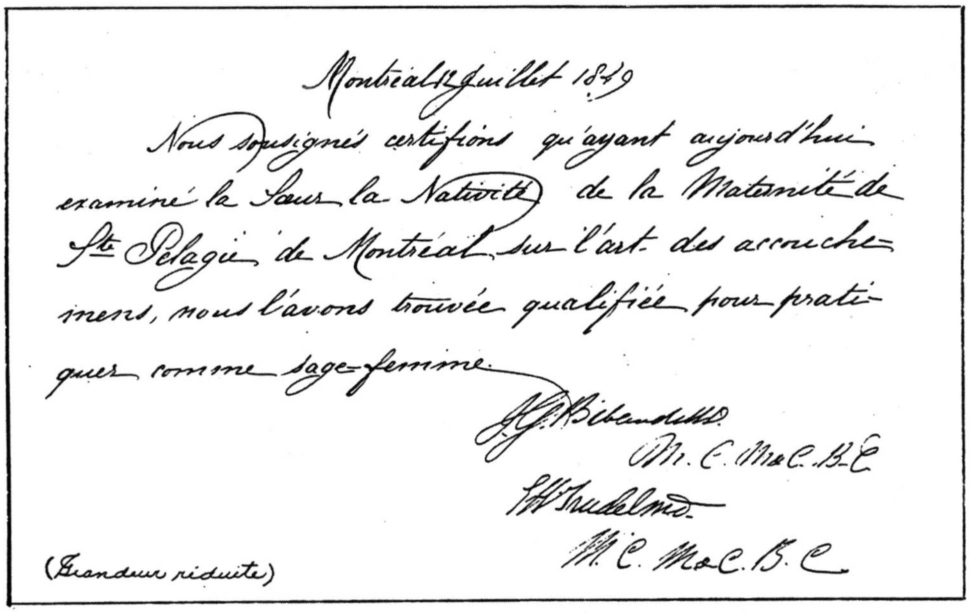
Montréal 12 juillet 1849

Nous soussignés certifions qu'ayant aujourd'hui examiné la Sœur la Nativité de la Maternité de Ste Pélagie de Montréal sur l'art des accouchemens, nous l'avons trouvée qualifiée pour pratiquer comme sage-femme.

J. G. Bibaud M.D.
M. C. McC. B. C.
F. X. Trudel M.D.
M. C. McC. B. C.

(Grandeur réduite)

Figure 8
Rosalie Cadron-Jetté's Midwifery Certificate
1849
Misericordia Sisters, Montreal

> In one case...a clerk conducted such a long and exhausting examination that the girl went into convulsions; the sisters asked him to finish, which he did not want to do; my sister Sept Douleurs came to get me, and it was with great difficulty that I was able to make him stop, although the girl's convulsions were still ongoing; the consequence was a great hemorrhage that almost caused her to die. Similar cases arose, and some of the girls were left with infirmities....
> A number of clerks wanted a number of times to have the patient take remedies to hasten the term of childbirth, and when we told them that this was against the normal procedure, they said that that many doctors did this and it was almost always when they were tired and wanted to leave; others [wanted] to give them remedies to lessen their pain and this way it would give them the time to go and take a rest; the sisters had a great deal of difficulty preventing them from doing this, as it would have been very detrimental to the patient.[28]

The obvious incompetence of the young doctors, and even certain professors, did not, however, keep the nuns from being shunted.[29] The final decision came from Rome. The axe fell on their practice in 1865, when the Congregation for Institutes of Consecrated Life and Societies of Apostolic Life forced the Misericordia Sisters to revise their constitution and abandon the fourth vow, which was considered unbecoming to their virtue. From then on, they had to use the services of physicians and lay midwives. A third (lay) order, the Daughters of St. Thais, eventually renamed the St. Margaret's Daughters, replaced the midwife sisters.

At first introduced as volunteers, the doctors at the Maternité de Sainte-Pélagie managed to gradually impose their directives and their way of seeing things on the nuns. Their contracts with the order eventually reduced the nursing sisters to a secondary role assisting the doctors. Finally the nuns were squeezed out of the obstetrical universe altogether, no longer being allowed to preside at deliveries or train future midwives.

Epilogue

In 1880, when the Grey Nuns of Montreal became fully engaged in hospital work, the order's involvement in Notre-Dame Hospital, an institution started by a group of physicians, is explained by a logic that had been in place since 1639. In effect, one could not envisage the foundation of such an institution without the support of a female religious order that had acquired long experience in the organization of care and the preparation of medications. The contribution of the order's members also enabled the operating costs to be greatly reduced, since the community asked only for minimal wages. In addition, the nuns' participation added great legitimacy to the charitable vocation of an institution that had to seek funding through subscriptions, bequests, and private donations.

When the new hospital was founded, the Grey Nuns community assigned 14 nuns to the care of patients, including a superior and an assistant. As nurses and pharmacists, they served meals to patients, treated them, dispensed remedies, and staffed the dispensaries. They provided everyday care with relative autonomy, except when it came to medical actions, which were closely controlled by the physicians. Well trained to provide patient care thanks to solid hospital experience acquired at the Montreal General Hospital, the nuns also cared for souls. Although these objectives did not create a paradox, they were, nevertheless, "to achieve the salvation of souls...*to resign ourselves to satisfy the requirements of science*" (emphasis added).[30]

At the dawn of a second stage of expansion of the hospital network across Canada, which was accompanied by a redefinition of the institution, the elements that would lead to major transformations at the turn of the following century were thus already in place: A science swept up in the excitement of its discoveries, a medicine that openly proclaimed its faith in its final victory over disease — although it did not really foresee when this would happen — and whose practice was based on increasingly large financial and technical investment, a society in which the rise of industrialization required the efforts of a healthy workforce — all of this radically changed the old hospital order. The modern hospital, resolutely oriented toward efficiency and whose ambition now consisted of putting all patients back on their feet — rather than addressing only a poor clientele — thus was taking root at the turn of the twentieth century.[31]

In the final analysis, these changes in priorities can be traced back to conceptions of health, treatment, and prevention, and the premises on which they are based. Beyond a simple critique of the powers and privileges of medicine, experts in the history of health care have demonstrated that these concep-

tions were structured, with variants depending on the era, around four fundamental dualities: population/individual, magic/science and reason, spirit/body, and holism/technicism. Modern medicine, as it developed in the nineteenth century, tended to be situated at the extreme poles of these four dualities: the individual, science, body, and technique. The first term implies a concentration on the individual and healing to the detriment of populations and the preventive approach, while the three others imply that medicine is largely reduced to a physicochemical and fragmented art, to the detriment of a conception of the human being as a bio-psycho-social whole. Offering a point of view of the human being that claims to be objective, the biomedical model provides, rather, a reductive outlook. What is more, this scientific dogma has become popular belief, since medicine is part of positive scientism. In this view, science is equivalent to the "exact sciences" — that is, material, objective, and unassailable knowledge. Yet, "all scientific construction is arbitrary...[since] it is the conceptual and material tools that determine what one sees and hears of nature...and of the patient. A subjective and arbitrary point of view of the body and disease [would] thus [become] a scientific dogma and [a] popular belief."[32]

Under the pretext of healing the body, medicine has erected an immense apparatus of social control, the therapeutic effectiveness of which is contestable. Historians and experts on public hygiene and the social sciences have shown, for example, that curative medicine was not the main factor responsible for considerable gains in longevity that humankind realized during the nineteenth century. It was due above all to improvement in living conditions and the implementation of public hygiene measures advocated by reformers that infant mortality and mortality due to infectious diseases declined extraordinarily, illustrating ipso facto the overlap between social organization and health. Similarly, studies on obstetrical practices between 1900 and 1930 have demonstrated that the massive intrusion of physicians into this sector did not lower mortality rates. "On the contrary, it would even seem that these rates increased because of the type of intervention practised by physicians who were still technically inexperienced."[33]

Thus, for the Catholic church's power over and discourse on the definition of the first Catholic hospitals in Quebec — as religious places in their origin and their purpose — were substituted those of the medical establishment, which from then on ensured that the biomedical model had primacy. If, in the short term, the religious orders that owned hospitals managed to maintain the upper hand in the operation of their establishments, the College of Physicians and Surgeons of Lower Canada, more or less supported by faculties of medicine, was constituted as the only repository of medical science and the sole guardian of health. By depriving the nuns of part of their authority, the physicians later came to control the operation of hospitals and to relegate the religious institutions to administrative tasks.

CHAPTER 5

The Nightingale Influence and the Rise of the Modern Hospital

Kathryn McPherson

For more than a century, Canadians have relied on hospitals to provide the facilities, equipment, and personnel central to scientific medicine. As elsewhere in the Western world, Canadian hospitals were "reformed" in the late nineteenth century, so that rather than being charitable institutions dedicated to serving the poor, hospitals began serving patients from all classes of society. Whether general hospitals or specialty institutions, and whether administered by Catholic orders, Protestant denominations, community volunteers, or government officials, hospitals have not only provided care, they have also played important educational functions, training new generations of health care practitioners, especially nurses. This chapter explores the evolution of the modern hospital in Canada with particular focus on the symbiotic relationship between health care institutions and the nurses who staffed the wards or learned their trade there. As part of this discussion, the chapter assesses the influence on Canadian hospitals of health care's most famous reformer, Florence Nightingale.

Nurses and the Pre-industrial Hospital

Throughout the colonial era of Canada's history, hospitals were familiar elements of the "pre-industrial"

urban landscape. Institutions like Montreal's Hôtel-Dieu constituted vital components of the civic infrastructure.[1] Like their counterparts in Britain, Europe, and the United States, the hospitals of eighteenth and nineteenth century New France and British North America were charitable institutions, administered by local elites fulfilling their social obligations to their community's destitute and poor. Medical and nursing staff laboured to alleviate the suffering of patients, but early Canadian hospitals were primarily custodial, rather than therapeutic, institutions.

As the number and size of Canadian cities grew in the nineteenth century, so too did the number of hospitals. Indeed, because hospitals symbolized the established social relations of giving and receiving charity, building a hospital appeared almost "necessary" for fledgling towns aspiring to become cities. Many of these institutions grew out of pressing local needs. Rapid population growth often spawned outbreaks of diseases such as typhoid, which spread before city leaders could get effective sanitation measures established, or rashes of industrial accidents among the throngs of workers who literally were building the city.

Like their predecessors, the hospitals of industrializing Canada continued to serve the poor, transient workers and newcomers without familial resources. Patient fees represented a very small percentage of

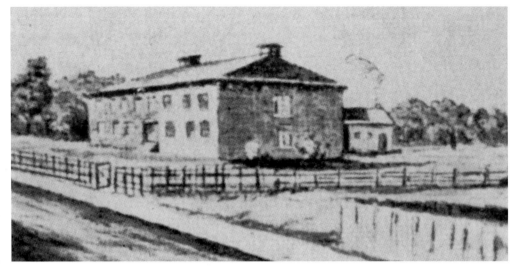

Figure 1
The York Hospital, forerunner to the Toronto General Hospital
1819
JM Gibbon & MS Mathewson, *Three Centuries of Canadian Nursing*, Toronto: Macmillan, 1947

nineteenth century hospitals' income, with municipal and provincial grants and significant charitable fund-raising providing the vast majority of institutional budgets.[2] That local elites understood hospital care to be part of the provision of charity was exemplified in Moncton where in 1897 the town fathers turned down a proposal to build a new hospital and instead decided to renovate the top floors of the local almshouse for the accommodation of hospital patients.[3]

Given the elite nature of hospital governance, it is not surprising that on the wards of these nineteenth century hospitals one of the highest priorities was patient discipline. As historian Jim Connor argues, social elites linked moral values with therapeutic need: "...those in power determined who deserved their charity: not the lazy or destitute; not those with chronic, infectious, or terminal disease; and, in the case of women, not the pregnant."[4] For those patients deemed worthy, rules of institutional behaviour underscored the link between health and morality: patients were prohibited from smoking, using abusive language, or socializing too intimately with patients of the opposite sex. Hospital administrators and the local elites who served on hospital boards expected hospital staff to create an orderly, disciplined, and clean environment, wherein even the roughest of patrons would experience the environmental balance needed to regain good health and even improve their own morality.

By the late nineteenth century, institutions' dedication to charitable care was being challenged by

dramatic new developments in scientific medicine. Biomedical advances, especially the germ theory of disease conceived by researchers such as Pasteur and Koch, the development of anesthetics, and Lister's method of antiseptic surgery, confirmed for many Canadian doctors that hospitals could and should be sites of therapeutic, not custodial, care. Not surprisingly, those seeking to reform the hospital quickly turned their attention to the quality and quantity of nursing care provided in these institutions.

As Judith Young and Nicole Rousseau discuss in chapter 1 of this volume, assessing the real character of hospital nursing in nineteenth century Canada is difficult given the paucity of primary documentation. What emerges from the available evidence is that hospitals relied on a wide range of caregivers, male and female, religious and lay, paid and unpaid, skilled and unskilled.[5] As late as 1893 officials at Vancouver's city hospital acknowledged that during the day nursing attendance was fine, but at night the lone man assigned to oversee three wards "is accustomed to get the worse for liquor and go to sleep."[6]

Complicating our understanding of nineteenth century nursing is the fact that some of our most evocative descriptions of nineteenth century hospital nurses come from twentieth century observers reminiscing about the bygone era of the "old style nurse." In doing so, those observers often reproduced the potent cultural iconography of figures such as Sairey Gamp, the slovenly, drunken night watcher of Charles Dickens's novel *Martin Chuzzlewit*.[7] For example,

Canada's most famous physician, Sir William Osler, recalled in 1913 that during his training at the Montreal General Hospital (MGH) in the 1860s the nurses "were generally ward servants who had evolved from the kitchen or from the backstairs into the wards.... Many of them were of the old type so well described by Dickens...."[8] Other commentators noted the absence of any kind of nursing care. *The Canadian Nurse* editor and international nursing leader Ethel Johns described the early days of the Winnipeg General Hospital in her 1953 history of that institution. Johns reported that Winnipeg's first hospital, established in the city's north end in 1873, included a building with no plaster on the brick walls or ceiling. City doctors attended the patients, but "the thought was that those who by misfortune got knocked out by sickness were lucky to have this primitive hospital to receive them. The patients would care for each other when able to do so, assisted by any help that could be obtained."[9] Images of shoddy nursing became part of twentieth century narratives of progress, as commentators contrasted the worst of the slovenly, old nurses with the new, trained personnel of the "modern" hospital. But the popularized image of the "Gamp" may also have made a one-dimensional character out of a much more complex and uneven range of pre-industrial ward attendants.

The International Campaign for Nursing Education

Whatever the quality of the nursing, there is no doubt that by the 1870s and 1880s many Canadian hospitals sought reform, and nursing was a central part of the reform agenda. Canadian doctors and medical administrators joined the international movement advocating trained nursing staff and in doing so endorsed the blueprint for change most potently argued for by British reformer Florence Nightingale.

Florence Nightingale is one of the most famous women of her day, second only to Queen Victoria. While many of the details of Nightingale's career may have faded from public memory, her name recognition has not. She remains an icon of nursing, invoked in almost every discussion of nursing history — or even contemporary issues.

Born in 1820 to an upper-middle class family, Nightingale grew up in a world where nursing was deemed the domain of working class women — certainly inappropriate for someone of Nightingale's classical education and class status. In spite of this, as a young woman Nightingale declared nursing as her chosen vocation. Eventually overcoming her family's objections, in 1853 Nightingale assumed the position of superintendent at London's Harley Street Home for Ill Gentlewomen. There she gained her first administrative experience and used her familial and social ties to build professional relationships with medical and political leaders of her day. When the Crimean War erupted in 1854, British military authorities faced public criticism for failing to provide a military nursing corps comparable to that of the French and Russian armies. In response, Britain's Secretary of State at War, Sidney Herbert, called on his friend Florence Nightingale. Nightingale recruited 38 nurses, organized equipment and provisions, and set off for Scutari, Turkey, to take charge of the military hospital there.[10]

There is no doubt that Nightingale embraced her mission with zeal. She secured medical supplies, improved the hygiene of the army hospital, visited patients at night — thereby earning the title "lady with the lamp" — travelled to the military front, and won the begrudging respect of the medical officers. Important as those tangible achievements were, Nightingale's more substantial accomplishment was the indirect result of new telegraph technology. The telegraph permitted journalists, for the first time, to provide fast and extensive coverage of the war, offering the daily newspapers in Britain and much of the English-speaking world up-to-date stories from the front. In the midst of regular reports of military blunder, Nightingale's outstanding efforts on behalf of British troops propelled her to heroic status throughout the Western world.

Back at home, Nightingale's friends and supporters decided that her work needed appropriate recognition. They agreed to solicit donations from the public to support a fund through which Nightingale could promote the education of nurses. British citizens responded with enthusiasm, joined by contributors from as far away as Australia. By 1856 over £44 000

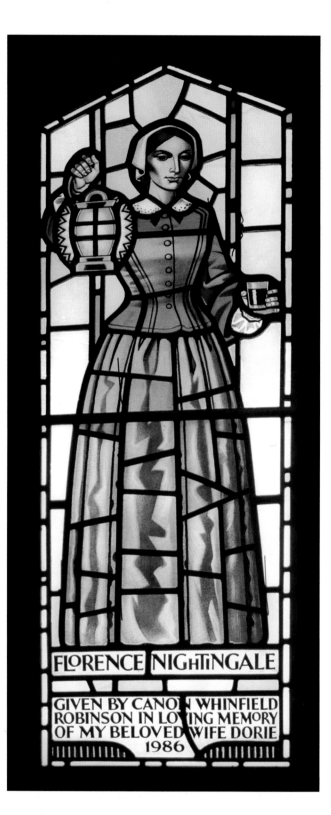

FLORENCE NIGHTINGALE

GIVEN BY CANON WHINFIELD
ROBINSON IN LOVING MEMORY
OF MY BELOVED WIFE DORIE
1986

had been donated. When informed of the fund, Nightingale's only stipulation was that she, and the fund's trustees, would control its use.[11]

At war's end, Nightingale returned to England, struggling with a chronic health problem that had developed in Crimea. Her first priority was to lobby for a government inquiry into army medical and sanitary reform, a subject that sustained her attention for much of her life. Not until the 1860s did Nightingale and the Nightingale Fund trustees finally establish a use for the fund, in the form of a nursing school organized in conjunction with London's St. Thomas's hospital. Establishing the school required delicate negotiations. The educational system had to be grafted onto the existing hospital staffing model, and nurses had to be trained even as the usual number of patients was admitted, treated, and discharged. Given those tensions, the matron, Mrs Wardroper, was given the dual role of continuing in her duties as matron, overseeing the day-to-day functioning of the hospital, and also becoming lady superintendent, managing the education of the pupil nurses. Wardroper's students were paid a small sum, learned as they worked on the wards, and upon completion of their training were contractually bound to take a position at the hospital for a set period of time. Although working class women were the target group of recruits, St. Thomas's also made room for "lady pupils" from the middle and upper class, who paid for, rather than were paid for, their training and who were groomed for assuming supervisory roles. The graduates of the school were dubbed "Nightingale nurses" and the educational program soon came
to be known as the "Nightingale system."[12]

Hospital and nursing reformers in North America watched these developments closely, and there is no doubt that Nightingale's high profile activities focused attention on the question of nursing education. By 1900 hospitals around the globe were educat-ing nurses and employing trained nurses. Assessing the extent to which Nightingale can be credited with this revolution in nursing is a complicated matter, for in many ways she was just part of a more complex set of changes occurring in health care. For example, Nightingale was by no means alone in her quest for better quality nursing. In England, medical and hospital reformers had been lobbying for improved nursing since at least 1800,[13] and in the 1840s two training institutes had been established in Britain: Elizabeth Fry's Institute of Nursing in 1840 and the Anglican sisters' St. John's House in 1848.[14] Nightingale herself visited and drew inspiration from the deaconesses at Germany's heralded Kaiserwerth. American historians Vern and Bonnie Bulloch emphasize that in the United States feminists played key roles in organizing nursing training programs, such as Dr Elizabeth Blackwell who opened a nursing school in 1857 at her New York Infirmary. Scholars have also shown the pivotal role the civil war of 1860–1865 played in generating medical enthusiasm for nursing education within the United States.[15]

If Nightingale was not alone in identifying the need for trained nurses, nor were her graduates directly responsible for transporting the Nightingale system overseas. True, a few Nightingale nurses did travel to points in the British Empire, but their numbers were small and their influence questionable.[16] Nightingale nurse Lucy Osburn was dispatched to the infirmary in Sydney, Australia, with five pupil nurses in 1867, but shortly after her arrival in Sydney she made a diplomatic error that Nightingale never forgave. Although Osburn remained as the superintendent of the Sydney hospital for 25 years, the "Nightingale nurses" who travelled with her lasted less than three years, Osburn never again benefited from the Nightingale Fund, and Osburn's relationship with Nightingale was never repaired.[17]

In Canada, the MGH administration, determined to introduce "a system of trained hospital nurses such as approved of in England," appealed to the Nightingale trust for St. Thomas's graduates who could establish a nursing school at MGH. In 1875, Nightingale's friend and pupil Maria Machin was dispatched there with four other nurses, but soon after, one of those nurses had died and one had left to be married. Within a year, Machin was at odds with the hospital administration, in part over her ongoing conflicts with staff nurses, and by 1878 Machin had resigned.[18] It was, instead, a graduate

of the New York Hospital Training School, Nora Livingston, who took over the MGH program and guided it for more than 30 years.

Even though Nightingale's alumnae themselves had little direct effect in North America, was the Nightingale "system" influential nonetheless? Here again, the evidence is mixed. It is true that many Canadian hospitals introduced nursing education programs akin to St. Thomas's. Those programs brought pupil nurses into the hospital to learn as they worked. The pupils received board and room and a small stipend. Many hospitals emphasized that they wished to recruit a "better class" of girl, though no Canadian hospital endeavored to establish a two-tiered student group, with daughters of the upper-middle class being labelled "lady probationers," like the system that was in place at St. Thomas's. The most critical difference lay, however, in the authority of the lady superintendent. Most Canadian hospitals did establish an autonomous reporting structure where nurses reported to more senior nurses, not to doctors. In this, Canadian programs remained true to Nightingale's vision. But no Canadian hospital had independent funding, akin to the Nightingale Fund, through which the nursing program could wield some leverage in negotiations with the institution. Rather, nursing schools were caught in a web of dependency with their institutional homes; the hospital relied on the inexpensive and relatively skilled labour that nursing students offered, while the nursing educators were dependent on the legal, administrative, and financial authority of the institution. And while medical and nursing authorities both answered to the hospital board of directors, in many cases the nursing superintendent had far less access to the board, and boards regularly appointed doctors to them, while only rarely did nurses hold a seat.

The history of early hospital administration, then, is filled with tales of lady superintendents doing battle with medical doctors, hospital administrators, and boards of directors all to sustain their authority over the nursing realm. For example, in 1896, the lady superintendent of Halifax's Victoria General Hospital had to face a commission of enquiry. The complaints directed at superintendent Elliott revolved around her insistence that female nurses assist male patients

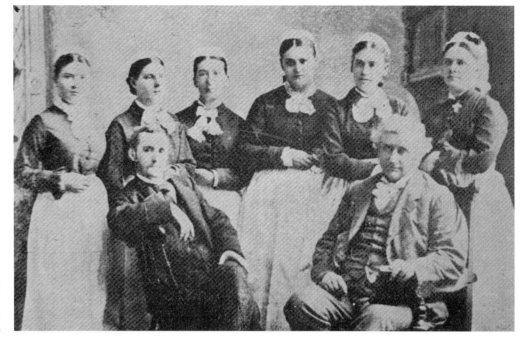

Figure 3
First graduating class and staff of the Mack Training School for Nurses
St. Catharines, Ontario
1878
Library and Archives
Canada, e002414894

with baths and bedpans and even administer catheters or suppositories. The commission stepped in to chastise the students who had complained, but reserved their most biting indictment for the superintendent, concluding that she displayed a vital lack of tact and gentility in her handling of the situation.[19] In other situations superintendents of nurses had their authority usurped by medical administrators, as in the conflict that erupted in 1914 at St. John's Newfoundland's General Hospital. When medical superintendent Lawrence Keegan began hiring staff nurses directly, nursing superintendent Mary Southcott and her nursing staff protested so vigorously that a Royal Commission was struck to investigate the administration of the hospital. The end result saw the power of the nursing superintendent diminished and Southcott dismissed.[20] At the Vancouver General Hospital, lady superintendent Helen Randal resigned her post in 1916 when medical superintendent Malcolm MacEachern ignored her recommendation for a replacement during her leave.[21] And nursing superintendents had to walk a fine line with their own students and staff, maintaining discipline but also loyalty; there were numerous instances where nursing students or staff complained to the medical superintendent or the board about the nursing superintendent, and in most cases the female

administrator was found at least partly to blame.

Clearly, nursing superintendents in Canada rarely achieved the administrative autonomy or authority envisioned by Nightingale, and nursing schools continued to suffer from the absence of any secure financial basis. What came to be called the Nightingale system was in fact a hybrid, in which the key element of nursing control over education was missing. Where we may see the strongest evidence of Nightingale's influence, then, is not in the direct application of the Nightingale blueprint, but in the ideological power of Nightingale's publicly articulated vision for nursing education and in her ability to champion nursing as a respectable occupation for women.

Cultural theorist Mary Poovey has addressed this point most forcefully. Poovey interrogates the production of "normative" gender roles in Victorian Britain, arguing that in the nineteenth century a new ideology of separate spheres defined the "normative (working) man" against the "normative (nonworking) woman." Working women, Poovey claims, threatened to disrupt this "symbolic economy" by exposing "the artificiality of [its] binary logic." Nightingale neutralized this disruptive potential by putting nursing on the public agenda but then firmly tethering the occupation to conventional gender roles, emphasizing nurses' nur-

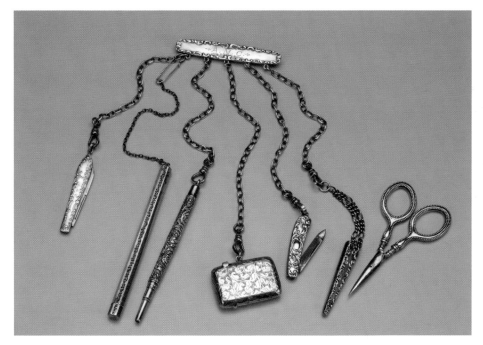

Figure 4
Nurse's chatelaine
ca. 1900
Photographer: Doug Millar
Alumnae Association of the School of
Nursing, Toronto General Hospital
Collection
Canadian Museum of Civilization,
2003.44.19

*Often given as a graduation
present, the nurse's chatelaine
pinned onto the skirt,
suspending useful items such
as a pen-knife, thermometer
holder, pencil, match case
and scissors.*

turing work, their management of sanitary conditions, and their ability "to make the hospital a home." In the process, Poovey states, Nightingale was able to "enhance the reputation of an activity that had been degraded because it was traditionally women's work."[22] One might add that Nightingale's success in reframing nursing's social status — what Poovey defines as dulling nursing's potentially disruptive effect in Victorian society — lay in Nightingale's command of print culture. Unlike most women of her day, Nightingale had the education, time, and economic contacts needed to write and to have her written work published. Her most famous work, *Notes on Nursing: What It Is, and What It Is Not*, first appeared in 1859, and within a month had sold 15 000 copies. *Notes on Nursing* was published in the United States in 1860, and was reprinted at least 50 times over the next 100 years.[23] In addition to her published work, Nightingale was a prolific letter writer, communicating with friends and colleagues around the world. Connected to the major artists and thinkers of her day, Nightingale was integrated into the cultural production through works such as Longfellow's 1857 poem about Nightingale, "Santa Filomena."[24] Over the next 100 years, Nightingale's historical contribution was articulated and re-articulated in biographical studies of her and in medical and nursing history

textbooks used to educate new generations of practitioners.[25]

In this way, Nightingale served as a touchstone and source of inspiration for nursing reformers around the globe, suggesting an influence that is hard to calibrate or quantify. Whatever tensions working nurses, students, and their supervisors might have experienced within institutions, a wider social endorsement of nursing as important social work was available in the form of Nightingale's published work and publicized efforts.

The Trained Nurse and the Modern Hospital

Nightingale and her contemporaries reformulated nursing into a respectable occupation for women, but in doing so they were also the architects of an educational model that inextricably linked nursing to hospitals. Nurses relied on hospitals to provide recognized training programs, but hospitals came to rely on nursing students to staff the hospital wards. In the late nineteenth and early twentieth century, hospitals in all industrial nations established training schools, eliminating the "old style" nurses of the pre-industrial institution and producing a relationship of mutual dependency between the "trained nurse" and the

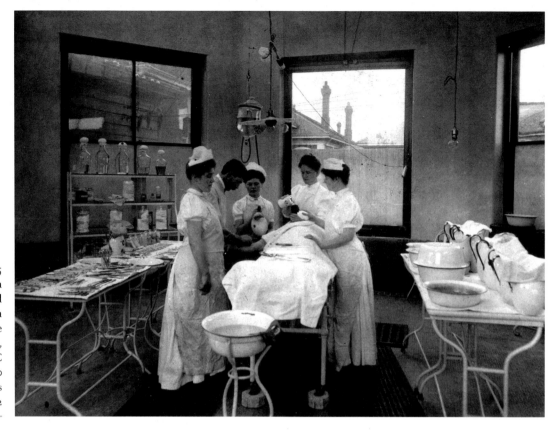

Figure 5
**Pemberton
Memorial
Operating Room**
Royal Jubilee
Hospital,
Victoria, BC
ca. 1900
BC Archives
Collection, B-09492

modern hospital that created her. St. Catherine's Marine and General Hospital was the first Canadian institution to open a nursing training program with its 1874 Mack's Training School. Over the next two decades, major urban hospitals across the nation followed suit, founding programs such as the Winnipeg General School of Nursing (1887), Halifax's Victoria General School of Nursing (1890) and Toronto's St. Michael's Hospital School (1892). By 1909, 70 hospital schools were in operation, and by the 1920s there were over 200.[26]

Growth in the number and size of hospital nursing education programs was part of a larger expansion in the number and size of hospitals, specialization within and among hospitals, and the increasingly diverse class background of patients using hospitals during the period from 1880 to 1930. Patients from all classes, all ethnic groups, and all regions came to depend on hospitals to provide the latest surgical and medical interventions that scientific medicine had to offer. The ability of institutions to respond effectively to this demand was due, in no small measure, to the workforce of student nurses who staffed hospital wards.[27]

Each year, hospital schools admitted a new class of students. If these probationers survived their first three months of training, they stayed on as juniors, then intermediates, and then seniors, assuming more responsibility for ward supervision and specialty care as they advanced. Upon graduation, most nurses left institutional service and sought their fortunes in private duty work or on public health nursing staffs. Few remained in hospitals, and those who did were employed as nursing instructors or supervisors, overseeing another cohort of pupil nurses. This model of institutional staffing became known as the apprenticeship system, and it remained the dominant mode by which Canadian hospitals staffed their wards until well past the Second World War.

The advantage of this system to hospitals was unequivocal. By relying almost exclusively on the labour of student nurses, hospitals enjoyed minimal staffing costs. Pupil nurses earned a small monthly stipend — for example, $8, $10, and $12 per month for juniors, intermediates, and seniors, respectively[28] — and were provided with board and room. In return for this modest payroll, hospitals acquired

Nurses' Residences: Recognition and Respectability

Dianne Dodd, Parks Canada

The Ann Baillie building, erected in 1903–4 as a home for nurses at the Kingston General Hospital in Kingston, was one of a number of impressive, domestic structures that began to appear in English Canada in the early twentieth century. Physicians, nursing leaders, and hospital administrators hoped that these buildings would attract respectable, middle class young women to the field of nursing and assure their parents that their daughters would be adequately supervised. These homes were certainly a step up from the early days when student nurses — who trained in the hospital as apprentices, providing hospitals with their principal nursing workforce — were often forced to live in hospital wards. There they faced not only strenuous demands but possible contagion from close proximity to patients. One of the earliest nurses' residences, the Baillie Building was designed as a home. Later residences had a more institutional flavour. They were larger and included classrooms, labs, and elaborate recreational facilities for the student nurses, reflecting the increasing emphasis on formal education.

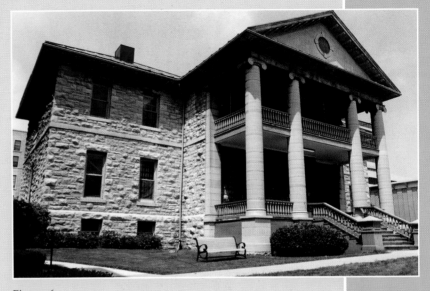

Figure 6
The Anne Baillie Building, former nurses' residence
Kingston General Hospital
Kingston, Ontario
Photographer: James De Jonge

By contrast, in French-speaking Canada, nurses' residences did not play such a prominent role. There simply was no need to elevate the status of nursing in the French Catholic hospital system, which had developed much earlier, and relied upon women in religious congregations for much of their nursing. These women already held highly respected positions within the community and church. Neither was there as pressing a need to find accommodation for hundreds of lay nurses until much later in the century, as religious women were housed in their convent buildings.

The Baillie Building, along with four other nurses' residences in Canada, was recognized as a national historic site by the Minister of Canadian Heritage in 1998. The others are Hersey Pavilion, Victoria Hospital, Montreal; Begbie Hall, Royal Jubilee Hospital, Victoria, BC; Pavilion Mailloux, Hôpital Notre-Dame, Montreal; and St. Boniface Hospital School of Nursing, Winnipeg, Manitoba. They are symbols of the nursing profession's struggles for recognition and nurses' contribution to health care in the community and the hospital.

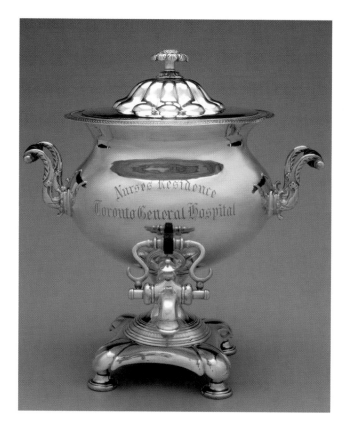

Figure 7
Tea Urn
Toronto General Hospital Nurses' Residence
early 20th century
Photographer: Doug Millar
Alumnae Association of the School of Nursing, Toronto General
Hospital Collection
Canadian Museum of Civilization, 2003.44.4

a disciplined and dependable workforce. Students lived and worked in the institution. Except for short annual holidays and a half day off on the weekend, students were under the direct supervision of hospital administrators at all times. And the student-nursing workforce appeared almost infinitely expandable. Hospitals recruited new pupils from among local families — welcoming young women from skilled working class and middle class families alike — but also drew heavily upon the surrounding countryside. By the 1920s between one-third and one-half of apprenticing nurses hailed from Canada's rural communities. Cheap, subordinate, and plentiful, the workforce of pupil nurses was also skilled. Chapter 6 of this volume explores the expertise nurses offered Canadian medical science over the past century. Within hospital nursing schools, student nurses acquired these skills as they advanced through the various levels of their apprenticeship so that by their senior year they were proficient in direct patient care and ward supervision.[29]

The apprenticeship model of hospital staffing and of nursing education offered institutions many advantages. The benefits to nurses and nursing are less clear. Many nursing historians have emphasized the exploitative nature of apprenticeship education. They point to hospitals' minimal investment in instructors or educational facilities and argue that in most schools education was haphazard, uneven, and always subordinated to other institutional demands. In addition, the students worked exceptionally long and hard. Student nurses worked 12-hour shifts, either days or nights, at least six days per week. At anywhere from $8 to $12 per month the stipend was token at best. In the 1920s and 1930s many schools implemented an 8-hour day for students and introduced more instructors but shift work with only a day off per week remained the norm. Not surpris-

ingly, then, some students succumbed to chronic diseases — most seriously tuberculosis — and many others struggled with more acute work-related health problems including burns, cuts, infections, and collapsed arches.[30]

Other historians acknowledge these problems, but also note the advantages that apprenticeship education offered Canadian women. Unlike universities, hospital schools of nursing cost only a modest tuition fee (usually $25 plus a small cost for the uniform), offered a small monthly stipend (which meant that students did not have to rely on their families for spending money), and provided residence accommodation. The latter element of apprenticeship education was particularly important for rural women who faced limited occupational choices in their home communities but whose families balked at permitting their daughters to move into the city unchaperoned. Indeed, for most women in modern Canada, nursing education, however gruelling, was no more demanding than factory work or domestic service (which remained the leading employer of Canadian women until the Second World War). And at the end of their

On All Frontiers

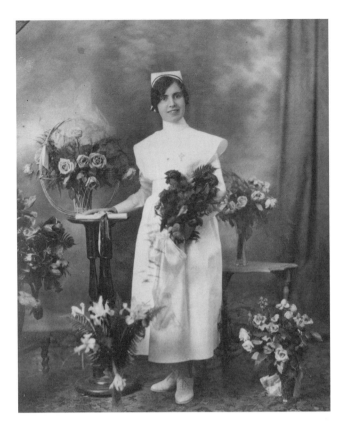

Figure 8
Graduation portrait of Isabel Hornby
Holy Cross Hospital, Calgary, Alberta
ca. 1920
Glenbow Archives, Calgary, Alberta, NA-35719

social role for trained nurses, the occupation had to be differentiated from other kinds of caregivers in the health care market. By defining nursing as a "woman's occupation," nurses distinguished themselves and their work from the male-dominated medical profession. But to claim a public face for trained nurses, the occupation also had to draw a firm boundary between itself and other women in the community who tended the sick. That group included midwives, untrained nurses, domestic servants, and female kinfolk, all of whom continued to provide important health care services even after trained nursing had been established. To draw that boundary, trained nursing staked a claim to an image of female respectability that rested on the deportment and etiquette of white bourgeois femininity.

Canadian hospital nursing schools insisted that students be single or widowed and between the ages of 18 and 35. Prospective recruits had to achieve a base level of education, which increased from grade 9 in the late nineteenth century to grade 11 or 12 by the 1920s. Applicants had to speak either English or French fluently, thus eliminating from consideration many first-generation immigrants to Canada. And, regardless of their educational achievement or language skills, no African-Canadian or First Nations applicant was admitted to a Canadian nursing school before the 1940s. Only a few students of East Asian ancestry were admitted.[33] Nursing schools thus used educational, linguistic, and racist barriers, along with marital status and age, to define nursing as an occupation of relative privilege. Nursing was defined as different than domestic service, then, in part by the composition of the workforce.[34]

From the earliest days of their nursing education program, students were immersed in the rules and deportment of respectable femininity and constrained sexuality. Whether in residence or on the wards,

three-year apprenticeship, "graduate nurses" left the tightly regulated world of hospital education for work in public health or private duty nursing. There, practitioners could boast a significant set of skills, formal certification, substantial geographic mobility, and membership in an occupation strong enough to nurture local, provincial, and national associations. For these reasons, nursing joined teaching and secretarial work at the pinnacle of the hierarchy of female-dominated occupations in late nineteenth and early twentieth century Canada.[31]

In his assessment of the material advantages that the apprenticeship system of nursing education and hospital staffing offered, historian of medicine Charles Rosenberg has pointed to the "economic logic" that drove the nursing–hospital relationship. He writes: "Both hospitals and prospective nurses were capital poor: it was only natural for the two parties to barter: work for diplomas."[32] But accompanying this "economic logic" was also a "social logic" that revolved around the issues of gender, race, and respectability.

Hospital administrators, nursing leaders, and working nurses agreed that to carve out a unique

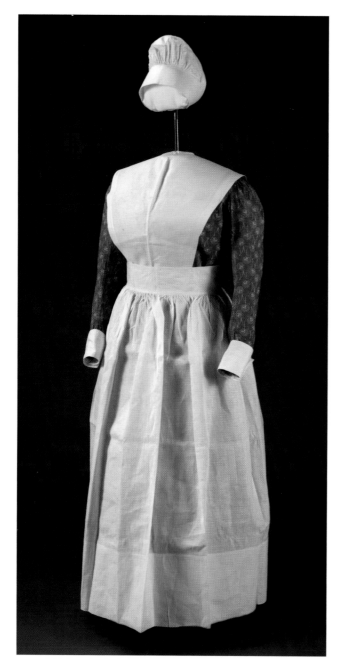

Figure 9
Student Uniform, Edna Muir
Western Hospital, Montreal, Quebec
1916–1920
Photographer: Doug Millar
Canadian Nurses Association Collection
Canadian Museum of Civilization, 2000.111.421

the apron had to be impeccably clean, and the cap firmly secured and at exactly the right angle on the head. Morning inspection of uniforms underscored the importance of professional dress. Not all students conformed to these codes of behaviour. Nursing supervisors were vigilant in their supervision of student behaviour, reprimanding their pupils for smoking, missing curfew, and, as the twentieth century progressed, kissing boyfriends too close to hospital grounds.[35]

For some students, the bonds of respectability were too constraining and they left, or were asked to leave, their hospital school. But most apprentice nurses conformed sufficiently to complete their education, knowing that at the end of their three-year apprenticeship they could leave the strict regime of the hospital. Once in private duty, though, graduate nurses found the image of social and sexual respectability a valuable feature of their professional status: as respectable white women traversing the countryside or travelling the city streets alone by day or night, the image of "nurse on duty" proved potent defense against the appearance of sexual impropriety — and even against possible sexual assault. The economic logic that drew young women and growing hospitals together — Rosenberg's "work for diplomas" — was cemented into a wider social accord by the image of white, bourgeois, female sexual respectability that hospital schools of nursing claimed for their apprentices. From the 1870s to the 1940s, hospitals and their apprenticeship staff claimed a privileged place for nurses within the female world of work, while at the same time fostering the public image of respectability for the hospital that was needed to recruit middle class patients into the "modern hospital."

Hospital Nursing and the Biomedical Revolution: From 1945 to the Present

In the years after World War II, the nurse–hospital relationship changed dramatically. True, hospital schools of nursing continued to educate a large percentage of Canadian practitioners and, as a result, apprentice nurses continued to be a vital source of institutional labour: students still worked while they

students were forbidden from flirting, gossiping, indulging in liquor or tobacco, from being rude and insubordinate, and from staying out past curfew. The nurse's uniform physically represented this ideal: the uniform skirt had to be a fixed length off the floor,

learned. It was not until the 1980s that community college and university nursing education programs superseded hospital-based schools. But in the 1940s and 1950s, Canadian hospitals began adding large numbers of RNs to their staffs; these new RNs provided patient care directly, rather than simply supervising apprentice nurses as had been the case before.

The reasons for this shift in institutional staffing patterns are complex. In the Depression of the 1930s, the old system of staffing hospitals almost entirely with apprentices began to break down when graduate nurses found they could not support themselves in private duty care. Out-of-work RNs turned to their alma maters, prompting superintendents of nursing to use their positions of authority to help alumnae survive the economic crisis; superintendents began to hire RNs as staff or general duty nurses to work alongside rather than just supervise apprentice nurses. Then, in the post–World War II years, Canadian hospitals began to grow in size and complexity, so that the student nurse workforce could not adequately service institutional needs. Biomedical advances inspired the creation of new medical specialties and new hospital wards and units; hospital and health insurance programs made institutional care affordable for a greater number of patients; and federal hospital construction grants helped municipalities expand health facilities. New, more technical, tasks were assigned to nursing staff, and nursing "specialties" began to proliferate. Student nurses were neither skilled enough nor plentiful enough to meet these new institutional and therapeutic demands.

But were there enough RNs available to sustain hospital growth? Nursing leaders and hospital management across Canada struggled in the 1950s through 1970s to expand the nursing workforce. Married women — even married women with children — were recruited back into paid labour as the old restrictions on admissibility to the profession began to break down. A small number of male nurses were integrated into a profession that for nearly a century had been designated "women's work." And racist barriers that had kept visible minority women out of nursing were eliminated.

These changes to the composition of Canada's nursing workforce did not occur without struggle, as the example of African-Canadian nurses reveals. Throughout the 1940s, black women in communities across Canada applied for admission to hospital nursing schools and, when they were denied, worked with local activists and political leaders to challenge racist exclusion. Immigrant nurses faced additional barriers. As scholars Agnes Calliste and Karen Flynn have both shown, in an era when the Canadian government was welcoming white immigrants with open arms, Afro-Caribbean nurses had to endure a lengthy and difficult process of demonstrating their credentials and employability to federal officials, who were carefully screening migrants from non-white nations. Regardless of birthplace, black nurses often faced discrimination on hospital wards, confronting racist slurs or "jokes," being assigned the "heaviest" patients, or being denied promotion to leadership or managerial positions. Even when the institutional setting was supportive of black nurses, those practitioners had to face racism of the wider society: in 1950 a student nurse in Windsor, Ontario, could not attend the graduation dance for her hospital school because the hotel in which the dance was being held refused to serve black customers.[36]

By the 1980s, discrimination based on race, ethnicity, sex, or sexuality was being directly challenged, as most practitioners recognized that diversity among Canadian nurses made the occupation stronger. But nursing faced other kinds of divisions too. In the post–World War II era, continued shortages of RNs and the seemingly incessant demand for hospital services had prompted the introduction of a range of subsidiary patient-care personnel — attendants, nurses' aides, licensed practical nurses, registered practical nurses, and nursing assistants began to assume tasks that had once been delegated to nursing students or staff. Auxiliary or "non-professional" nursing staffs were characterized by greater gender and racial diversity than even the "professional" staffs of RNs: indeed, many immigrant nurses ended up working in "non-professional" nursing positions when their educational credentials did not conform to Canadian licensing standards. Differences among nurses were further complicated in these years by the promotion of many RNs into hospital management at the same time that RNs working on wards

Charlotte Edith Anderson Monture (1890–1996)

John Moses, Canadian Museum of Civilization, grandson of Edith Monture

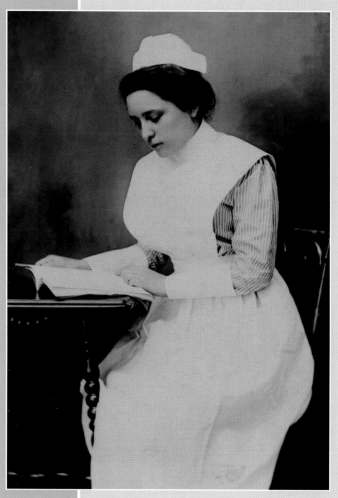

Figure 10
Charlotte Edith Anderson Monture
1914
Courtesy of John Moses

Edith Monture (née Anderson) was an exceptional woman for her time. A member of the Upper Mohawk band from the Six Nations of the Grand River Reserve near Brantford, Ontario, she was among the first of her generation to leave the reserve to pursue a career.

Anderson had attempted to undertake nurses' training in Canada during an era in which the federal *Indian Act* placed restrictions upon the pursuit of higher education by status Aboriginals. Her attempts to gain admission to a number of Canadian nursing schools having been denied, Anderson met with greater success within a more progressive and welcoming American system. She graduated first in her class from the New Rochelle Hospital School of Nursing, north of New York City, in 1914. Living and working as a public health and school nurse in New York City as the United States entered the First World War in 1917, she volunteered for duty as a Nursing Sister with the American Expeditionary Force's Army Medical Corps.

Her wartime journal reveals her as a warm and compassionate woman who was deeply touched by the suffering of her patients. After the death of her "pet patient Earl King the boy who adopted me for his big sister," her journal entry for 16 June 1918 briefly recounts: "My heart was broken. Cried most of the day and could not sleep...."

Following her service overseas at US Army Base Hospital 23 in Vittel, France, Anderson returned home to the Six Nations Reserve in 1919. Here she married Claybran Monture, raised a family, and continued working as a nurse and midwife at the Lady Willingdon Hospital on the reserve until her retirement in 1955. Charlotte Edith Anderson Monture died on the Six Nations of the Grand Reserve in 1996, shortly before her 106th birthday.

Source: Charlotte Edith Anderson Monture, *Diary of a War Nurse* (Ohsweken, ON: privately printed, 1996), 27.

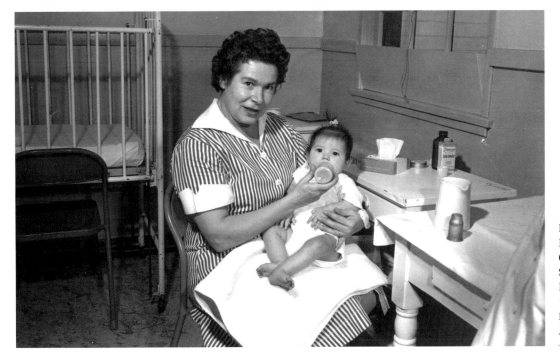

Figure 11
**Practical Nurse
Course, Vocational
School**
Nanaimo, BC
1962
British Columbia
Archives, 1-24276

began forming unions to represent their interests. In Catholic hospitals, especially in Quebec, the administrative work of nurses took a very different turn during the 1970s. In that decade, as historian Aline Charles has shown, female religious lost their unique roles as administrators and workers within Catholic hospitals.[37]

Conclusion

Canadian nurses have a long and complex relationship with our nation's hospitals. Throughout its transition from a custodial to a therapeutic institution, nurses have helped define and build the modern hospital. In the 1870s, when nursing education programs were first established, hospitals were still defined as a popular class institution — a site where the social relations of charity could be acted out. But as hospitals grew and their therapeutic repertoire expanded, hospitals began to draw upon patients from all social classes. Respectable Canadians turned to hospitals to provide what scientific medicine promised. Hospitals met this new demand through new medical-scientific techniques, through the training of physicians and surgeons, and through the building

of more genteel accommodation. But in many ways the new system of nursing education and staffing was the lynchpin. Inexpensive, disciplined, skilled, and respectable, apprenticing students and their supervisors offered hospitals what their pre-industrial predecessors could not. The transition in the 1940s to hospital reliance on graduated rather than student nursing staff and the introduction of auxiliary categories of nurses meant that hospitals now relied on a whole range of categories of caregivers, but the hospital–nurse relationship remained strong. Whether students learning as they worked, RNs providing general or specialized care, or administrators overseeing the educational and therapeutic services, hospital nurses have provided services essential to modern medical care. In turn, hospitals have proved formative in shaping Canada's nursing workforce, serving as a key educational institution and the dominant employer of RNs. Florence Nightingale and her contemporaries in the nursing reform movement of the nineteenth century could not have imagined how central skilled nurses would become to health care in the twenty-first century or the long journey that hospitals and nurses would take together.

CHAPTER 6

"Body Work," Medical Technology, and Hospital Nursing Practice

Cynthia Toman

Nurses have been predominantly associated with hospitals for the greater part of the twentieth century, whether as students in training or as graduate nurses upon completion of their training. Within hospital settings, they engaged in a wide variety of activities that involved "body work" — I use this term to refer to both the treatments and procedures that nurses performed on patients' bodies, and the skilful use of nurses' own bodies in the performance of patient care. Body work frequently required the skilled and timely use of equipment and machines, as well as the technological knowledge that went with it. Historian Kathryn McPherson has pointed out how the mastery of specific nursing skills served to clearly differentiate trained nurses from lay health care providers while creating an occupational space and legitimacy for nursing as paid women's work. Nurses have consequently valued skills highly; indeed, the possession of skills became central to their collective identity.[1]

In this chapter, I examine the evolution of body work as performed in Canadian hospitals by nurses from the late nineteenth century to the end of the twentieth century. During that time it shifted in nature from simple work that nurses shared with lay care providers to highly specialized technological care requiring advanced training. Changes in the nature of body work and in who performed it have had signifi-

cant implications for nurses and for the nursing profession. Hospitals, professional organizations, and nurses themselves learned to capitalize on the need for technological skills related to patient care. Although the combined influence of body work, medical technology, and hospital expansion created new employment opportunities for nurses, it also fragmented the profession. On one hand, nurses typically perceived technology as a desirable and positive component of patient care that provided possibilities for advancement at the bedside. On the other hand, many felt ambivalent about the effects of technology on patient care and on their own roles as nurses. Debates within the profession increasingly divided nurses into two groups: "technicians" who remained at the bedside and "professionals" who moved away from the bedside (and from body work) into positions of leadership, management, and education. These debates led to further controversies, creating hierarchies among nurses and disagreements about how and where nurses should be educated.

From Shared Work to Nursing Technique

Nurses engaged in body work and used medical technology in various ways. Prior to the early 1900s, for example, much of their work involved tools,

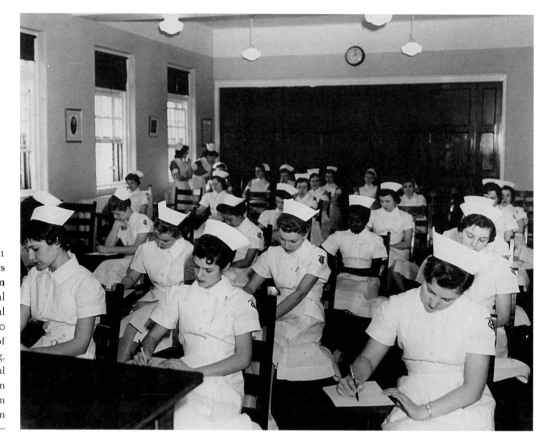

Figure 1
Nursing students in classroom
Toronto General Hospital
ca. 1950
Alumnae Association of the School of Nursing, Toronto General Hospital Collection
Canadian Museum of Civilization

treatments, and medications that were commonly available and could be used by both lay and trained healers alike in caring for the sick. They did not perceive themselves as having special ownership of the technology or its associated knowledge since they shared equipment both with physicians and with other untrained or semi-trained care providers. During the first decades of the twentieth century, however, body work became associated with increasingly specialized knowledge and language, as nurses' training emphasized the scientific principles of antisepsis and asepsis, the measurement of bodily functions and medications, and the routinization of nursing care under the rhetoric of scientific management or efficiency nursing.

Although hospitals needed students primarily for their labour, student nurses entered hospitals to acquire marketable skills that would equip them for independent or semi-independent private duty nursing practice. Their work consisted of a range of activities referred to variously as techniques, procedures, or "nursing arts," which have been classified into six cat-

egories. Administrative activities included labelling and storing patients' belongings on admission; charting and recording treatments, medications, and tests; and stocking hospital supplies. Assisting with diagnostic tests included preparing patients and equipment; collecting samples; delivering samples to the lab; and recording results. Assisting medical and surgical personnel included assistance with examinations, surgical procedures, treatments, and dressings for incisions or wounds. Therapeutic nursing duties involved a range of tasks that nurses performed alone such as giving medications, enemas, douches, and lavages as well as plasters, foments, and poultices. Maintenance of the hospital ward and equipment included cleaning and organizing it so that sufficient supplies were always available when needed. Personal service tasks involved a multitude of activities performed for the benefit and well-being of patients such as bathing, feeding, and assisting them with toileting, dressing, and ambulation as needed.[2]

Indeed students spent the greatest portion of their training in the perfection of these techniques,

On All Frontiers

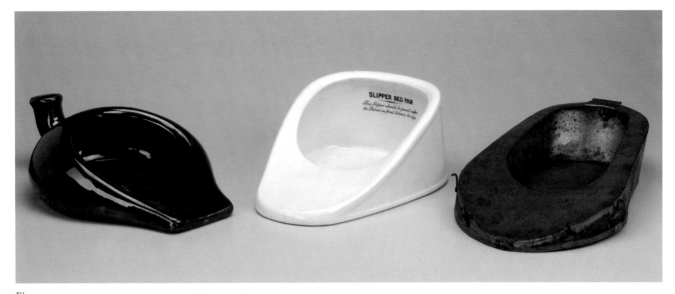

Figure 2
Bedpans
ca. 1850–1920
Photographer: Doug Millar
Canadian Museum of Civilization, D-2697; Gift of Mrs. John Outram, F-10150, F-10166

Nurses take care to maintain privacy and dignity during their intimate relations with patients.

which became standardized and hospital specific. Skills were a source of pride associated with training in certain prestigious hospitals. For example, Gertrude Fawcett was a 1934 graduate of the Montreal General Hospital who described how to distinguish a graduate of her hospital from a graduate of the rival Royal Victoria Hospital: "There [were] procedures to do everything...making the bed without the patient; making the bed with the patient; bathing the patient; mouth care; getting the patient up; walking with them — they all had a procedure." Fawcett declared you could tell where a student trained by how she made her beds: "[It was] a case of folding along the linens a certain way.... When it came time to make the corners, why we made the corners and tucked them in...like an envelope. Well theirs, instead of being on the slant, hung straight down."[3]

One early textbook for student nurses (1914), describes eighteen types of baths including: a vapor (steam) bath, a starch bath, a drip-sheet bath, and an "affusion" which is described as "wrapping the patient in a sheet and placing him on a canvas cot, and then sprinkling him with water from an ordinary watering-pot." The same textbook describes ten kinds of enemas, including a "nutritive enema," in which extracts of beef, beef juice, eggs, and milk were introduced into the bowel to provide nourishment for patients who were unable to retain food orally.[4]

Nurses were also responsible for keeping records on patients' nutritional intake, knowing the appropriate diets for different illnesses, preparing these diets, and devising ways to ensure that patients took as much of them as possible. Their training included weeks spent in the hospital kitchen where they learned to prepare different types of diets. Long before the discovery of insulin and its subsequent use in diabetes during the 1920s and 1930s, for example, nurses' knowledge, skills, and teaching abilities formed key components of the strict dietary management on which diabetic patients relied for survival.

By the 1930s, several provinces had asylums and mental hospitals that also operated training schools for nurses. The Ontario Hospital, for example, was a network of training schools in several cities

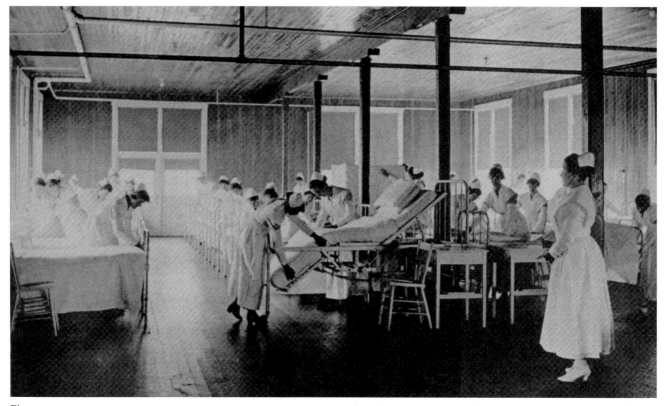

Figure 3
Students and bed-making in the Heather Pavilion
Vancouver General Hospital
1918
Photographer: Stuart Thomson
City of Vancouver Archives, CVA 99-857

throughout the province. Students typically spent part of their training at an affiliated teaching hospital such as the Toronto General Hospital, in order to complete medical-surgical components of their training and gain experience on general wards. They assisted in a variety of bath treatments and hydrotherapies, learned how to produce quiet/restful environments as therapies, assisted with electric shock treatments and insulin shock therapy, and supervised the regimentation of daily activities for mental patients. Nurses at the Brandon Hospital for Mental Diseases in Manitoba performed tasks associated with insulin shock therapy such as "the regular taking of pulses and temperatures, drawing blood samples and monitoring patients after they emerged from their comas...injecting the insulin and inserting the nasal alimentary tubes through which the glucose solution which brought the patients out of the coma was

given." They also "worked outside the hospital to perform clinical outreach work such as administering intelligence tests at mental hygiene clinics in the schools." [5]

Another area of early body work that consumed much of nurses' time and energy was the prevention and control of infection. Antisepsis, disinfection, and the perfection of standardized techniques[6] were especially significant prior to the development of major antibacterial and antibiotic drugs. Patient survival depended partially, or perhaps mostly, on "good nursing" before the introduction of various sulfa and penicillin preparations during the 1930s and 40s. The principles of antisepsis applied equally to the care of patients, the equipment, and the environment. Nurses sterilized equipment and supplies and followed elaborate instructions for isolating infectious patients with diphtheria, scarlet fever, cholera, smallpox, typhoid

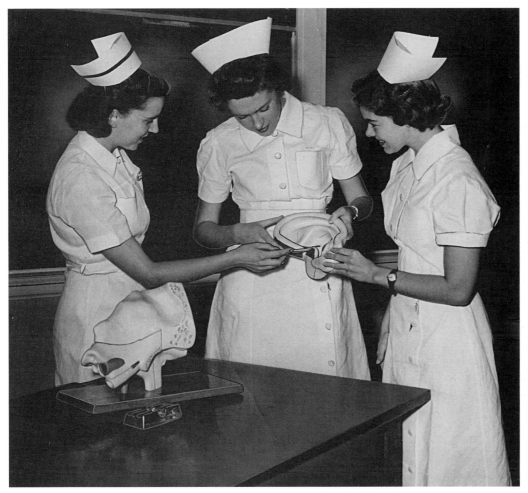

Figure 4
Student nurses examining anatomy model
Toronto General Hospital
Alumnae Association of the School of Nursing, Toronto General Hospital Collection
Canadian Museum of Civilization

fever, and tuberculosis. Jean Milligan, for example, described cleaning needles, glass containers, and rubber tubing for the administration of blood transfusions while she was a student nurse on night duty. Students typically cleaned this equipment by hand on the wards. After supervisors inspected it thoroughly, it was packaged, sterilized in autoclaves, and reused. Milligan vividly recalled the difficulty of cleaning various small parts:

> The big job that we all "loved"...was cleaning these sets afterwards — to send them up, to get them ready for the next [transfusion]...cleaning the tubing and these long flasks. You couldn't even get your hand into them, they were so narrow. There couldn't be a mark on them anywhere. They [the night supervisors] used to hold these flasks up to the light, and look at them before they'd roll them up to go to the OR to be autoclaved for the next

person. You just had to wash and shine these, and make sure there was nothing left.[7]

Students perfected hundreds of techniques. They prepared and applied poultices, stupes, foments, and hot packs. They cleaned, irrigated, and drained various body cavities using syringes, catheters, and solutions. They systematically changed a wide variety of dressings specific to different therapeutic requirements from surgical incisions to extensive burns. A major part of student learning involved the preparation and administration of a variety of medications by different methods such as oral, injection, topical, and inhalation routes. They gave different types of therapeutic baths for fevers and skin diseases. Tours of duty in the delivery room and the operating room, where they performed hundreds of pre- and post-operative procedures, were fundamental parts of every nurse's training. Nurses also prepared all the

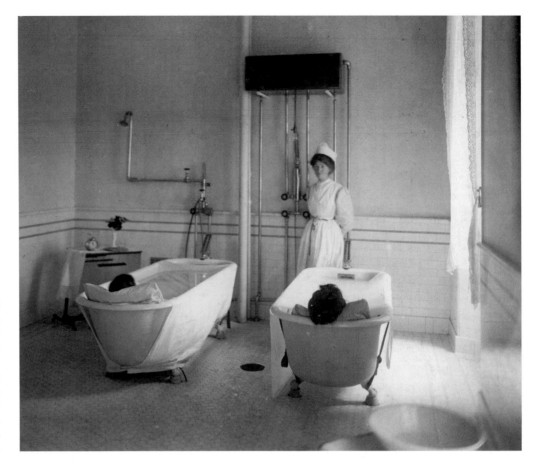

Figure 5
**Student nurse
and patients,
continuous water
bath treatment room**
Hospital for
the Insane
Kingston, Ontario
1907
Archives of Ontario,
RG 15,E-7 Vol. 20

necessary equipment and solutions to assist physicians with a multitude of diagnostic tests and treatment procedures such as lumbar punctures and transfusions.

Prior to 1900, students learned these techniques primarily through demonstrations and lectures. They had to make meticulous handwritten notes based on the lectures and submit them to the instructor for correction. The "Rules for Nurses" of the Lady Stanley Institute for Trained Nurses at Ottawa made it clear that lecture notes "must be written out fully and placed in the Lady Superintendent's office for correction within forty-eight hours after each lecture." Notes accumulated during training provided them with valuable, basic reference material for their subsequent practice in private duty. Accuracy and completeness was therefore important to safety, as well as the pride associated with a particular training school. At the Winnipeg General Hospital between 1924 and 1928, student notebooks contained a 17-step process

for preparing and administering a hypodermic injection using an alcohol lamp.[8]

Textbooks on nursing practice began to replace handwritten notebooks as reference material around the turn of the century. Bertha Harmer, a graduate of the Toronto General Hospital School of Nursing and Columbia University in New York, returned to Toronto General as an instructor and later taught at both the Vassar Training Camp in New York and St. Luke's Hospital School of Nursing in New York City. She was assistant professor at Yale University School of Nursing prior to becoming director at the School for Graduate Nurses at McGill University. Harmer wrote one of the best-known textbooks of the period, *Principles and Practice of Nursing*, which became the classic text used in Canadian schools of nursing, published in five editions between 1922 and 1942.[9]

Hospitals also developed in-house procedure books to standardize techniques and treatments

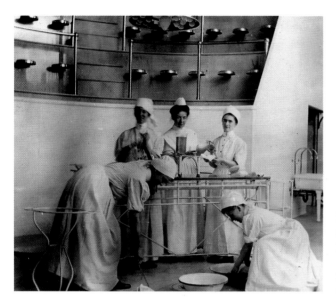

Figure 6
Cleaning up the Operating Room
Montreal General Hospital
1900
McGill University Archives, PU023847

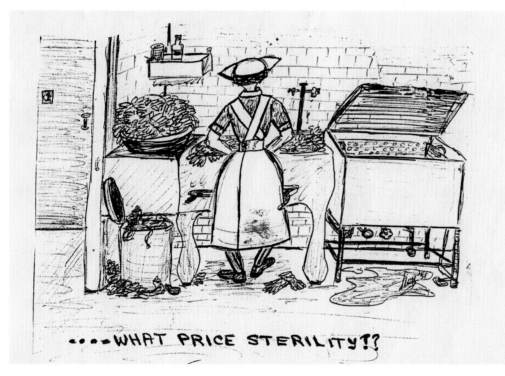

···WHAT PRICE STERILITY?!

Figure 7
Cartoon
Artist: Shirley Stinson
1951
Courtesy of Shirley Stinson

Nursing student at the University of Alberta Hospital, Shirley Stinson sketched this comment on the drudgery of washing and autoclaving hundreds of rubber gloves every day.

within their own facilities. Procedure manuals existed as early as the 1920s and served as one way to deal with the constantly changing novice workforce. They guided students when instructors were not available, established boundaries of safety in practice, and could be used as legal documents establishing expected standards of care, as during a judicial inquiry at Ottawa during 1949. By mid-century, procedures were increasingly complex with elaborate step-by-step instructions and lists of required equipment.

Oxygen therapy was one technique taught to nursing students in 1914. One textbook describes oxygen administration as follows: "If the patient is strong enough he inhales the gas through a glass nozzle placed between his teeth, but for unconscious and very sick individuals a funnel is held over the mouth and nostrils."[10] By 1939, oxygen administration included nasal and oral catheters, inhalers, face masks, oxygen tents, and oxygen chambers or respirators.

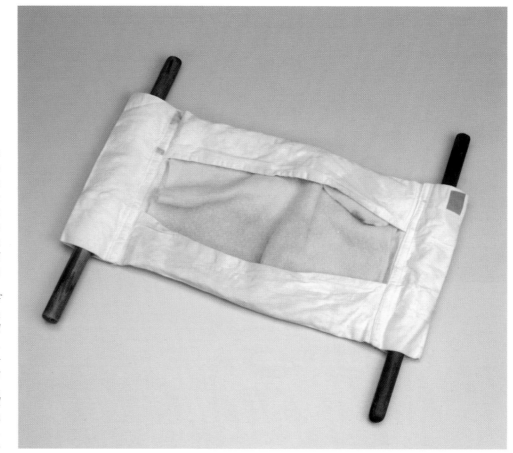

Figure 8
Fomentation Stupe
1920s–1930s
Photographer: Doug Millar
Public General Hospital
Chatham Nurses Alumnae
Association Collection
Canadian Museum of
Civilization, 2004.13.55

A stupe consisted of strips of woollen cloth in a linen bag attached to wooden handles. Nurses lowered everything but the handles into boiling water, wrung out the cloth, and then placed the stupe on the infected site.

Nurses were admonished to monitor the patient, humidify the oxygen, take precautions against fires where oxygen was in use, "crack the valve" (described as "open the valve on top of the oxygen cylinder slightly and close it quickly") to release any dust particles prior to administering oxygen to patients, and most of all, to prevent the cylinder from falling over.[11] The respirator, also known as an iron lung, was possibly the greatest nursing care challenge during these years of widespread polio epidemics. Patients who were placed in iron lungs were totally dependent on nurses for all of their physical and psychological care as well as the ability to breathe. When electricity failed, nurses and all available hospital staff had to maintain the cyclical pattern of breathing for each individual patient by means of hand or foot pumping until the power returned. Little wonder, then, that military nurses were posted to Manitoba to care for whole wards of patients in iron lungs during the 1953–1954 polio epidemic.

Delegation of Medical Technology to Nurses

Although hospitals were the primary training grounds for nurses during the first half of the twentieth century, few trained (or graduate) nurses either desired or found permanent paid employment there prior to the 1940s, when a combination of conditions made hospital work more attractive. The Great Depression of the 1930s was especially devastating for nurses and many found it necessary to combine nursing with non-nursing employment. Dorothy Grainger, for example, worked in private duty and construction, writing: "Business was slow in Calgary so I combined a labourer's job with private nursing…. I applied and was soon on the job learning the skill of laying steel re-enforcements for concrete. Blueprints were easy to read and my male boss was impressed with my progress. Wages were much higher than the $5.00 offered RNs for a twelve-hour shift."[12]

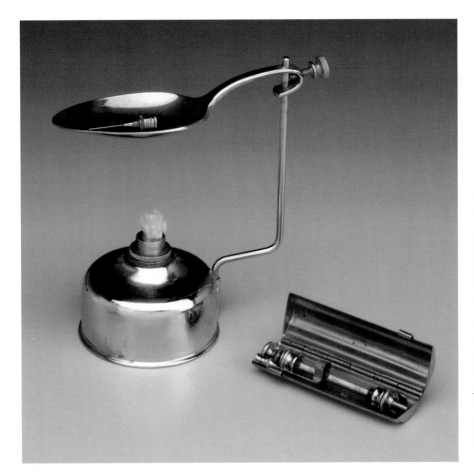

Figure 9
Alcohol lamp, needle, and syringe
1920–1930s
Photographer: Doug Millar
Public General Hospital Chatham Nurses
Alumnae Association Collection
Canadian Museum of Civilization
2004.13.23

The needle was placed on a spoon in boiling water (heated by the alcohol lamp) to sterilize both. The water was then discarded, fresh water boiled, and medicinal tablets dissolved on the spoon and drawn up into the syringe. The process, though tedious, reduced the high risk of infection.

During the 1940s, nurses took advantage of an emerging nursing shortage that was partially related to the Second World War, the increased use of medical technology in hospitals, and a gradual shift from a student workforce to a graduate nurse workforce — to build long-term careers within hospitals. By the middle of the decade, there were many more nursing vacancies than nurses who wanted to fill them — a dramatic reversal from the conditions of the 1930s. The Registered Nurses' Association of Ontario (RNAO) Placement Service, for example, reported only 54 employment inquiries in relation to 672 nursing vacancies advertised in Ontario during March 1946.

Hospitals had become increasingly important as central locations for medical technology that was too expensive for individual physicians to own, too seldom used by individual physicians, or too difficult to transport to private homes, as was common prior to the 1900s. Initially physicians were the primary users of X-ray machines, anesthetic and surgical equipment, and equipment for the analysis of blood and urine. But soon the operation of X-ray equipment became the responsibility of a nursing supervisor or specially-hired graduate nurse, and student nurses incorporated technological responsibilities into their every-day workload. As procedures became more routine, student nurses prepared both the equipment and the patients for a variety of medical tests and procedures; they assisted physicians during these procedures and cleaned up following them.

When hospitals expanded in number and size during mid-century, nurses' skills enabled the proliferation of medical technology within patient care. Physicians generally introduced new technologies and were responsible for them until the volume of treatments increased or became burdensome to the medical staff. At that point, hospitals typically hired a few graduate nurses whom physicians trained to perform specific isolated skills, such as giving blood or starting intravenous infusions. Physicians

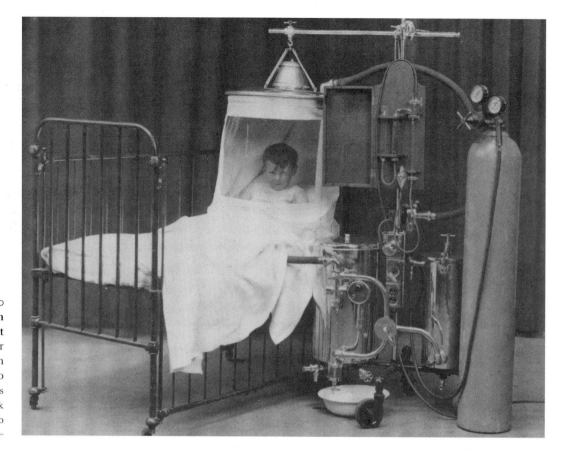

Figure 10
Child in oxygen tent
Hospital for Sick Children
Toronto, Ontario
Hospital Archives
The Hospital for Sick Children, Toronto

retained the power to "order" the medical technology but nurses often became the primary, and more proficient, users of it. They formed the human interface between medical technology and patients, particularly as physicians transferred more and more procedures. Indeed, these special teams became so successful that as one hospital reported, "the work increases as fast as suitable nurses can be secured."[13] According to the hospital annual report, medical technology invested nurses with professional status even though it was second-class:

> Granted the doctor comes first always when we think about the healing of the sick. But those of us who are much around hospitals place the nurse up very close to the doctor. The duties and responsibilities of a nurse have been expanded immensely by the new methods of healing. She has now to be expert and knowledgeable in many things. She has become a high-class technician and nursing is a real profession.[14]

Blood transfusion, for example, was a complex procedure during the 1930s, when donation and transfusion were surgical procedures often performed at the same time and in the same or adjacent rooms.[15] The nurse collected special equipment from the training school office, the operating room, and the drug room to add to the "blood tray" prior to the procedure. She prepared basins of warm water to hold beakers of donated blood and saline solution for the infusion process. She also fetched an ounce of whisky or brandy for the procedure tray although the step-by-step instructions did not specify who should use it — patient, physician, or nurse. While one nurse set up equipment and assisted the physician collecting the blood from a donor, a second nurse maintained the appropriate pressure for blood flow by pumping air into a blood pressure cuff around the donor's arm. The first nurse held the collection beaker, stirred the blood with a glass rod to keep it from coagulating, and then placed the full beaker covered with a sterile towel into the basin of warm water. The physician "scrubbed" again, inserted a needle and started the saline intravenous for the blood recipient. The nurse poured and strained the donated blood through a

A Life of Sacrifice

James Wishart, Carleton University and Queen's University

The costs of economization by hospitals and health systems have often been dispropor-tionately borne by nurses and nursing students who have felt compelled to sacrifice their own physical and mental health for the welfare of their patients. "Helen" (a pseudonym), a student at Kingston General Hospital in the early 1930s, tells the story of being left alone on night duty in charge of a 26-patient medical ward in her second year of training:

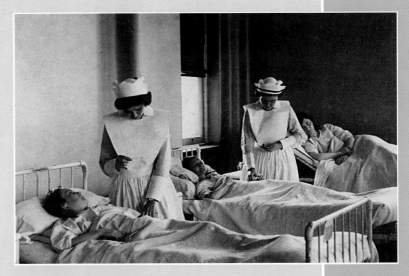

Figure 11
On morning rounds
St. Michael's Hospital, Toronto, Ontario
ca. 1924
St. Michael's Hosptal Archives

Of these 26 patients, there was one very ill man — he was in his late 30s — with pneumonia. In those days there'd be no antibiotics, so we had to treat pneumonia with a mustard plaster every fifteen minutes, and linseed poultices. So that was just one patient out of 26. [There were] six typhoid patients in two rooms...you couldn't go into their rooms until you scrubbed thoroughly and put a gown on, using complete Isolation technique. And most typhoid patients were delirious. They'd be getting out of bed and following you and touching you. And you couldn't leave the one isolation room and go to the other without a complete five-minute scrub. In another room next to the Isolation was a lady who was hemorrhaging. I couldn't get to her — we lost her. That is a memory that will never leave me. You could only be one place at a time. And another man, in another room, in a cast, with a broken back, had gotten the bed side down and had fallen on the floor, and there he was. Plus all the other patients that needed care. You had to go through and struggle with it. You were all by yourself — you couldn't get help. I nearly left training that next morning.

The anguish Helen felt at having lost a patient to understaffing was still keen 60 years after the fact.

Source: "Helen," RN [pseudo.], interview with James Wishart, 15 Nov. 1996, Kingston, ON.

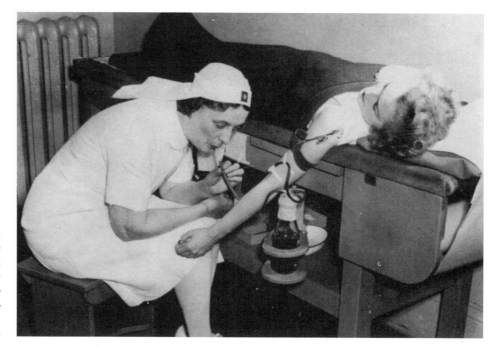

Figure 12
Red Cross nurse provides the suction for a blood donation
Norman Miles Guiou, *Transfusion:*
A Canadian Surgeon's Story
in War and in Peace
Yarmouth, NS: Stoneycroft, 1985

gauze placed over the top of a glass cylinder. She capped, inverted, and hung the cylinder on a pole from which blood infused into the recipient by gravity.

Nurses were also responsible for observing patients' status throughout these procedures, maintaining the arm position so that the needle did not become dislodged from the vein, and making sure that the tubing did not run dry between cylinders or flasks of blood. When technology changed so that blood could be refrigerated for later use, timing was critical as it had to be warmed immediately prior to administration. Students were often assigned the care of eight to sixteen patients where, as Milligan said, "it always seemed to us that [transfusions] were in the [far opposite] end rooms so you were running from one to the other. You didn't dare phone an intern and say that I let this run dry." Nurse Patricia Crossley recalled that "when you had a large room with twenty patients in it...you could go into a room and at a glance you could see it [the transfusion running]. But as you changed to semi-private and then private [rooms], you really had lots of walking to do to make sure the blood was alright."[16]

As nurses assumed increased responsibility for medical technologies, they found that some skills were contingent on the time of day, week, or year.

Hospital policies frequently "permitted" them to perform skills after hours, on weekends, and during holidays that were prohibited when physicians or interns were readily available. For example, medical interns gave the relatively few intramuscular injections prescribed during the 1930s and early 40s. When penicillin became available for civilian use, the initial formulations were neither very potent nor long-lasting within the body, and treatment required injections every three hours. Interns could no longer keep up with the increasing use of the drug by the end of the 1940s and intramuscular injections became a standard nursing skill. Similar policies during the early 1950s clearly stated that only "specially trained" nurses could take blood pressures, and then only under specific circumstances: "Nurses may take blood pressure readings on skull or accident cases at regular intervals after midnight...." But by 1954, blood pressure measurement was also a standard skill expected of all nurses.[17]

Physicians increasingly relied on nurses' constant presence at the bedside, their greater familiarity with equipment, and the proficiency gained through frequent performance of skills and procedures. As one astute nurse leader wrote, "It would have been very inconvenient for all concerned if the nurses had not known a good deal about the

On All Frontiers

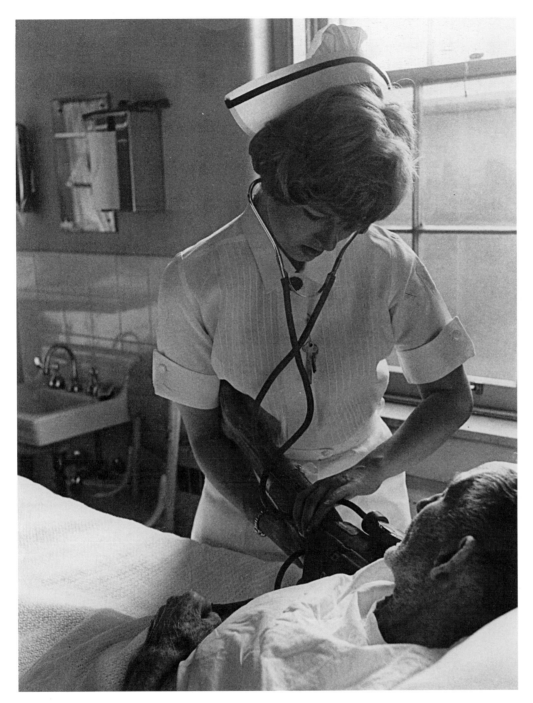

Figure 13
Nurse at bedside taking patient's blood pressure
Toronto Western Hospital
ca. 1970
Photographer:
James H Peacock,
Department of
Photography, Toronto
Western Hospital
Toronto Western Hospital
Nurses' Alumnae
Association Archives,
Photograph Collection

apparatus used…. But the fact that they did know was probably never noticed."[18]

Hospitals and physicians soon recognized that widespread use of medical technology was contingent on the availability of reliable skilled nurses. The shortage of 2000 physicians, for example, prompted Ontario hospitals to establish "intravenous and blood infusions" as the first act "delegated" to nurses in 1947. The College of Physicians and Surgeons of Ontario (CPSO) restricted this act to specially trained nurses only, because it "did not believe these responsibilities should be included in the regular duties of a nurse."[19] Physicians and hospitals developed a formalized process known as "delegation" that included specific training, testing, certification, and periodic re-testing for specific skills to be transferred to nurses. By 1972, there were 22 delegated medical acts plus 11 additional acts for nurses in specialty areas, including external cardiac massage, hemodialysis, epidural analgesia, gastric and tracheotomy tubes, and defibrillation. Delegation was not, however, a smoothly flowing transfer of roles and responsibilities across disciplinary boundaries. It shaped a gendered division of labour, provided impetus for a shift from a predominantly student workforce to a graduate nurse workforce, and exacerbated ideological differences between leaders and bedside nurses while also differentiating among nurses on the basis of technological skills.

When the CPSO approved tuberculosis tests and immunization injections for administration by nurses in 1957, the RNAO protested it had not been consulted. They based their arguments against this delegation on lack of training and legal protection, insisting these procedures were outside the scope of nursing practice. They also argued these added responsibilities imposed an unacceptable burden during a period of nursing shortage. A year later, the RNAO opposed the delegation of intravenous medications but later compromised with the CPSO. In a jointly issued statement, both organizations reinforced the administration of intravenous medications as a medical act, to be performed by nurses only in situations where physicians were unavailable. When the College of Nurses of Ontario became the regulatory body in 1961, it took a stance that the medical profession could delegate acts, but the nursing profession would decide whether to accept or reject that delegation.[20]

Delegation also had unintended consequences. Some physicians and interns, for example, found there were fewer opportunities to develop needle-insertion techniques once nurses assumed those responsibilities. Perceiving a loss of skills, one hospital assigned interns to work on the "Blood Team" with nurses for a period of time, to compensate for decreased practice experiences — a case where physicians learned from nurses.[21]

Other unintended consequences included unacceptable nursing workloads and substandard patient care. Two *Ottawa Citizen* editorials precipitated a judicial inquiry into the state of patient care at the Ottawa Civic Hospital in 1949 at which patients, families, and ordinary citizens testified there were not enough nurses "to keep up with the pace of technological change." They described long waiting periods, inexperienced nurses, dirty wards, prolonged pain and suffering, medication errors, and lack of observation during post-anesthetic recovery. One patient reported the need to monitor her intravenous infusion closely through the night since she would have to get "another needle in because the next bottle of intervenous [*sic*] wouldn't run…. They wanted me to watch the intervenous [*sic*] all night, and I had to stay awake to watch it, otherwise it would run dry…I was too scared to sleep." In his final report, Judge McDougall noted an 86 percent staff turnover during the previous year, and declared the hospital to have a severe nursing shortage with existing staff "very, very seriously overworked." He found the causes to be a rapid expansion of facilities and services following the war, a shortage of both interns and nurses, and an inexperienced student work force unable to keep up with increasingly technological care. As a result, the hospital's Medical Advisory Board recommended hiring additional nurses "regardless of cost."[22]

Over the next two decades, Canadian hospital administrators tried a variety of means to produce more graduate nurses, to retain nurses in practice, and to restructure roles for better utilization of nurses. One strategy included elimination of the marriage bar so that nurses would no longer have to resign when they married. Other strategies included a reduction of the work day to 8-hour shifts, the introduction of flexible and split shifts for married women, and refresher courses for nurses returning to active practice. The use of auxiliary personnel such as nursing assistants and orderlies expanded during the 1950s and 60s along with the active recruitment of men and immigrant nurses to fill vacancies in hospital staff nursing positions. Yet, there never seemed to be enough nurses. Hospitals struggled with a persistent nursing shortage as more and more women moved away from restrictive careers and practice environments, taking advantage of new work opportunities opening up to them. As Dr Lorne Gilday of the Western Division of the Montreal General Hospital summarized, "Nurses come and nurses go, and more seem to go than come."[23]

Skills and Differentiation between Nurses

Hospitals began to experiment with another strategy during the 1950s, in the search for greater efficiency and continuity in the care of patients with intensive nursing care needs. They clustered specialized equipment and nurses with specialized skills into small patient care units such as recovery rooms, dialysis units, intensive care units, and coronary care units. Emerging specialty units challenged nurses with new equipment such as oscilloscopes for monitoring heart rhythms, Bennett and Bird respirators, transducers for arterial and venous pressure measurements, manometers for central venous measurement, defibrillators, and various catheters and drainage tubes. Nurses' vocabularies soon incorporated terms such as "pistons, valves, switches, magnets, inspiratory and expiratory time, Cournand's curve, proximal airway pressure, pressure gradients and peripheral lung pressures, alveoli-capillary blocks, shunting, and hyalinization."[24] Nurses even referred to themselves in technological terms as human "thermometers, barometers, monitors, information processors, and human/machine interfaces" when articulating their roles and responsibilities within hospitals.[25]

Delegated skills took on added significance within these new environments by differentiating among nurses based on technological skills. Nurses were no longer identical or interchangeable, and some nurses were able to capitalize on delegated skills to secure work in specialty units where technological competence was a key condition of employment. As one nurse said, "You always knew that would get you into the critical care areas because critical care areas are about machines and equipment.... Nurses always liked skills and psychomotor tasks. It felt like they were getting into the physician's domain. It made it a little bit more challenging for them, and a little more interesting, and they always wanted to pick up the technology."[26] The acquisition of special restricted skills also created a

hierarchy among practice nurses themselves. Nurses who worked on the frontiers of medical technology in cardiac surgical units of the 1970s, for example, recall feeling "special" and being treated as "special" because their knowledge and skills were essential to the functioning of these units. But they also recall a perception of resentment from general duty nurses.[27]

Specialty units facilitated a blurring of traditional lines between nurses and physicians. Nurse Pat Doucett described how collegial relationships developed as they learned from one another through the care of critically ill patients and the abundance of emerging medical technology in one early cardiac surgical unit. When cardiac surgery was relatively new in 1968, one cardiac surgeon preferred to stay by his patients through the first post-operative nights. He had abundant opportunities to observe nurses and their work at the bedside during this time. Many years later, he stated, "I always felt that probably the most vital thing for a patient was the nurses' knowledge.... Because there were a thousand things that the nurse was seeing and monitoring that she wasn't reporting and charting...just from her experience. And the patients were totally dependent on them, particularly in the early days."[28] Part of that collegiality involved humour and creativity. In the same cardiac surgical unit, nurses waited outside the operating room doors, ready to receive the patient as soon as he or she passed through the doors. One anesthetist sent poems to the waiting nurses to indicate the approximate time of the patient's arrival. The following poem predicted the arrival time for a man who had undergone the replacement of two heart valves, and according to the poem, he needed special attention paid to his lungs and breathing during the immediate recovery period:

Lub dub and clickety clack
This double valve we're bringing back.
His lungs are full of fluid and air
And of them you must take good care.
IPPB and Mucomyst
TLC we do insist.
Hold his hand and mop his brow.
Nurse him like only you know how.
In one hour, we'll be through the doors
And from then on, he is all yours.[29]

Nursing specialties developed in parallel with medical specialties during the 1950s and 60s. As nurses worked closely together over time within specialized units, they developed increased expertise and nursing knowledge related to these groups of patients who shared similar illnesses and/or surgical trajectories. However, nursing specialties soon began to develop in areas specific to nursing, and by the end of the century there were nurse specialists in skin care, pain management, and palliative care, as well as coronary care nurses, dialysis nurses, and recovery room nurses.

Advanced education and training for nurses during the period from the 1920s to the 1950s had focused primarily on supervision, administration, teaching, and public health. By the 1960s and 70s, however, nurses also sought advanced education related to clinical practice areas and programs that prepared them as nurse practitioners and clinical nurse specialists. Relatively few advanced practice nurses found long-term positions within hospitals, however. Those who did struggled to remain in practice at the bedside. Rosemary Prince Coombs, for example, completed a master's degree in clinical practice at the University of Washington in Seattle. She was hired in 1968 specifically to organize and lead the nursing component of a newly formed cardiac surgical unit. Based on her experiences there, she described advanced practice nursing within hospitals in an article for *The Canadian Nurse Journal*. Coombs envisioned an expanded scope of practice and increased autonomy for nurses with advanced practice expertise but she found that hospitals were unable, or unwilling, to use them effectively.[30] In a similar manner, Wendy McKnight reflected on her role as Clinical Nurse Specialist in the Emergency Department during the early 1970s. As she recalled,

> It was a shame the role ended when it did...because I really didn't want to leave.... There was a review of positions done here at the hospital...no one really understood the role. They basically said there was no room for one-of-a-kind positions, and "You are more valuable in an education position." And I said, "No, I want to be more involved in patient care and influencing practice...." I have always looked back and

thought, "You never know what your career might have been, eh?"[31]

For the most part, these early advanced practice roles disappeared during the 1980s — partially due to funding and legal issues, and partially due to a lack of acceptance by physicians and hospitals. Most Canadian programs closed until the mid-1990s, when nurses rallied once again, moving into expanded practice roles to help meet the "crisis" of physician shortages in underserved areas.

Summary

Body work, medical technology, and hospital nursing intersected to create new employment opportunities and occupational spaces for nurses while creating divisions within the profession based on technological skills and knowledge. Women in the early 1900s used skilled body work to legitimate nursing as paid work, and perceived hospitals as a place of training and preparation for roles that they would assume in private duty. Hospitals capitalized on student nurses as a reliable source of cheap labour during this period and partially contributed to the devastating conditions nurses experienced during the Great Depression. As hospital nursing shortages emerged during and after the Second World War, nurses looked increasingly to hospitals for reliable, steady employment opportunities. Indeed, hospitals became the primary employers of nurses in Canada as demands for technological care influenced a gradual shift from a student to a graduate nurse workforce.

On one hand, medical technology legitimated the employment of graduate nurses within hospitals. Nurses comprised an expandable workforce with basic scientific knowledge and skills that positioned them well as the human interface between medical technologies and patients. They were frequently called upon to interpret technology to patients and their families, as well as to ensure compliance with related procedures. They monitored the technology, reported results and problems with the equipment, and adapted procedures to individual patient needs as necessary. Nurses used their constant presence at the bedside to negotiate for better working conditions, more autonomy, increased status within the profession, and a measure of job security as they became an increasingly essential component of hospital work.

On the other hand, medical technology served to create divisions within nursing related to questions about professional and/or technical status. By the 1970s, considerable debate emerged regarding nurses and technological skills that paved the way for multiple levels of nursing care providers: were nurses technicians based on skills or were they professionals based on a distinct body of knowledge? Some leaders suggested a need for two levels of nurses, with technical nurses to be educated within hospitals and community college programs and professional nurses to be educated within universities. Many leaders expressed considerable concern that medical technology simply comprised "junior doctoring" rather than nursing, with downloading of work from physicians to nurses when the technology no longer held associated power or prestige. These debates continue as the profession struggles to clarify the levels of knowledge and skill associated with diverse nursing practices, such as clinical nurse specialists, advanced practice nurses, nurse practitioners, nurse clinicians, specialty practice nurses, registered nursing assistants, and patient care assistants. An understanding of nurses' historical relationship to hospitals and medical technology has significant implications for the emerging nursing shortages of the twenty-first century.

CHAPTER 7

Public Health Nursing

Marion McKay

On 15 April 1950, in a public ceremony sponsored by the federal government and the province of British Columbia, Aileen Bond and Amy Wilson received Distinguished Service Medals for "...personal sacrifice and personal risk above and beyond the call of duty."[1] This heroic chapter in the history of Canadian public health nursing began in late December of 1949 when Wilson, an Indian Affairs public health nurse stationed at Whitehorse, received a call for help from Halfway Valley, an isolated First Nations community near the Alaska Highway. As she made preparations to travel to the community, Wilson could only speculate about the nature of the medical emergency. She gathered as many supplies as she could carry, including a borrowed tracheotomy tube. "Inclusion of this little tube" she wrote, "suddenly made me realize how very much on my own I would be."[2] Braving −50°F weather, Wilson and a male guide arrived several days later to find a community devastated by starvation and, as Wilson had correctly surmised, a diphtheria outbreak. She quickly realized that she would need more help. Her request for assistance was received by Aileen Bond, the senior public health nurse at the Peace River Health Unit in Dawson Creek, BC. Bond left Dawson Creek on Christmas Eve, making her way by bush plane, horse sleigh, and snowshoes to join her colleague. In her official report, she stated: "The Indian camp where the diphtheria raged was discovered by spotting a funeral fire on a nearby hill."[3] Forty-eight of the 52 inhabitants of the community were ill. Five died.

Working in complete isolation and under extremely primitive living conditions, the two nurses cared for the sick and dying. They strapped the diphtheria antitoxin and penicillin to their bodies to keep it from freezing. Only broth, hot brandy, and sugar were available to feed the patients until food was dropped by an airplane several days later. Once the epidemic was under control, Wilson and Bond remained in the district for ten more days to immunize almost one thousand individuals who lived within travelling distance of the highway.

Although public health nurses are proud to claim these two heroic women as their colleagues, Wilson and Bond's experience might well have been recounted by a district nurse in northern Alberta or by an outpost nurse in Labrador. Because the needs of the community often shaped the roles and responsibilities of the community-based nurse, the boundaries between district, outpost, and public health nursing have always been blurred. Public health nurses, however, focused their efforts primarily on prevention of illness and promotion of health rather than on the provision of direct nursing care.

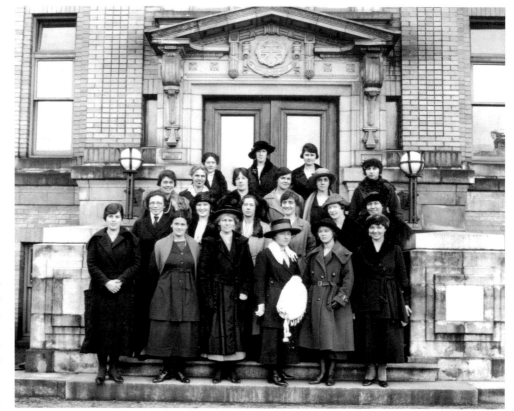

Figure 1
University of British Columbia public health nursing class
Vancouver, BC
1921
British Columbia Archives,
E-02369

After the First World War, the Canadian Red Cross provided funding to support post-diploma programs in Public Health Nursing at five Canadian Universities.

This chapter traces the history of public health nursing in Canada. It briefly describes the origins of this form of nursing practice, its incorporation within civic and provincial health departments, and changes in the nature of the practice throughout the twentieth century.

An Elite Calling

In the late nineteenth and early twentieth centuries, nursing was one of the few careers that offered the prospect of an independent life for ambitious young women. Public health nurses were counted amongst the profession's elite. Employment in this speciality practice required clinical skills beyond those obtained in hospital training programs. Particularly after the First World War, community health agencies and public health departments sought nurses with post-diploma training in public health from a university or other recognized program. Public health nurses tended to remain in their practices longer than those employed in hospitals or as private duty nurses. They also enjoyed greater financial stability and higher salaries.[4]

Public health nurses actively sought opportunities that combined challenging work with travel and adventure. Amy Wilson wrote that when she was offered the position of Alaska Highway Nurse in 1949, she could not resist the prospect of being responsible for an area covering roughly 200 000 square miles.[5] Other public health nurses wrote of their eagerness to find a place where they would be challenged to the limits of their knowledge and skills. Still others sought a practice free (or at least more distant from) the hierarchy and constraints of supervisors and large institutions. Bessie J Banfill, who worked in rural Saskatchewan, found that her work amongst the settlers, many of whom were immigrants from Eastern Europe, fulfilled a deep personal need. "...[I]mpulsive by nature, and restless and dissatisfied with hospital routine and nursing patients surrounded by luxury, I longed for more challenging adventure and freedom."[6] Many genuinely enjoyed interaction with people, and embraced opportunities to learn about other cultures.

Whether working in urban slums or isolated districts, public health nurses encountered significant

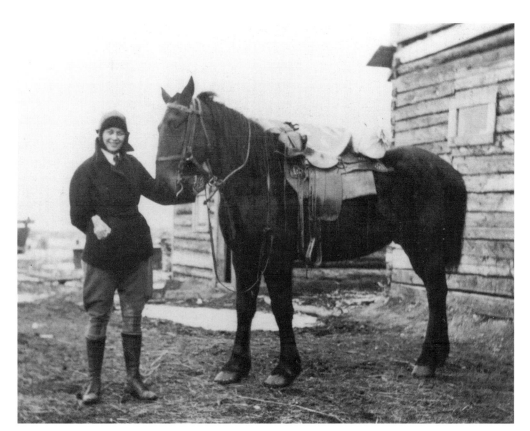

Figure 2
**Jean Morton,
District Nurse**
Worsley, Alberta
Glenbow Archives, Calgary,
Alberta, NA-3942-3

When roads were non-existent or impassable, nurses used other modes of transportation to travel about their districts.

challenges in the course of their work. Not the least of these was the problem of getting to their patients in the first place. Urban public health nurses, particularly in the early years, walked many miles to conduct home visits. In 1908, a Winnipeg General Hospital nursing student described the rigours of travel to the home of one patient.

> Let us accompany a nurse who has received an early morning call to a hitherto unheard of street in Elmwood. She sets out in the twinkling starlight of a frosty winter morning, and stands shivering for the first street car at the CPR depot. Some time elapses before the car appears, but at last her patience is rewarded, and she is soon on her way to her destination. But suddenly a halt is called, and alas for the nurse's hopes. There is a car straight ahead athwart the track, and the only remedy is to get out and walk…. The Louise Bridge is crossed — always a cold spot in the winter, the wind coming in gusts off the frozen river — and then the search begins for the patient's abode…. After a scramble across open drains, and piled up heaps of clay, the desired haven is at last gained.[7]

This was not work for the faint of heart or the frail of body.

First hand accounts of early rural public health nurses also contain vivid descriptions of the various modes of transportation used in the course of their work. Nurses travelled on foot, by car, on horseback, by dog sled, on airplanes and trains, and on snowshoes. They braved dangerous road and weather conditions to travel to families in need of care.[8] Olive Matthews, describing her work as a child welfare nurse in rural Alberta, reported: "I have a car for my school inspection, given voluntarily by Argyle and Clear Lake districts. It is the only way of covering 925 miles twice a year and paying home visits."[9] Apparently, she was fortunate to have one. Dorothy Priestly, recalling her early years as a public health nurse, wrote:

> I was the first public health nurse in Prince Rupert, called a school nurse by everyone but myself. I arrived on Sept. 1st, 1937 and was taken to the City Hall where I was greeted by a small pair of foot scales and one of the old black record books, quite empty…. An office to work in never

entered the picture, or a car.... From that time I scrounged a little space here and there when school opened. Never did I get transportation and I walked for 5 1/2 years.[10]

Their sense of adventure, independence, courage, and humanitarianism led Canadian public health nurses to serve in Canada's poorest urban districts and most isolated rural communities. These qualities also placed them at the forefront of efforts to make health care accessible to all Canadians.[11]

Public Health before the Nurses

In late nineteenth and early twentieth century Canada, public health departments were often temporary bodies organized during communicable disease outbreaks and dismantled as soon as the crisis was over. Although legislation permitting the formation of health departments was enacted by provincial governments, most were organized at the local level. The first health departments were established in major cities, where funding was available to support their operations. Operating under sanitarian principles, early health departments devoted their energies to the construction of water and sewage systems, the creation of sanitary waste disposal strategies, the regulation of food and milk supplies, and the control of communicable diseases such as smallpox, typhoid fever, and tuberculosis. All other matters related to health were the responsibility of the individual or family. Those who were unable to provide for themselves either went without or, if sufficiently desperate, turned to local welfare agencies and charitable organizations for assistance.[12]

The first generation of "trained" Canadian nurses exhibited a lively interest in the potential roles that they might play in the community. Although the development of public health nursing in Canada initially lagged behind Great Britain and the United States, Canadian nurses were well aware of the work being accomplished in other parts of the world. Early editions of The Canadian Nurse carried news from sister nursing associations around the world and regularly printed articles about the various roles undertaken by public health nurses. There was also no doubt that the need existed. The problem, it

seemed, was the lack of political will to fund similar programs in Canada. As the editor of The Canadian Nurse observed in September 1907, the slow development of medical inspection programs in Montreal schools could be attributed to the fact that "...their first report showed that there was such overwhelming evidence that it was needed." School health programs, the editor went on to say, were an appropriate field for "...intelligent, well educated, tactful and progressive nurses...because...no system of medical inspection of schools has yet been satisfactory or successful unless the aid of the nursing profession was enlisted."[13] The lack of public funding resulted in many public health nursing programs being pioneered by local charitable organizations devoted to the alleviation of the suffering of the poor. These programs clearly demonstrated that health education and prevention of illness played an important role in improving the overall health status of the community. However, the takeover of these programs by public health departments was often undertaken with considerable reluctance and only after charitable programs had foundered in the face of overwhelming need and inadequate financial resources.

Gaining a Foothold as Civil Servants: Public Health Nursing in the First Two Decades of the Twentieth Century

Although the exact chronology varies from one jurisdiction to another, the first nurses employed by health departments were specialists responsible for either tuberculosis control, child hygiene programs, or school inspection programs. As medical officers of health and political leaders became convinced of the value of having nurses on the staff of health departments, additional specialized programs were quickly added. By 1920, a typical urban public health department had nurses employed in at least these three speciality areas.

Tuberculosis Nursing

At the beginning of the twentieth century, tuberculosis was the leading cause of death in Canada. It was a particular problem amongst the urban poor, where

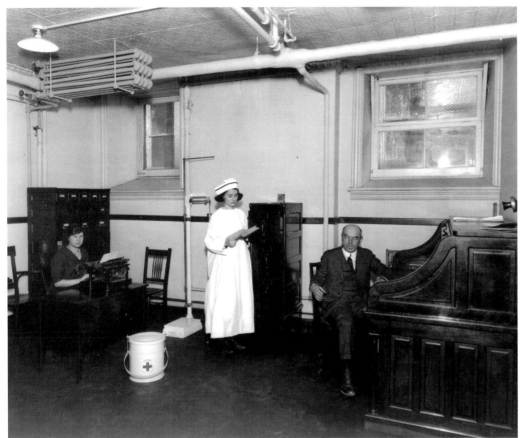

Figure 3
**Staff of the
Tuberculosis Clinic**
Hamilton, Ontario
Department of Health
1919
Archives of Ontario,
RG 10-30-2, 1.13.7

chronic undernourishment and overcrowded living conditions contributed to the rapid spread of the disease. First Nations people were also extremely susceptible to tuberculosis, which had only been recently introduced to North America by European settlers. Tuberculosis often rendered entire families destitute when the primary wage earner either became too ill to provide for the family or was forced to leave work to care for sick family members. Often, their only recourse was to turn to charitable organizations or the health department for help. Health department reports contain graphic descriptions of the circumstances in which some families were found. In 1911, Charles Hastings, Toronto's medical officer of health, reported that a public health nurse had "… found a woman whose hair and bedclothes were matted with sputum, being cared for by her husband, who was also working half-time and trying to look after their three small children." A similar event was documented the following year when another Toronto public health nurse discovered an abandoned woman

suffering from tuberculosis who had received no care or assistance for three days.[14]

Eradication of tuberculosis became a major focus of early twentieth century reformers. In Canada, two national voluntary organizations were formed to combat the disease. Local anti-tuberculosis societies mounted intensive public education campaigns about the prevention of tuberculosis and the safe care of its victims. Nurses were soon employed by these societies because they could freely enter private homes to convey, in a more personal and detailed way, the information that anti-tuberculosis campaigners were anxious to disseminate. They instructed family members about the physical care of patients, emphasizing the use of aseptic techniques to prevent the spread of the disease within the household. Patients were encouraged to remain outdoors as much as possible, and tents were provided so that they could sleep outdoors. Sputum cups, medications, food, and clothing were donated by voluntary societies and distributed at the nurses' discretion. As well as convincing

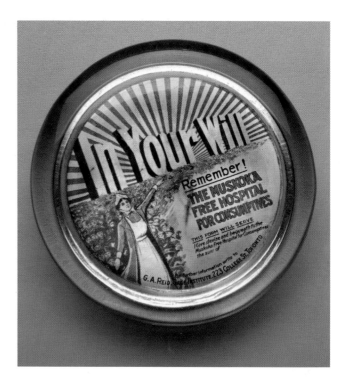

Figure 4
Paperweight
ca. 1900
Photographer: Doug Millar
Canadian Museum of Civilization, 985.10.2

*Such paperweights were
presented to donors to the
Muskoka Cottage Sanatarium
(tuberculosis hospital).*

patients and their families to follow conventional
medical therapies, tuberculosis nurses also endeav-
oured to convince private physicians that the reporting of tuberculosis cases was in the best interest of
both the patients' and the public's health.[15]

Coordination of the health education and health
visiting programs of the anti-tuberculosis societies
with the sanitation and inspection programs of the
local health departments provided gratifying results.
However, anti-tuberculosis society nurses could not
compel patients to follow their instructions. Lack of
regulatory authority and a desire to have tuberculosis
programs centrally coordinated ultimately resulted
in the transfer of tuberculosis nurses to civic health
departments. For example, in 1914, Winnipeg's
medical officer of health requested that the anti-
tuberculosis society's nurse, Miss Rathbone, be made
a civic employee because this would enable her "...to
have the power to make people carry out our regulations where at present persuasion and argument are
about the only weapons she can personally use."[16]

According to *The Canadian Nurse*, Ottawa was the
first Canadian city to boast a tuberculosis nurse. Miss
Rayside was employed by the Ottawa Anti-Tuberculosis
League in 1905 to visit in the homes of tuberculosis
patients. Between 1907 and 1914, similar programs
were established in Montreal; Winnipeg; Colchester
County, NS; and Vancouver. The first tuberculosis
nurse known to have been employed by a local health
department was Christina Mitchell, who was hired in
1907 by the Toronto Health Department. However, she
had previously been employed as a tuberculosis nurse
by the Toronto General Hospital with funding donated
by a concerned citizen. When this arrangement ended,
Toronto's city council agreed to include her salary in
the Health Department's budget.[17]

By 1950, the campaign to control tuberculosis
was considered a virtual success. Improved housing,
nutrition, sanatorium care, and case follow-up had
interrupted the chain of disease transmission in the
community. Newly developed antibiotics offered the
promise of cure. Once the most feared disease in
Canadian society, by 1950 tuberculosis had been relegated to the backwaters of the health care system.[18]

School Health Nursing

In some Canadian cities, the first public health nurses
were employed to preserve and promote the health of
school aged children. Political and economic developments at the end of the nineteenth century had rede-
fined the nature and purpose of childhood in
industrial society. These changes had a particularly
significant impact on working class and immigrant
children who, until that time, left school at a very
early age to seek employment. Their wages were
essential to the family's economic survival. As children were gradually removed from economic production and placed in the public school system, the
significant health problems from which they suffered
became impossible to ignore. Undiagnosed and
untreated physical problems interfered with their
ability to learn effectively. Communicable diseases,

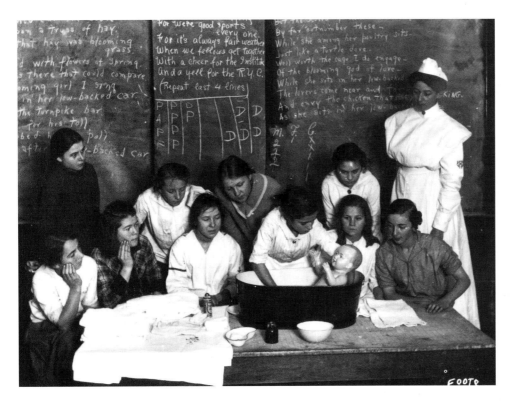

Figure 5
Public health nursing demonstration
Winnipeg, Manitoba
1916
Manitoba Archives
Foote Collection, N2663

As well as assessing the health of school children, nurses provided basic instruction in hygiene, nutrition, and the care of infants.

particularly diphtheria, scarlet fever, and measles, spread rapidly in crowded and sometimes unhygienic schools and spilled out of this setting to infect others in the community. Standards of personal hygiene practised by immigrant and working class families shocked middle class teachers and social reformers. Thus, in addition to communicable disease control and physical inspection of school children, another initiative mounted within the school setting was the education of school girls in domestic skills such as food preparation and infant care. Teaching these children in the school setting, it was hoped, would facilitate the dissemination of middle class standards of personal and household hygiene to working class and immigrant homes.

Provincial legislation was necessary to allow physicians and nurses to enter public schools to examine the children. In 1906, Montreal became the first Canadian city to institute the medical inspection of school children. This program, like others subsequently organized in other major urban centres, fell under the jurisdiction of the school board. Efforts to control communicable disease outbreaks in the schools were coordinated with the local health department. Because many families could not afford the

treatments recommended by the school nurse or physician, local welfare agencies and charitable organizations also became involved in supporting school health programs. Ultimately, most school health programs were taken over by local or provincial health departments as public health programs were gradually consolidated under one jurisdiction.[19]

Initially, only physicians were involved in school inspection programs. However, because home visits were often required to educate the parents about their child's problem and to ensure that all recommendations to rectify it were followed, nurses were soon employed to undertake this aspect of the work. Nurses found their work challenging, and sometimes heartbreaking. A great deal of time was spent securing charitable assistance to augment the meagre financial resources of the family. As one Vancouver school nurse reported, "...although a great deal of [sic] parents are unable to afford even the simplest of treatments, we are able to a certain extent to overcome this difficulty through the kindness of the different specialists in the city." Another Vancouver nurse reported discovering that a family of seven that had been referred to her shared their two small rooms with three boarders. Bridging the chasm between their middle class Western European customs and those of the families they visited challenged the tact and adaptability of many school nurses. Reporting that she had never been asked to afternoon tea, one school nurse recounted that she had, however, been offered a beer "...at an Italian's house in the afternoon."[20] School children were often reluctant participants in the process of enhancing their health. Mona Gleason's study of school medical inspection in British Columbia includes the stories of children who vigorously resisted the school's efforts to improve their hygiene, who skipped or ran away from school during immunization campaigns, and who bitterly resented the patently unfair comparison of their general state of cleanliness with classmates who came from wealthier families. Despite all of these challenges and difficulties, the role of the school nurse became an integral part of most Canadian public health nursing programs.

Child Welfare/Child Hygiene Nursing

Infant mortality rates in Canadian cities began to rise in the late nineteenth century and continued to climb until well into the second decade of the twentieth century. This development created tremendous concern amongst social reformers, who believed that healthy children were an essential component of a modern industrial nation. Canadian programs to reduce infant mortality were initiated by philanthropic women. In the early twentieth century, they established milk depots to provide safe infant formulas for women who were unable to breastfeed and could not afford pasteurized milk for bottle feeding. In addition, they provided health education to new mothers. Nurses were employed to staff the milk depots, conduct well baby clinics, and carry out home visits in the community. By 1910, a variety of women's groups, settlement houses, and church missions had established well baby clinics for Toronto's poorest citizens. In Winnipeg, a child hygiene program was founded by the Margaret Scott Nursing Mission, with funding from the city's health department, in 1910. The Mission encountered major financial difficulties and could not continue the program. It was taken over by the city in 1914. A similar pattern of municipal takeover of voluntary programs occurred in other Canadian cities. Public health nurses took the place of visiting nurses in the delivery of child hygiene and milk depot programs.[21]

Although voluntary child welfare programs were generally well received in Canadian cities, the establishment of *gouttes de lait* in Montreal became a source of contention between women associated with the Fédération nationale Saint-Jean-Baptiste (FNSJB) and a coalition of physicians and clergy. Efforts on the part of the women to establish child welfare programs were resisted by physicians, who feared that these programs would interfere with their medical practices, and by members of the clergy, who believed that women should be relegated to an advisory role in any program that aspired to enhance the growth and vigour of Quebec's francophone population. Until 1916, the FNSJB resisted opposition from these two groups and successfully established several *gouttes de lait* in Montreal. However, the loss of effective leadership within the organization enabled a coalition of physicians to gain control of the funding for the city's *gouttes de lait*. This arrangement lasted until 1953, when the city council ceased funding physician controlled *gouttes de lait* and assumed control of them itself.[22]

As was the case with school nurses, child welfare nurses carried out their work under very difficult conditions. Barriers of language and custom hampered their efforts to educate mothers of young children. Many families lacked even the most basic supplies for their newborn infants and improvisation became the order of the day.

"Perhaps one small, shallow pan is all the house can boast...in it the bread is made..., the water boiled, faces washed, and floors scrubbed. A nurse, who has always been in a hospital, with everything to work with, cannot realize what it means to be out in the world, until she enters homes of this kind."[23]

It was little wonder that the commodious black bags carried by public health nurses contained, in addition to medications and nursing supplies, infant layettes, bottles of soup, eggs, and other items to assist destitute families. Many small children also believed that the family's newborn infant arrived in the same receptacle.

On All Frontiers

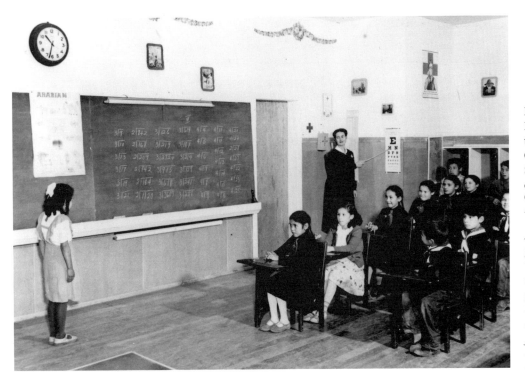

Figure 6
**Public health nurses
testing eyesight**
Cumberland House,
Saskatchewan
ca. 1940
Glenbow Archives, Calgary,
Alberta, NA-339-4

*An important part of
public health nursing
was the detection
of significant health
problems, that
interfered with the
child's ability to
function in the
school setting.*

Consolidating the Practice and Opening New Frontiers: Public Health Nursing between 1920 and 1950

Between 1920 and 1950, urban public health nurses reshaped their practices from a specialist focus in a single program to a generalist practice where individual nurses were assigned to specific districts and provided a variety of services as required by individuals and families residing in that district. At the same time, rural and remote areas of the provinces began to develop the basic infrastructures to deliver public health programs to their citizens. Nurses were often the first public health professionals to set up practice in these areas. Both developments solidified the role of the public health nurse as an essential element of Canada's health care system.

Urban Public Health Nursing

By 1920, public health nursing was well established in Canada's major cities. New responsibilities were assigned to them, including venereal disease control, the administration of immunizing agents, the inspection of preschool children, prenatal classes, home

nursing instruction, health teaching to community groups, and the prevention of chronic diseases such as cancer and cardiovascular disease. In some jurisdictions, industrial (occupational health) nursing was also included in their mandate.

The major innovation during this era was the transition from specialist to generalist practices. Toronto's health department pioneered this change. By the second decade of the twentieth century, the city's public health system had evolved into a confusing mix of programs under the auspices of a variety of private and civic organizations. Health care officials also feared that too many health visitors, acting in an uncoordinated manner, might be visiting a single household. In 1914, the health department amalgamated the child hygiene and communicable disease programs at the service delivery level. Each public health nurse provided direct care in the home for both programs. "We decided to specialize in homes rather than diseases," wrote Eunice Dyke of this innovation, "and to safeguard the interests of the medical specialist by office organization rather than multiplication of health visitors."[24] The generalist role of the public health nurse expanded throughout this era as public health programs administered by other

Jean Cuthand Goodwill

Lesley McBain, University of Saskatchewan

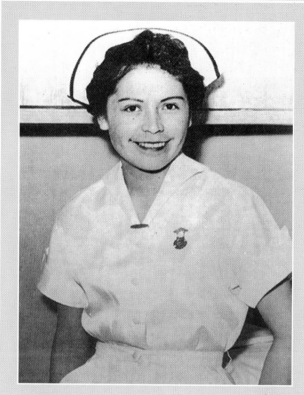

Figure 7
Jean Cuthand Goodwill
1957
Indian Health Nursing Station, La Ronge, Saskatchewan
Department of Indian and Northern Affairs

Jean was a Cree woman from Little Pine Reserve in Saskatchewan and was the first Aboriginal to complete nurse's training in Saskatchewan. She spent much of her life helping to bring positive change for northern people. She graduated from the Holy Family School of Nursing in Prince Albert in 1954, and then nursed at Lac La Ronge, Saskatchewan, and later in Bermuda. She worked with the Indian and Metis Service Council and in 1963 was appointed director of the Indian Metis Friendship Centre in Winnipeg. She was a founding member in 1974 and served as president (1983–1990) of the Registered Nurses of Canadian Indian Ancestry, now called the Aboriginal Nurses Association of Canada. She was involved in the establishment of Aboriginal nursing programs and received an honorary doctorate of law from Queen's University in 1986, and a national excellence award from the National Aboriginal Achievement Foundation in 1994.

When Jean worked in the North she spoke the language (Cree) and understood the Native way of life. She knew the harsh conditions and commended the non-Native nurses for their work. In an 1984 editorial in *The Canadian Nurse*, Jean stated, "To some extent the terrain, the scenery, the midnight sun, the serenity of the silence and the purity of the air comfort the nurse who tries to deal with the human devastation that has resulted from imposition of another way of life on Canada's native people." She strongly believed that in order for northern communities to become "modern" it was not enough to simply transfer southern customs to the North. Northern communities needed the infrastructure of indoor plumbing, running water, and decent housing to overcome health problems and to prepare them for modernization. Health care could best be served by combining Aboriginal traditions with modern nursing techniques, but only when Aboriginal people themselves were ready and involved in the process.

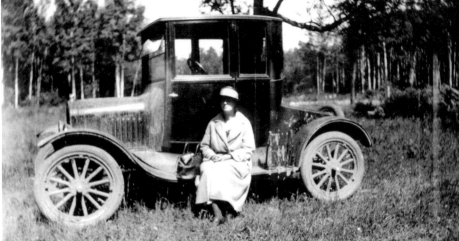

Figure 8
Public health nurse sitting on a car at South Gillies
Thunder Bay District, Ontario
1923
Archives of Ontario,
RG 10-30-2, 2.20.1

By the 1920s, the ability to drive a car was an essential skill for many public health nurses. In their memoirs, public health nurses referred to their vehicles with great affection.

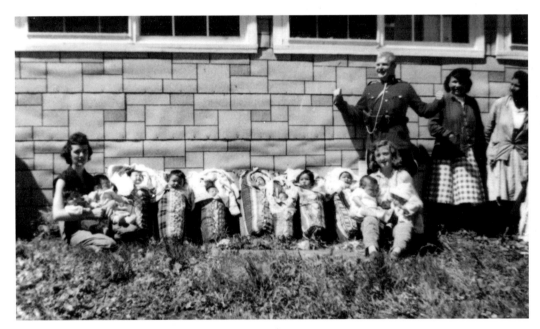

Figure 9
Nurses with Naskapi babies at child health conference
Sandy Lake, Manitoba
1950s
Glenbow Archives,
Calgary, Alberta, NA-3040-17

Some nurses successfully bridged the gap between European and Aboriginal health care practices and customs and others found the cultural differences too difficult to traverse.

jurisdictions, such as school boards, were brought under the control of the health departments, and as new programs were developed within health departments.

Public Health Nursing in Rural and Northern Canada

Renewed interest in the role that nurses could play in improving the health of all Canadian citizens emerged in the aftermath of the First World War. The post-war reconstruction era was characterized by a determination that Canadians would be as healthy and productive as recent advances in medical science could make them. Particular concern was expressed about the state of health of populations living in rural and remote areas of the country where the development of public health programs had lagged behind that of urban areas. Several factors had contributed to this state of affairs. The sparse population in non-urban Canada made the logistics of establishing effective public health programs difficult. A severe shortage of appropriately prepared nurses in the immediate post-war era made it nearly impossible to secure the necessary workforce. The need for primary care in rural and isolated areas also limited the successful establishment of public health programs. Many communities wanted visiting nurses who provided bedside nursing care, rather than public health nurses who focused on health education and prevention of illness. However, the most significant obstacle to the permanent establishment of public health nursing programs in rural and remote areas was the lack of local funding. The precedent of having public health services organized through civic or municipal departments of health, which had been established in Canada's major cities, could not be replicated in more sparsely populated areas of the country. Many provincial health departments struggled to establish local health departments in the interwar years, and their development was slow and uneven. Often, funding from the Red Cross or the Rockefeller Foundation was used to initiate the establishment of a local health department. However, ultimately most provincial health departments were forced to finance their programs themselves in order to sustain them.[25]

The first public health nurses employed in rural and northern Canada faced significant obstacles. They often worked alone and the magnitude of the task assigned to them sometimes seemed overwhelming. Mona Wilson was employed as Prince Edward Island's second child hygiene nurse. Her biographer eloquently describes the situation in which she found herself:

> When Mona arrived in Prince Edward Island in 1923 she faced a daunting task. Partly because of the province's poor financial situation, there were virtually no public health facilities.... After meeting with the Red Cross board of directors and learning how wide ranging her responsibilities were, Mona felt like weeping and by the end of the day she was ready to return to Toronto.[26]

Once public health nurses actually arrived in their rural districts, they faced even greater challenges. Because of the large districts to which they were assigned, the time available to provide follow-up in complex situations was significantly constrained. They were more likely to be called out on medical emergencies, which interrupted more routine public health programs and sometimes took the nurse away from the community for several days.

Meryn Stuart's study of the Rural Child Welfare Project in northern Ontario (1920–25) leaves little doubt that public health nurses were often in "...a difficult and sometimes impossible situation."[27] The provincial government hoped that local governments would establish permanent health units after the Child Welfare nurses demonstrated their value in protecting and enhancing the community's health status. As it turned out, local governments were happy to accept these services as long as they were funded by the provincial government, but much less enthusiastic about making the financial commitment to continue them. The Rural Child Welfare nurses, having struggled to establish a foothold in a new district, knew that more often than not their reassignment to another community meant the termination of public health programs in the community they were currently serving. As well, local citizens and many (but not all) local physicians did not support the program. To some extent, this problem arose because of personal and professional differences of opinion about the prevention and treatment of illness. Ethel Johns, soon to be appointed as head of the first baccalaureate nursing program in the British Empire, had this advice for the readers of *The Canadian Nurse* in 1918:

> Granted, co-operation will not be easy; it is barely possible that without meaning to do so you may offend the village oracles, even (under my breath I say it) the local doctor. He may consider your ideas on infant feeding as a trifle highfalutin. He may even characterize your treasured child welfare ideals as tommyrot, but be patient with him; remember he isn't as young as you are and hasn't had your advantages, and remember that he has served his generation well on many a long freezing winter drive....[28]

Some physicians also opposed the placement of public health nurses in their communities because they feared that the nurses would compete with them for both patients and income. It took considerable effort on the part of the nurses to assuage these concerns. One of the strategies employed to mute these protests was to refer all individuals found to have "abnormal" conditions to the attending physician for

On All Frontiers

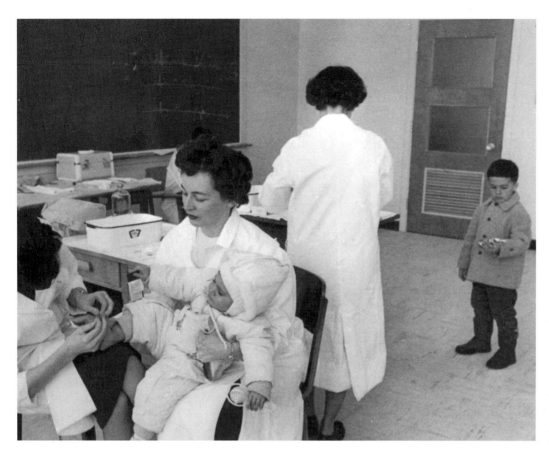

Figure 10
Public health nurses administering polio vaccines
Wedgeport, Nova Scotia
1961
Photographer:
Bob Brooks
Yarmouth County Museum Archives,
Album 86

follow-up, even in cases where the nurses had the knowledge and skills to provide this service themselves. Thus, went the joke circulated in the Ontario Health Department, a public health nurse, upon being asked if she thought the weather was nice, referred the individual to a physician for an opinion.[29]

Unlike their counterparts in urban settings, the first rural public health nurses were often generalists. They delivered programs in health education, dental health, communicable disease control, pre- and post-natal care, prevention of chronic illness, and medical/surgical nursing. In addition, they delivered babies and provided emergency medical, dental, and even veterinary assistance on the frequent occasions when these professionals were not available. Although the work was arduous and never-ending, the sense of satisfaction in both a career and a way of life was sufficient reward for many nurses. Reflecting on her early years of public health nursing in the Peace River District of northern Alberta, Amy Wilson wrote:

I enjoyed the work in this area; first aid, home nursing classes, immunizing the children, attend-ing maternity cases, trying to be counselor [*sic*] and friend as well as nurse to these people whom I understood and respected. From them I learned many things about homestead life: where not to ride a horse in that muskeg country, how to shoot, how to prepare and cook wild game and how to improvise.[30]

The skill of improvisation may have been the most useful lesson of all.

Public Health Nursing in the Last Half of the Twentieth Century

The general contours of public health nursing were firmly established by the end of the Second World War. However, specific details of the practice have shifted in response to changes in the composition of the Canadian population, differences in provincial programs, and the changed patterns of disease both within Canada and globally.[31]

Roles and responsibilities in the area of communicable disease control have been transformed as the

Alberta's Travelling Medical Clinics

Jayne Elliot, RN, PhD (History)

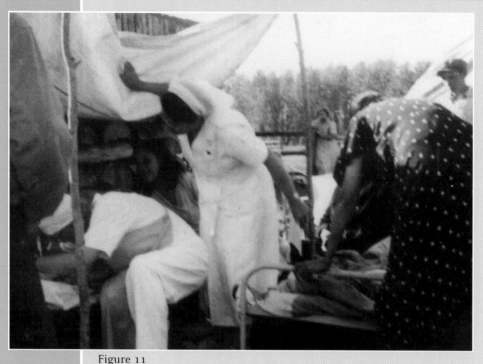

Figure 11
Dr Gardener and Olive Watherson examining patient
Pipestone, Alberta
1939
Glenbow Archives, Calgary, Alberta, A 3145-26

Travelling medical clinics supplied some of the amenities of urban health care and medical treatment to people who were unable or unwilling to travel out of their rural areas. With the exception of two years, the Department of Health in Alberta conducted an organized system of travelling clinics to rural communities from 1924 to 1942. The clinic team usually consisted of a physician, a surgeon, two dentists, three nurses, and a medical and dental student as assistants and truck drivers. They carried out medical and dental examinations and performed minor surgery. In 1935, for example, the clinic team saw 5105 children, performed 888 operations, undertook 2149 dental examinations, and extracted 2238 teeth.

The clinic travelled during the summer months, spending approximately two days in each community. On the first day, parents brought their children for medical checkups and immunizations. Surgical procedures such as the removal of tonsils and adenoids and dental work took place on the second day in a church or hall that had been freshly cleaned by community members. Patients recovered from their operations in tents set up nearby. Parents who had travelled great distances camped until their children were able to tolerate the drive home. After cleaning and repacking, the clinic moved on to the next site on the third day.

Although it was an itinerant and usually enjoyable summer for the nurses, they worked hard. Just moving the clinic from place to place was a challenge when the roads were sometimes in such poor condition that the trucks became bogged down in mud. They were also involved in all aspects of the clinics, from helping to set up the tents and equipment, assisting the physicians, surgeons, and dentists in their work, to nursing the recovering patients, and sterilizing and repacking the supplies at the end.

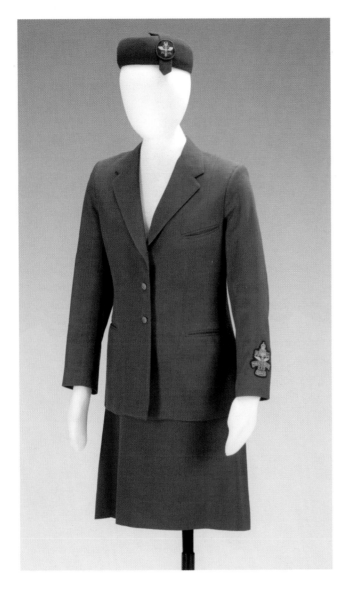

Figure 12
Public health nurse's winter uniform
British Columbia
1948–1970
Photographer: Doug Millar
Canadian Museum of Civilization, 2004.97.5; 2004.91.4; 2004.45.1
Gift of Shirley Jones, Lorna Storbakken, Vicki Anderson

communicable disease control programs in the face of public complacency and decreased public funding.[32] Recent tragedies, such as the E. coli 0157:H7 outbreak in Walkerton and the SARS outbreak in Toronto have put communicable disease control back on the public agenda. All Canadians have been reminded that communicable diseases can and will exploit weaknesses in the public health system.

Public health nurses continue their involvement in promoting the health of mothers and newborn infants. Earlier discharge of postpartum women and newborn infants, a trend that began in the late 1980s, has resulted in a much closer working relationship between the hospital and community sectors of the health care system. Highly efficient referral systems, and the implementation of seven day a week postpartum programs in many Canadian communities have enabled public health nurses to provide timely assessment of the postpartum family's progress in the community.

The prevention of chronic illnesses such as cancer, cardiovascular disease, and type 2 diabetes has increased in importance over the past 50 years. As well as health teaching to individuals and families, public health nurses have been in the forefront of efforts to direct preventive programs to at-risk populations though community development initiatives and health education in settings such as the public school system, the workplace, seniors' housing developments, and community clubs. Public health nurses have also provided leadership in efforts to move beyond a focus on the prevention of specific diseases and, instead, to create the mechanisms necessary to promote the health and general well-being of the total population. This change in emphasis has led to a renewed interest in the role that the environment plays in the creation of health, to the establishment

list of reportable diseases requiring public health follow-up lengthened with each passing decade. For sexually transmitted diseases, the original emphasis on the control of syphilis and gonorrhea has enlarged to include many other infections, including AIDS, hepatitis B and C, and chlamydia. Tuberculosis, considered to be virtually under control by the mid-twentieth century, re-emerged in the 1990s as one of the leading threats to global health. Imported communicable diseases continue to threaten public health, but in the twenty-first century, public health nurses anticipate and plan for imported cases of tropical diseases, SARS, and influenza rather than cholera, smallpox, and typhoid fever. Since the 1970s, public health nurses have struggled to maintain the integrity of

Street Nurse and Activist, Cathy Crowe

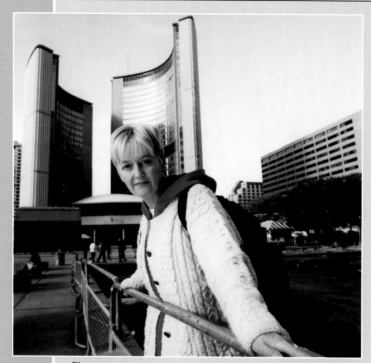

Figure 13
Cathy Crowe in front of Toronto City Hall
2002
Courtesy of Cathy Crowe

Christina Bates, Canadian Museum of Civilization, and Cathy Crowe

Some public health nurses have turned to social activism to address the needs of their communities. Armed with her bulging backpack full of the necessities of health care, Cathy Crowe has reached out to the homeless in Toronto on sidewalks, in tent cities, and in shelters since 1987. While working in an exclusive doctor's office after graduating from the Toronto General Hospital School of Nursing in 1972, she decided she wanted to do something more meaningful with her nursing. She left the nine-to-five job and began work in various downtown community health centres, meanwhile earning a degree in nursing, then a master's in sociology.

As a nurse, Cathy Crowe brings expert knowledge and research methods to the understanding of the devastating effects of homelessness, such as the growing spread of tuberculosis, HIV/AIDS, and hepatitis. Combining respect and great empathy for her patients with political savvy and ruthless determination, she, along with other committed people, founded the Toronto Disaster Relief Committee, dedicated to having homelessness in Canada declared a national disaster, and the One-Percent Solution, a proposal that all levels of government spend an additional 1 percent of their overall budgets on housing.

Cathy Crowe counts her patients as some of the best lobbyists for housing. James Kagoshima was a homeless person who joined her at many rallies. In her own words, this is Cathy Crowe's eulogy for James:

I first laid eyes on James Kagoshima at a national housing rally — outside Toronto's City Hall. He was in the front row, fully appreciating the music and speeches. He was laughing, chanting slogans. Many times I have seen him pounding the pavement giving out leaflets and 1% buttons to homeless people and speaking at press conferences and vigils. At one press conference, he impatiently threw his hat down on the ground and stepped on it, indicating his shame at our country's track record on housing. James attended to many homeless people sleeping outside that I never could have reached. He brought them sleeping bags, food, and friendship.

Years later, incapacitated by pitting edema and confined to a wheelchair in a homeless shelter, James agreed to aggressive treatment so that he could keep fighting homelessness. Before long he was walking again, and speaking out. Sadly, his recovery was shortlived. On the day he died the kind ICU nurses allowed me to pin a 1% button on his hospital gown before life supports were ended.

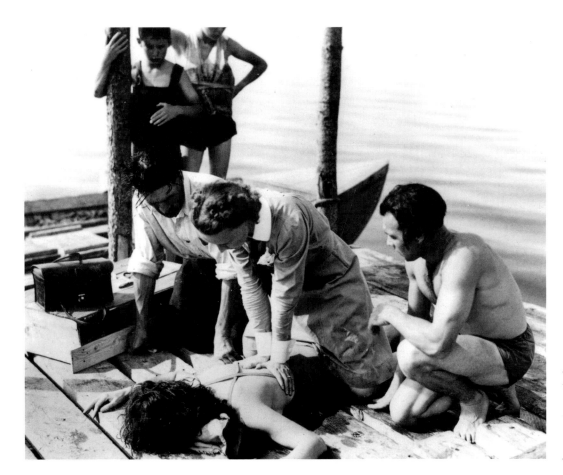

Figure 14
Public health nurse demonstrating artificial respiration
Slave Lake, Alberta
Glenbow Archives,
Calgary, Alberta,
NA-3948-2

of intersectoral initiatives to promote health, and to active collaboration between health care professionals and lay people in the development of community-based health promotion strategies.

In some ways, the practice of the public health nurse has come full circle. The early public health nurse was concerned about the safety of a community's water and food supply. The early twenty-first century public health nurse is similarly preoccupied. Pioneer public health nurses depended on the support and assistance of their communities for the successful implementation of new programs. Contemporary community development programs require the same kind of cooperation and support. The threat of epidemic diseases overshadowed the beginning and marked the end of the twentieth century. Public health nurses in both eras shaped their practices in response to this reality. Finally, as in the beginning, the specialist role for the public health nurse has again emerged. Although the vast majority of public health nurses still work as gener-

alists, the increased complexity of the programs they deliver demands specialist support at both the service delivery and administrative level. This support is provided by nurses with advanced preparation in specific aspects of public health nursing practice.

Conclusion

The first century of Canadian public health nursing has been marked by significant achievements and dramatic transformations in the health needs of Canadians. The first generation of Canadian nurses recognized that a career in public health offered them autonomy, challenge, and, perhaps most important of all, an opportunity to make a difference in the lives of the people they served. They argued passionately that the state had a responsibility to provide health care to its citizens and that nurses could make a significant contribution to this endeavour. Those who followed in their footsteps have seen that vision fulfilled.

CHAPTER 8

Religious Nursing Orders of Canada: A Presence on All Western Frontiers

Pauline Paul

Most Canadians can identify a religious nursing order that has been involved in caring for their community. Many, however, do not realize the extent to which religious nursing orders played a leadership role in the development of nursing and health care services across Canada. Nursing sisters, as they will be generically referred to in this chapter, were often the first care providers on new frontiers and, although the number of sisters has been declining since the 1960s, a significant number of the health care institutions they created remain as evidence of their contribution to the development of Canada from coast to coast. This chapter undertakes to explore the legacy of religious nursing orders from 1760 to the present. But because this is such a huge task, it is impossible to do justice to all religious nursing orders and to explore their presence in all regions of our vast country. It was necessary to set limits and focus on specific geographical areas and religious orders.

Because the role of nursing sisters on new frontiers is of particular interest, we chose to focus on western Canada. Similarly, since Roman Catholic religious nursing orders have been the most prevalent in Canada, they will occupy centre stage. The magnitude of the role played by these sisters is evident when examining statistics published in 1947: At that time, Roman Catholic sisters operated at least 146 hospi-

tals, including 36 of the 66 large Canadian hospitals.[1] In addition, because French-Canadian orders were prevalent in western Canada and operated most of the large Roman Catholic hospitals of that region, we will give primary emphasis to them. Although most orders who came to western Canada, and most of the orders that operated hospitals in Winnipeg, Saskatoon, Calgary, Edmonton, and Vancouver, originated in Quebec, the contribution of these religious orders to the foundation of Quebec hospitals will not be our focus, since this subject has already been addressed in chapter 4. Rather, our purpose here is to explore how sisters from Quebec played a key role in spreading nursing across the West.

By examining how major French-Canadian religious nursing orders spread across the country, creating impressive networks of hospitals and dispensaries, it is possible to shed light on the overall development of religious nursing in western Canada. The French-Canadian orders had in common with nursing sisters of all denominations a fundamental belief that helping others was an important calling, as well as the common experience of being for significant periods of time the main — if not the only — providers of health care services to the populations they served. We can say, then, that the experiences of French-Canadian nursing sisters are probably fairly representative of the experiences of all nursing sisters

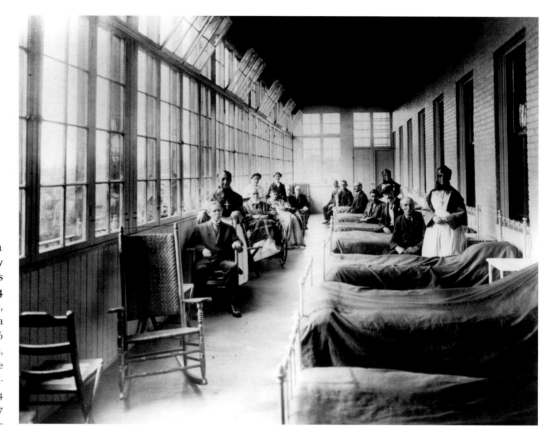

Figure 1
Sisters of Charity tending patients Taché Hospital, 4
St. Boniface,
Manitoba
1926
Manitoba Archives,
St. Boniface
Collection–Hospital-
Taché. Item #4
Negative 9367

in western Canada. It is also possible to say that the experiences of nursing sisters in the West were comparable to those of their counterparts in other regions of Canada; no matter where they were and when they devoted their lives to the care of others, nursing sisters faced certain common challenges related to geography, culture, and economics. At any given time in our past, nursing sisters have served Canadians of all origins across all regions of the country. This chapter, through an exploration of the experience of nursing sisters in the West, provides a snapshot of the leadership role Canadian sisters played in the development of nursing and health care services in our country.

Setting the Stage: Canada from 1760 to 1899

By 1760 Roman Catholic religious nursing orders had already established a network of hospitals in the part of New France that was later to become the province of Quebec. After 1760, Quebec Roman Catholic nursing orders continued to grow under the new British rule. Their existence was further assured by the 1774

Act of Quebec, which, among other things, gave French North American people religious freedom.[2] Without this freedom, nursing sisters would not have been able to pursue their activities and provide services that had no equivalent in other North American British colonies. It is important to recall that, at the time, organized nursing was practically non-existent in the English-speaking world, and that it would take another century before the first graduates from the British hospital nursing schools, subsidized by the Nightingale Fund, began to bring about the reforms from which modern nursing emerged.

Between 1760 and 1900, what is known today as western Canada was transformed from an area predominantly inhabited by Native and Metis populations to a territory where an increasing number of people from varied European origins were gradually settling to build a new life. At the beginning of this period, the fur trade was the main source of commerce, while by the end, it had been almost replaced by other economic activities, giving rise to the creation of larger towns and new provincial entities.

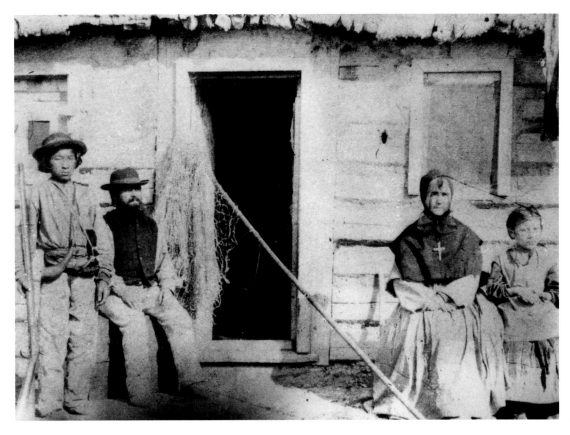

Figure 2
**Grey Nun
visiting a Metis
family at home**
Manitoba
Manitoba Archives
Stovel Advocate
Collection, 282
Negative 10201

Responding to Many Calls: Nursing Sisters Come to Western Canada

Conditions similar to those that had enticed French sisters to come to New France led French-Canadian sisters to the Prairies. In the early 1800s, the fur trade was still the main economic activity in western Canada and the Hudson's Bay Company had the monopoly on this activity there. Bishop Provencher had come to the region in 1818 at the request of the Company, which considered that the presence of the clergy might help to bring order to the population of the Red River region.[3] At the request of Bishop Provencher, the Sisters of Charity of Montreal, commonly known as the Grey Nuns, agreed to provide missionaries for the West. The development pattern, then, was not unlike that of New France: fur traders were the first to come, followed by missionaries, who, in turn, were followed by sisters. Similarly, the sisters came to serve quite a small population. In this case, however, one order, the Grey Nuns, had the dual responsibilities of providing nursing care and of

educating children. Seventeen of the 25 Grey Nuns of Montreal eligible for a mission in the West volunteered their services, but only four of them were selected. Sisters Valade, Lagrave, Coutlée-St-Joseph, and Lafrance were chosen because of the combination of skills they would bring to the mission: Sister Valade, who was to be in charge, had nursing experience and was a quarter Metis. It was thought that this latter attribute would help her better understand the Metis population to be served. Sister Lagrave, who was to be devoted to home visits, was considered particularly tactful. Finally, Sister Coutlée-St-Joseph was to be responsible for the future novices and teach the boys, while Sister Lafrance was to be in charge of the girls' education.

The sisters left Montreal in canoes on 23 April and finally arrived at the Red River in St. Boniface, Manitoba, on 21 June 1844. This event was to mark the beginning of a long series of expansions that brought the Grey Nuns of Montreal to what are now Saskatchewan, Alberta, and the Northwest Territories. Less than a century later they operated and/or owned

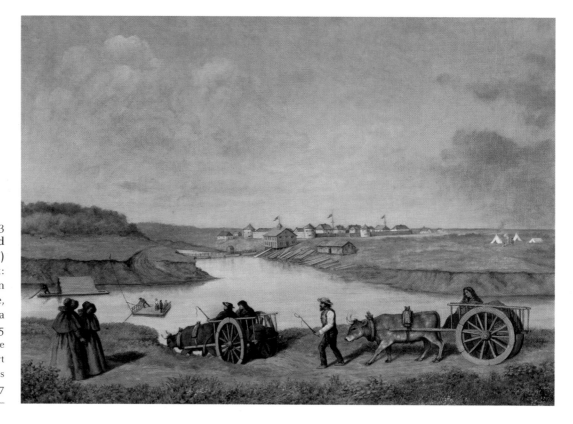

Figure 3
**Untitled
("The Forks")**
Artist:
W. Frank Lynn
St. Boniface,
Manitoba
1875
Collection of The
Winnipeg Art
Gallery. Gift of Mrs
J.K. Morton, G-70-7

15 hospitals in locations as varied as Ile à la Crosse (Saskatchewan), Edmonton (Alberta), and Fort Simpson (Northwest Territories).

Providing services prior to the arrival of most settlers and in remote areas often devoid of physicians required courage and faith. Sister Emery, one of the first Grey Nuns who settled at Lac Sainte Anne, the first Alberta mission, in 1859, provides a vivid description of a sister's life in the West: "Here one has to be a jack of all trades. A few days ago, I taught a poor man how to winnow barley; it was rather extraordinary to see a Grey Nun doing this...."[4] Eleven years later, after the mission had been moved to Saint-Albert (near Edmonton), Sister Emery wrote that during the last six months of 1870, nursing duties had included home visits to 36 families (a total of 692 visits), the provision of wound care to 22 patients, the vaccination against smallpox of 218 children and 133 adults, and the distribution of 392 meals.[5]

Similarly to the Grey Nuns, the Sisters of Saint Ann, founded in Saint-Jacques, Quebec, in 1851 by Esther Blondin, ventured to a number of areas of western Canada. In 1858, four of the 40 sisters of the

fledging order left for Fort Victoria, now known as Victoria. Sister Mary of the Sacred Heart (Salome Valois), Sister Mary Angèle (Angèle Gauthier), Sister Mary Lumena (Virginia Brasseur), and Sister Mary of the Conception (Mary Lane) left for the far away mission. After a six-week journey, first by train to New York, and then by ship along the Atlantic Coast, across Panama, and along the Pacific Coast, the sisters arrived at Fort Victoria. Although their primary mission was education, the Sisters of Saint Ann had recognized prior to leaving for Fort Victoria that nursing skills would be needed. For this reason, two sisters had been sent to the Hôtel-Dieu de Montréal to gain the necessary experience. Although the sisters did not open Saint Joseph's Hospital until 1876, they provided informal nursing care to the residents of Fort Victoria from the beginnng.[6] During the following decades these sisters expanded their missions to other parts of British Columbia, to Alaska, and to the Yukon.

The Klondike gold rush brought the Sisters of Saint Ann to Dawson, Yukon, on 11 July 1898. As was the case in many other missions, a Catholic missionary had requested the sisters' assistance. Reaching

Sister Lagrave and the Grey Nuns' Mission

Christina Bates, Canadian Museum of Civilization

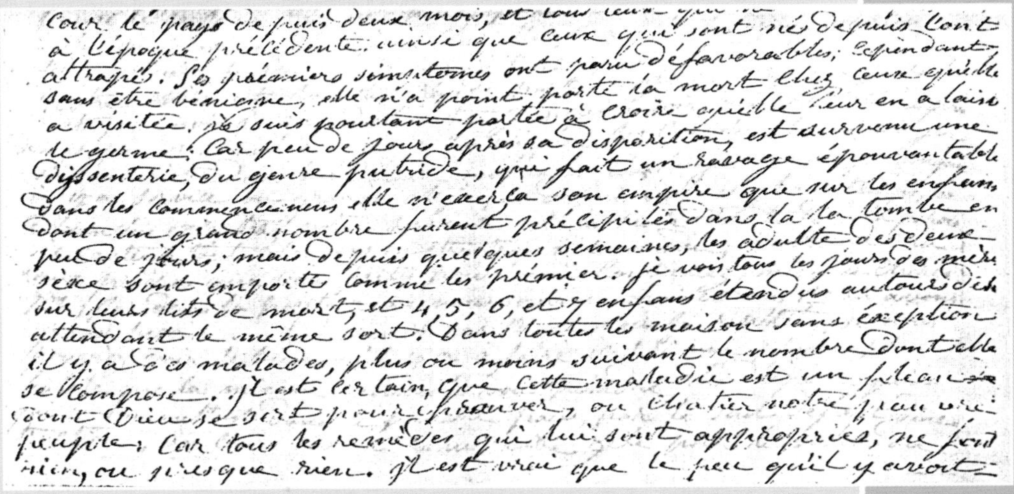
cour le pays depuis deux mois, et tous ceux qui ...
à l'époque précédente ainsi que ceux qui sont nés depuis l'ont
attrapée. Les premiers simptomes ont paru défavorables; cependant
sans être benigne, elle n'a point porté la mort chez ceux qu'elle
a visités. Je suis pourtant portée à croire qu'elle leur en a laissé
le germe; car peu de jours après sa disparition, est survenu une
dyssenterie, du genre putride, qui fait un ravage épouvantable
dans les commencements elle n'exerça son empire que sur les enfans,
dont un grand nombre furent précipités dans la tombe en
peu de jours; mais depuis quelques semaines, les adultes des deux
sexes sont emportés comme les premiers. Je vois tous les jours des mères
sur leurs lits de mort, et 4, 5, 6, et 7 enfans étendus autour d'elles
attendant le même sort. Dans toutes les maisons sans exception
il y a des malades, plus ou moins suivant le nombre dont elle
se compose. Il est certain que cette maladie est un fléau dont
Dieu se sert pour éprouver, ou châtier notre pauvre
peuple; car tous les remèdes qui lui sont appropriés, ne font
rien, ou presque rien. Il est vrai que le peu qu'il y avait

Figure 4
Sister Lagrave to her Mother House
St. Boniface, Manitoba
1846
Archives of the Grey Nuns of Montreal

When Sister Eulalie-Marie Lagrave and her three Grey Nun companions left Quebec's old-world culture for the harsh frontier at the forks of the Red River in 1844, they did not forsake their traditional values and world view. Sister Lagrave was the oldest of the group and most skilled in medical care. Most of her work involved going to remote regions to nurse the sick in their homes, travelling by Red River cart. Her letters sent home to her Mother Superior and convent sisters are evidence of the overriding sense of religious mission the sisters all shared.

Faced with epidemics, which hit particularly hard among the Metis and Aboriginals, as well as settlers with no prior exposure, Sister Lagrave was overcome with helplessness at her inability to prevent the illness or cure its victims: "The measles…has spread across the land for the last ten months.… Every day, I see mothers on their deathbed, with 4, 5, 6 or 7 children lying beside them, awaiting the same fate.… [A]ll the appropriate remedies produce no effect, or barely any." But caring for the body was secondary to caring for the soul. She retained the centuries-old belief that illness was an outer sign of a spiritual problem: "Surely this illness is a scourge employed by God as a trial or a chastisement of our poor people." Obtaining Catholic converts from the Aboriginal population was her most important mission, especially when they were facing death: "The illness has taken a terrible toll among the poor infidels and very few of them ask to be baptised. Several days ago, I went to their encampment to visit the sick; I discovered in their lodge a girl of 20 and two young children who were dying. I used all my knowledge and my limited powers of persuasion to convince [her] to be baptised, but to no avail."

Sustained by the certainty that their harrowing work was for a higher purpose, Sister Lagrave and the rest of the Grey Nuns are said to have made 6000 visits to the sick during their first decade at the Red River. The Grey Nuns went on to establish missions in the most remote regions of the West.

Sources: Archives of the Grey Nuns of Montreal, correspondence, Sister M E Lagrave to "Ma très chère Mère et mes bien aimées Sœurs," 1846, Maison Pv.SB. Historique, doc. 70; Estelle Mitchell, *The Grey Nuns of Montreal at the Red River*, 1844–1984 (Montreal: Éditions du Méridien, 1987); Sister Mary Murphy, *St. Boniface: Heroines of Mercy* (Muenster, SK: St. Peter's Press, 1944).

Dawson had not been easy; the sisters had left for the North in September 1897, but low water level made it impossible for the steamship on which they were travelling to reach its destination. Consequently, the sisters had to wait until spring 1898 to resume their journey. The first months in Dawson must have been difficult for Sister Mary of the Cross, Sister Mary Joseph, and Sister Mary John. Their initial accommodations consisted of a former cold-storage room with no windows. Saint Mary's Hospital, which had been built by Father Judge, was a two-storey log structure with little equipment, no running water, and sacks of sawdust in lieu of bed mattresses. Until the sisters came to Dawson, the hospital had provided services only to male patients. Their arrival meant that women would also be cared for, since they could be hospitalized in the convent. Dawson at the time of the gold rush was a true frontier town. Needless to say, there was no urban planning, and basic services, by then fairly common in the South, were notably absent. For example, there was no sewage system, and food was scarce. Considering the living conditions, it is not surprising that, in the fall of 1898, typhoid fever made necessary the admission of 150 patients. As well as running the hospital, the sisters were resonsible for fundraising, since the hospital was in debt and lacked some of the most basic resources. They did, however, benefit from some community support: In 1899, women from Dawson organized a Christmas charity bazaar in support of the hospital,[7] and miners also responded to the sisters' call for money. In addition to the health care services provided by the Sisters of Saint Ann, between 1898 and 1918, the Presbyterian Church also operated a small hospital in Dawson, the Good Samaritan Hospital, but decline in the town's population brought its closure. Nurses from the Victorian Order of Nurses also provided some services during the Klondike era. However, it was only the Sisters of Saint Ann who remained in Dawson once the gold rush was over and served the local population until the 1950s.[8]

Among the Roman Catholic orders of Quebec origin who participated in the development of modern hospitals in the West, the contributions of the Sisters of Providence, founded by Emilie Gamelin in Montreal in 1843, are particularly significant. Their missions in the West began in 1856, in the Washington Territory (later to become the American State of Washington), where Oblate priests had requested their presence. Like the Sisters of Saint Ann they reached the West Coast after a long sailing trip. Expanding northward from Washington, their first mission in British Columbia was established in New Westminster in 1886. In this location, the sisters operated a 15-bed hospital and also visited the sick in their homes. As in many other places, it took an epidemic to make the population realize the value of their services. After the typhoid epidemic of 1891, however, citizens gratefully rallied around the hospital and made donations. It was years, though, before the government began providing assistance with covering operating costs. Apart from their work in New Westminster, one of the most significant achievements of the Sisters of Providence was the opening, in 1891, of Saint Paul's Hospital in Vancouver, which was to become one of the major health care facilities of that city.

Although French-Canadian orders did predominate, orders of other origins also contributed to the development of health care and hospitals in western Canada. They usually settled in smaller centres, likely because the French-Canadian orders were already providing services in larger towns. For examples, the Sisters of Charity of Notre Dame d'Évron, a French community, established a hospital in Vegreville, in Alberta, in 1928. The Sisters of Saint Joseph of Peace, an order founded in England in 1884, operated a mining town hospital in Rossland, British Columbia. In 1938, the Sisters of Saint Joseph of Sault Sainte Marie, part of the Federation of the Sisters of Saint Joseph of Canada who played a significant role in Ontario, established a hospital in eastern Saskatchewan. And the Sisters of Saint Martha, an order founded in Nova Scotia in 1901, recruiting from the Gaelic-speaking people of Antigonish, began operating the Banff Mineral Springs Hospital in Banff, Alberta.[9]

Although immigrants who came to the West during the 1900s were from varied origins, it is interesting to observe that few religious nursing orders found their roots in cultural groups other than the two

Caroline Wellwood (1874–1947): Pioneer in Chinese Nursing Education

Janet Beaton, Faculty of Nursing, University of Manitoba

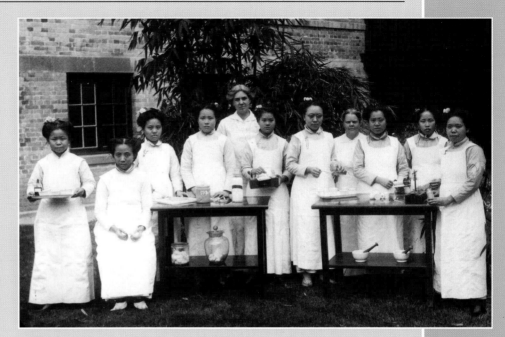

Figure 5
Nurses in hospital
Chengtu, China
ca. 1917
United Church of Canada, Victoria University Archives, Victoria University, Toronto, Ontario, 94.007P/19 N

Caroline Wellwood exemplifies those early Canadian nurses who, in response to the great missionary crusade of the late nineteenth and early twentieth centuries, set sail for Asia, Africa, or India to serve as medical missionaries. Born in rural Ontario in 1874, Wellwood, like many of her contemporaries, received her nurse's training in the United States. When she volunteered for service under the Woman's Missionary Society (WMS) of the Methodist Church of Canada in 1906, she could hardly have guessed she would spend the next 38 years of her life in China. The arduous five-month journey by land, river, and sea to the mission deep in the interior of southwest China tested her courage and called upon her keen sense of adventure and ability to adapt quickly to local conditions. Concerned about the treatment of Chinese women and children, Wellwood soon decided that the small hospital in Chengdu was inadequate to accommodate her vision for nursing in China. Deeply committed to her faith, to high standards of nursing care, and to improving the lives of Chinese women and children, she embarked on a vigorous campaign to establish a nurses' training school, a new phenomenon in China at that time. She also energetically lobbied the WMS in Canada for funding to construct a modern hospital for women and children. She succeeded in both these pioneering ventures, despite revolution, geographic isolation, and negative cultural attitudes toward nursing as a career for respectable young women. Although the 90-bed WMS Hospital for Women and Children was destroyed by fire in 1940, the nursing program, established in 1915, survives to this day at Sichuan University — as does her memory and the tradition of excellence in nursing education that she established.

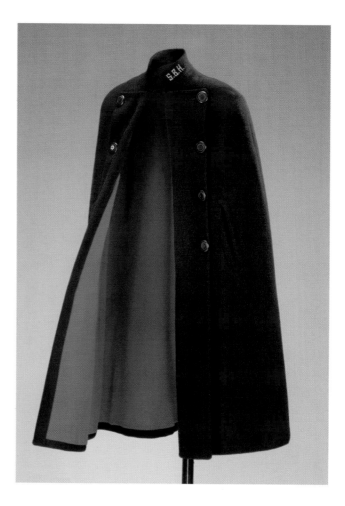

Figure 6
Nurse's cape, Anne Wade
St. Boniface Hospital, Manitoba
1947
Photographer: Doug Millar
Canadian Nurses Association Collection
Canadian Museum of Civilization, 2000.111.381

dominant French and English groups. Several factors contributed to this fact: Immigrants often had limited resources; they were also frequently, if not systematically, discouraged from maintaining their cultural identity; religious orders in their mother lands may have had little interest in migrating with them; and, finally, some immigrants came from regions of the world where the influence of nursing orders may have been limited. The order of the Sisters Servants of Mary Immaculate, part of the Catholic Ukrainian Church (a Catholic church of Eastern rite) is, however, one of those rare Canadian orders from neither French nor English cultural background. Founded in the village of Zhuzhyl in Ukraine in 1892, from the outset, among other activities, the sisters became involved in nursing. Lacking the resources necessary to build a hospital, they ministered to the sick in their homes. As we will see, nursing also became part of their early mission in Canada.[10]

The Sisters Servants of Mary Immaculate arrived in Edmonton in November 1902, after a long trip that took them by ship from Europe to New York, by train from New York to Montreal, and finally from Montreal to Edmonton. Why did these sisters come to Edmonton? Since the 1890s, a significant influx of Ukrainian immigrants had come to the Prairies and the Edmonton area. They were most of the time referred to as Galicians, Bukovinians, or Ruthenians, after the names of some of their Ukrainian regions of origin. Ukrainian immigrants had many hardships in Canada; settling the land required determination and patience. Although they were clearly needed to populate the West, they suffered many prejudices and were not considered to be as desirable immigrants as people of British origin.[11] After their arrival, the Roman Catholic clergy wanted to attract them to Roman Catholicism; however, the famous Father

Lacombe considered that such an attempt would not be successful and that it would be preferable to convince Ukrainian Catholic priests and sisters to come to the West. Lacombe was a persuasive man and first convinced Archbishop Langevin that Eastern rite clergy were needed. Having been selected as emissary to Europe, he was then able to secure the assistance of Basilian priests and Sisters Servants of Mary Immaculate for the Edmonton area. The first four sisters (Ambrose, Taida, Isidore, and Emilia) thus came to the new world. Significantly, Sister Ambrose had graduated from a school of nursing in Lviv, Ukraine. In July 1903, the sisters established their first mission in the Beaver Lake settlement, later to become the town of Mundare. Like the Grey Nuns before them, the sisters became involved in manual farm work; this was necessary to their survival. Sister Ambrose also immediately began her nursing duties:

In western Canada, at that time a doctor was a rarity, the sisters made sick calls at a moment's notice every day of the week. In this way their nursing skill, especially that of Sister Ambrose was put to practical use at once. If the sick could not be brought to the convent for treatment, the sisters travelled by wagon or cart to the farmhouses scattered throughout the district.[12]

More often than not when it was the mother who was ill, the sisters would also clean the house and prepare food for the family. Soon young Canadian women of Ukrainian origin would join the order and thus contribute to its expansion. In 1930, a long cherished dream of Sister Ambrose came to fruition when the sisters opened the Mundare General Hospital. It had taken years for the sisters to secure the needed funding. In the characteristic fashion of nursing orders, the Sisters Servants of Mary Immaculate had been planning ahead to ensure the success of their hospital; they had sent young sisters to nursing schools such as the Misericordia Hospital School of Nursing in Edmonton, Alberta, and the Grey Nuns' Hospital School of Nursing in St. Boniface, Manitoba, thus ensuring they would have a sufficient nursing workforce. The immediate admission of their new institution as a member of the American Hospital Association demonstrated their readiness to more formally enter the field of health care.[13]

As we can see, similar patterns occured in the establishment of the missions of the nursing sisters mentioned above: All of them first came to the West at the request of clergy. They founded their first missions where new frontiers were developing. They came early to serve the needs of Native and Metis communities and of the new settlers of western Canada. As the frontier became settled, the health care services that nursing sisters were able to offer developed along with their communities. In discussing the Sisters Servants of Mary Immaculate we have seen the foundation of their first hospital in Canada, a modern, American Hospital Association –certified institution. The next section will explore in more detail the involvement of religious orders in the foundation of many of the major modern hospitals that opened their doors when modern medicine and modern nursing were emerging throughout North America.

Religious Nursing Orders and the Development of Modern Hospitals: 1890 to 1970

Because of the significant experience they had gained in the operation of hospitals in eastern Canada and the centuries-old nursing tradition in the Province of Quebec, it is not surprising that, once the population of the larger western Canadian urban centres became sufficient to justify the creation of formal hospitals, French-Canadian Roman Catholic nursing sisters were among the first to take up the challenge. Although conditions were not identical from province to province and from city to city, the foundation of the Edmonton General Hospital (EGH) by the Grey Nuns is a fairly typical example of the role of nursing sisters in the development of modern hospitals.[14]

As we saw earlier, the Grey Nuns of Montreal established their first Alberta mission at Lac Sainte Anne in 1859. In April of 1894, six local physicians requested that the Grey Nuns establish a hospital in Edmonton, whose population had reached 1021 inhabitants. The physicians had pledged their support to the proposed institution. In addition, 850 individuals had petitioned the town council, asking them to financially assist the sisters; the number of petitioners certainly represented a vote of confidence. On its opening in 1895, the new three-storey 36-bed EGH was a large building for the small town. The first floor had two wards and two private rooms for women; men had similar facilities on the second floor, with the addition of a room for smokers. Finally, the third included a dressing room, three private rooms, and a state-of-the-art operating room.

Although all seemed to bode well for the new institution, the Grey Nuns soon experienced difficulties with some of the physicians who staffed the facility.[15] In 1899, four physicians decided to leave the hospital and organized a committee to examine the possibility of establishing a civic hospital. In 1899, in a letter to the *Edmonton Bulletin*, the Grey Nuns made public what they considered to be the cause of the physicians' departure. The letter indicated that the main irritant was that the physicians disagreed with the admission policies of the Grey Nuns. The fact that the sisters took the liberty of admitting those who

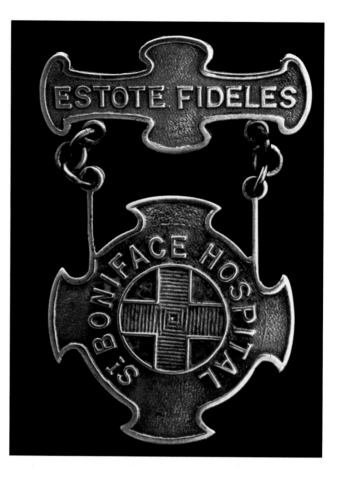

Figure 7
Graduation pin, E. Klassen
St. Boniface Hospital School of Nursing,
Manitoba
1934
Canadian Nurses Association Collection
Canadian Museum of Civilization, 2000.111.186

could not pay and that they expected physicians, on a rotating basis, to treat these patients was certainly a large part of the problem. Further correspondence and other evidence[16] indicate, however, that the authority of the nuns was also a key issue, that monetary considerations were also likely part of the equation, and that the conflict included religious overtones. Later that year, the physicians involved in the dispute, assisted by the Protestant clergy, convinced the city to create the Edmonton Public Hospital (EPH), which was to be a "non-sectarian" hospital.

The use of the term "non-sectarian" by the founders of the EPH was rather interesting considering the involvement of the Protestant clergy and of the local Masonic lodges. It is true that the EGH was clearly a Roman Catholic hospital, but it had always admitted patients without regard to denomination. In 1896, for instance, 494 Catholics and 450 Protestants were admitted. The sisters never considered sacrificing what they considered to be their moral duty to merely sectarian loyalties. Although the religion of the physicians who left is not known, it is clear that of the four who stayed two were certainly Catholic and French-Canadian.[17] In the year that followed, this rift affected the relationship between the EGH and the town council. However, the tension was short lived thanks to the Edmonton smallpox epidemic of 1901. Indeed, the victims of this epidemic would have been without care if not for the Grey Nuns, assisted by a lay nurse from the also-Catholic Misericordia Hospital. (Founded in 1900, the Misericordia Hospital was at the time primarily a maternity hospital and thus offered complementary services to those available at the EGH.) This episode at the EGH clearly demonstrates that the Grey Nuns considered it their duty to serve all those who were in need, irrespective of their creed or cultural background. This vision of

nursing was common to all religious nursing orders, for which the provision of care was a form of ministry. Indeed in all the years prior to the advent of hospital insurance, hospitals owned and/or operated by religious nursing orders served vulnerable populations without asking much in return. Although municipal hospitals provided some services to poorer individuals, it is fair to say that they did this to a lesser extent than did religious hospitals.

For all these religious orders, operating hospitals without much assistance from the state, while offering free services to large numbers of their patients, required ingenuity, determination, and faith. Nursing sisters found creative ways of keeping their hospitals alive at times of crisis. The dirty thirties were such a time, and the economic crisis threatened many institutions. In the case of the Grey Nuns of Edmonton, solvency was maintained by securing a provincial contract to take care of tuberculosis patients. Provincial grants were available for these patients, and this income compensated to some degree for the loss of "paying patients" who could now no longer afford payment because of the Depression.

Throughout the twentieth century western Canadian religious hospitals developed in parallel to their Eastern counterparts. By the 1970s, hospitals like the EGH or the Saint Paul's Hospital of Saskatoon, also operated by the Grey Nuns, and the Saint Paul's Hospital of Vancouver, operated by the Sisters of Providence, had grown into major urban institutions that provided all the services available regionally.

Nursing sisters were not only leaders in their own institutions but they also contributed significantly to nursing leadership in general and to nursing education. Although tensions have been documented between nursing sisters and the early nursing associations in Quebec,[18] sisters regularly served on the provincial councils of western Canadian nursing organizations. If Alberta is representative, nursing sisters also took a leadership role in Catholic Health Associations.[19] It is significant that the roles the sisters played in hospital administration made nursing present in many arenas where nurses would not have been represented. In general, nurses in lay hospitals had limited roles in higher administration; they were usually confined to nursing services. In contrast, sisters with a nursing background in Catholic hospitals were present in the administration of hospital departments and structures.

The Role of Religious Nursing Sisters in Nursing Education

Like their lay counterparts, nursing sisters' hospitals began to open schools of nursing in the early 1900s. These schools became increasingly important, since their students constituted a major workforce that could provide care and thus complement the services offered by the sisters. The number of Canadian nurses who were educated by nursing sisters is difficult to estimate. However, if one considers that the Grey Nuns of the EGH School of Nursing alone produced 1999 graduates between 1911 and 1973 (the year of its closure), one can extrapolate that the total number of nurses educated by sisters of all orders would be impressive.[20] Generations of nurses developed their nursing skills in religious hospitals from

coast to coast. The Grey Nuns of Montreal and the Grey Nuns of Ottawa also significantly contributed to the development of university nursing education, including the founding in 1934 by the Grey Nuns of Montreal, of the very first French-speaking university-level institution, l'Institut Marguerite d'Youville, which offered baccalaureate level nursing education.[21]

Language and Culture in the Community

As we have seen, the great majority of western Canadian nursing sisters were Roman Catholic and a large proportion of them were of French-Canadian origin. Although these sisters significantly contributed to the health of the population and were generally supported in their mission by those they served, tensions did occur. Some of these tensions have already been described in discussing the early years of the EGH, but other examples are found elsewhere in the history of that institution. Many of these issues surrounded the use of French. For example, in 1937, the local archbishop urged the sisters to officially recognize the EGH as an English-speaking institution.[22] Although this was not done, it is a good indicator that the issue of language was becoming problematic. Considering the nature of Canadian society at the time, it is more than likely that other nursing sisters in other locations would have had similar experiences. And tensions related to language did not only occur in the interaction between nursing sisters and the "outside" world, but also existed within orders. Sisters Cantwell and George Edmond, when writing about nuns of their own order (the Sisters of Saint Ann in Dawson), spoke about these tensions:

> Discordant views about the use of either French or English among the sisters were fraught with disruptive possibilities. Doctors and nurses, hearing the sisters speaking in French to each other, were uncomfortably suspicious of being discussed. The backgrounds of the sisters made the choice of either language unpopular, for some sisters were of French-Canadian descent; others, of British Columbian stock, or from various European cultures.[23]

WHMS Nurses in "Foreign" Settlements: The Ethelbert Mission

Ina Bramadat, Retired RN, PhD

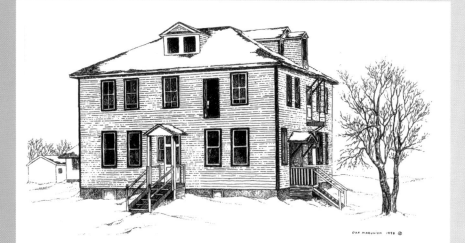

Figure 8
The Ethelbert Hospital, prior to demolition in 1983
Artist: Ora Maryniuk
United Church Archives, University of Winnipeg

In 1907, the Presbyterian Woman's Home Missionary Society (WHMS) answered an appeal from the Church to provide nursing services in Ethelbert, a community in the Ukrainian Dauphin Colony northwest of Winnipeg, the church's first "foreign" mission to new ethnic settlements on the Canadian Prairies.

WHMS nurses provided nursing care in the village dispensary and in settler's homes. Churches in more populated areas of the country sent bales of clothing and supplies to Ethelbert in response to WHMS reports of harsh frontier living conditions, isolation, and poverty. WHMS nurses were also trained missionaries. As part of the Church's mandate to integrate Ukrainian settlers into the culture of English-speaking Protestant society, nurses taught Sunday school, assisted with church services, and organized church groups. By 1915, the WHMS had built a 23-bed hospital with four nurses on staff. Although the hospital was not large enough to operate a training program, it provided practical nursing experience for girls from the local church boarding home.

By 1960, these local services were no longer needed. Paved highways provided ready access to larger facilities in Dauphin. The religious motivation that prompted the early nursing mission had lost its thrust, as the ideal of cultural assimilation changed to a vision of multiculturalism. As in other small communities across the Prairies, the Church's nursing mission was drawing to a close.

Today, the Protestant church stands alongside Catholic and Orthodox Ukrainian churches in one of the most vibrant centres of Ukrainian culture in Canada. Although the need for them has now passed, missionary nurses provided health care in the community for over five decades and were an essential part of Ethelbert's transition from frontier life to the present.

It is important to mention that the sisters were also active participants in the activities of the broader community. Their involvement would have been particularly important for their co-citizens when their ethnic group was in a minority situation, as was the case of the French-Canadians and Ukrainians. The sisters no doubt participated in church functions, but they were also found in community celebrations. For example, the Grey Nuns of Edmonton were involved in the planning of the French-Canadian celebration of Saint-Jean Baptiste Day. In 1928, the sisters assisted the Oblate Priests in the preparation of the June 24th picnic, and the hospital cafeteria was used to cook hams that had been purchased by La société Saint-Jean Baptiste. The sisters wrote: "We are happy to show our patriotism and to help the good Oblates."[24] Similarly, they made a point of being present at annual meetings of the French-Canadian association: l'Association Canadienne française de l'Alberta.[25]

Sisters from minority groups who shared the same cultural origin as their patients had first hand experience of this status and were likely better able to understand the needs of these patients than nurses who were members of the majority. The impact of this on the health of minority populations is difficult to evaluate. However, it is likely that simply being able to offer services in the mother tongue of their patients made a significant difference. Receiving care in one's own language would have been at least comforting.

Less Visible but Still Present: 1970–2003

The last three decades of the twentieth century brought significant changes that affected nursing sisters, gradually making them less visible. The advent of hospital and health care insurance, combined with the decline in religious vocations, presented major challenges. The more direct involvement of governments in hospital affairs meant changes in terms of policy, financing, and governance. And from the 1960s on, societal changes, including more opportunities for women and the advent of a more secular society, meant that recruitment into religious orders

was on the decline; a large proportion of nursing sisters were reaching retirement age and not being replaced. The aging of the nursing sisters workforce, coupled with the ever-increasing need for more hospital staff, made it difficult for religious orders to retain ownership of their hospitals. By the year 2000, the hospital landscape had dramatically changed, and, although many of the hospitals developed by the sisters continued to provide services, sisters themselves were no longer a constant presence. Yet to this day, there is something unique about these hospitals; a presence has remained as if sisters were still walking from ward to ward, providing some invisible comfort to the patients of today.

Conclusion

From the time of their arrival in western Canada around 1760, religious nursing orders made substantial contributions to the health care system in western Canada — and indeed across the country. Although their role in present years is now substantially diminished, their legacy is still very much with us. Nursing sisters were the first to provide health care in remote and frontier areas, and, when these areas became more settled, they were also among the first to establish and operate modern urban hospitals. Coming at the behest of clergy and initially serving the Native and Metis populations as well as early settlers, they stayed and continued to live by and spread their fundamental values of charity and faith, even as physicians, and later lay administrators, were gradually imposing their new scientific and more materialistic credo on hospitals and health care. Although French-speaking Roman Catholic orders originating in Quebec predominated, orders from other parts of Canada, as well as from England, France, and Ukraine, also made significant contributions. Religious nursing orders have also been significant contributors to Canadian nursing education, operating schools of nursing within their hospitals (such as the School of Nursing run by the Grey Nuns at EGH) and establishing university-level nursing programs. Generations of Canadian nurses were trained by nursing sisters, and countless health care institutions remain today as evidence of their years of loving labour. Although now aging, the remaining sisters continue to contribute to society; less involved in running major hospitals, they can now be found in other types of activities. Once again, they are seen providing food and shelter for those in need. No one can predict the future, but nursing sisters cared for generations of Canadians and that fact will always remain.

CHAPTER 9

Outpost Nursing in Canada

Dianne Dodd, Jayne Elliott, and Nicole Rousseau

Writing from her outpost nursing station in Atikokan in 1933, Red Cross nurse Maude Weaver described her previous week: Sunday night she admitted a woman who had had a stroke and was recovering but who had required "private duty nursing" in the two-bed outpost for the week. On Monday she stabilized an "acute abdomen" and put the patient on the train to Winnipeg. Wednesday morning she sutured a gash in a child's ankle. She boiled up "lots of things and put some cocaine in with a hypo needle above [the injury] and then put four stitches in with silk." That afternoon she arrived in time for the "last spasm" of a man who had suffered a fatal heart attack while out cutting oats. She called the coroner and signed transportation permits and other forms as proxy for him and the medical officer of health. Having no doctor meant that you "pretty well have to be undertaker along with everything else on this job," she wrote. The next morning as she accompanied the body to the train for shipment out to Fort William, the railway dispatcher told her she was needed fifteen miles down the line to attend to a sick woman. After rushing home for her bag, she boarded the train to Iron Spur "without even a hat." There she found a woman with a high temperature whom she suspected of having "gyn [*sic*] trouble," gave her an enema, a sponge bath, and the drugs codeine and aspirin. When her temperature jumped again in the afternoon, she contacted the railway dispatcher to stop the incoming freight train so she could send the woman to Port Arthur. Nurse Weaver summed things up: "It was a good sort of day for it seemed like a job worth doing, and my patient and her husband were so grateful."[1]

As Maude Weaver's account suggests, outpost nursing required independence and adaptability in order to care for patients in conditions that were far removed from those found in large, urban hospitals. No matter what the organization employing them, outpost nurses across the country confronted special challenges brought by working on the edges of settlement. Transportation and communication, for instance, posed their own sets of problems. And nurses often undertook tasks that went beyond the official bounds of their profession, as sanctioned by their nursing leaders, the medical profession, and legislative authorities. Those who succeeded in coping with these exacting demands gained considerable personal satisfaction and the respect of their communities.

Outpost nursing gained momentum in the 1920s, but began as early as the 1890s, and continues to the present day in some regions. Outpost nurses supplied professional expertise to populations who had little access to medical care. As public health teachers, the nurses undoubtedly reflected urban, white, middle class standards, which their patients were often

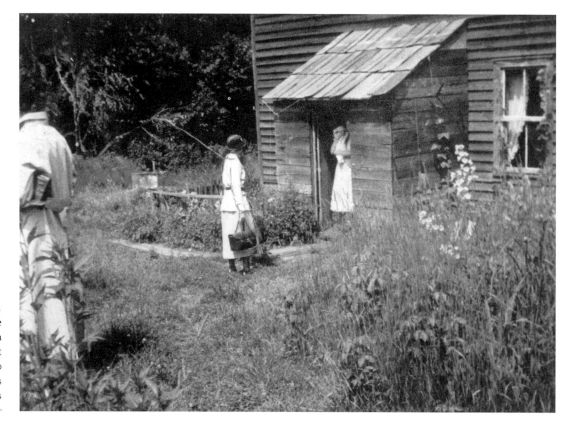

Figure 1
**Outpost Nurse
making a
home visit**
ca. 1920
Canadian Red Cross
Society Archives

unable or unwilling to meet. Nonetheless, their work had a significant impact on the health and welfare of isolated populations and helped to sustain and expand colonization efforts. Maternity care was one of their most important functions, and countless women without any other knowledgeable help available at delivery benefited from the skilled aid of their local outpost nurse. As well, by demonstrating the need for health care, outpost nurses promoted community and government support for the growing twentieth century health care infrastructure, thereby helping to build the social welfare state.[2]

The Origins of Outpost Nursing: The Victorian Order of Nurses

By the early twentieth century, physicians had more or less solidified their dominant position in the health care field. They enjoyed a monopoly on a fee-for-service basis for the provision of medical services, including maternity care. Until the introduction of universal hospital and medical insurance in the late 1950s and 60s, only the well off or steadily employed could afford to purchase health care protection offered through private insurance companies. Organized health care services for the truly indigent were managed through various municipalities or through private charitable groups. Entitlement to aid varied from place to place, however, and especially vulnerable were those living in the municipally unorganized rural and remote districts of the country. Responding to these conditions, several groups sought to provide health care services to isolated populations.

The route that brought Maude Weaver to her remote community began with the organizing efforts of the National Council of Women of Canada and the wife of Canada's Governor General, Lady Ishbel Aberdeen, who founded the Victorian Order of Nurses (VON) in 1897. Convinced that the lack of medical and nursing services for pioneer women contributed to a high maternal and infant mortality rate, they were angered by the refusal of the federal government to do anything despite its aggressive promotion of settlement. Thus, the VON sought to provide pre- and postnatal care for expectant mothers by establishing small cottage hospitals in communities throughout western and northern Ontario.[3] The vast geographic

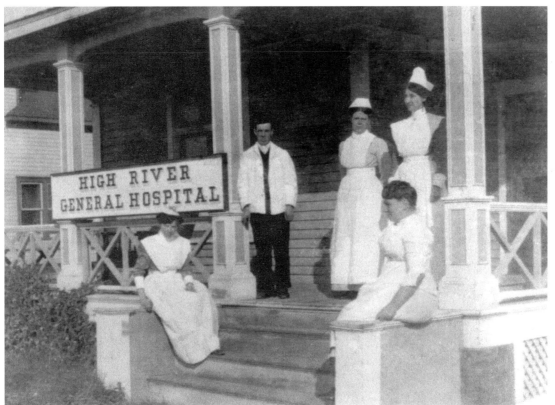

Figure 2
High River General Hospital and Staff
High River, Alberta
ca. 1914
Museum of Highwood, High River, Alberta

territory and sparse population in these areas made the cottage hospital program expensive. Small communities of struggling farmers and workers were hard pressed to provide even minimal support for medical and nursing facilities. Lady Minto, who succeeded Lady Aberdeen in 1900, embarked on a massive fundraising drive to finance the cottage hospitals, but the fund was soon exhausted, and the VON turned its attention to keeping existing hospitals open. The VON also offered visiting nurse services in "country districts," and by 1915, 19 districts had been established. Geography and insufficient community support again doomed the rural visiting nurse program to failure, although the VON's urban work gained momentum. This pioneering work demonstrated the need for health care and convinced medical officials that nurses were effective ambassadors of health, able to gain the confidence of women in the home who were responsible for the family's health care.[4]

The Impact of the Great War

Only in the aftermath of the First World War was the work of the VON finally recognized. The tragedy of untreated and preventable childhood illnesses, which had led to the rejection of high numbers of potential recruits, drove home the message that young Canadians were not very healthy. With the close of hostilities, ex-soldiers returned to Canada bearing not only physical and emotional scars, but also harbouring tuberculosis and venereal disease. With so many young "future fathers" lost in the war, maternal welfare took on a new significance in terms of rebuilding the nation.[5]

Responding, among other pressures, to the emphasis on health care directed at mothers and children, particularly among soldiers' families, the federal government established the Department of Health in 1919. A year later it organized a Child Welfare Division under Dr Helen MacMurchy. These events gave tacit recognition to the revolutionary notion that health care might now be both an entitlement of citizens and a responsibility of the state. The health department received requests for information for outpost mothers who feared that medical and nursing aid might not be available at the time of birth. Many of these requests came through the Home Branch of

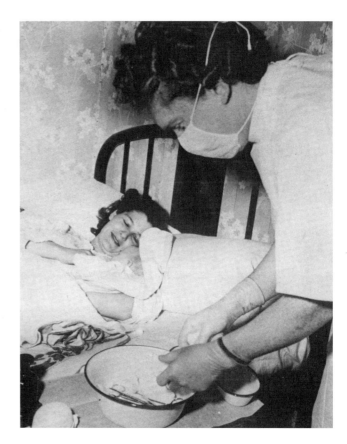

Figure 3
Laura Attrux, Home Delivery
Slave Lake, Alberta
1953
Irene Stewart, *These Were Our Yesterdays*,
Friesen: Altona, Man. 1979

the Soldier Settlement Board, which was helping to settle 25 000 ex-soldiers on "surplus" lands in the western provinces. "Discovering" that pioneer women lacked maternity care — a problem that the VON had brought to light decades earlier — MacMurchy wrote a special supplement to the *Canadian Mother's Book* in 1923, explaining the labour process in considerable detail and giving some practical advice on how to handle an "emergency birth." Still, the book was no substitute for medical care, and only served to highlight the frightening implications of facing childbirth without professional care.[6]

Outpost Programs across Canada: From the Voluntary to the Professional

As a more effective strategy, public health officials were already turning to programs providing nurses for isolated communities. These nurses maintained clinics and sometimes hospital wards in their homes, and supplied a generalized nursing service to residents of their remote districts. The work begun by the VON was adopted and expanded by better-financed provincial governments and quasi-official organizations, such as the Canadian Red Cross (CRS), in the interwar period. The program with the widest national coverage during these years was a chain of outpost nursing stations and hospitals established by the Canadian Red Cross Society (CRCS). Others included the Newfoundland Outpost Nursing and Industrial Association (NONIA), the International Grenfell Association (also in Newfoundland and Labrador), the Alberta District Nursing Service, and the Quebec government's Medical Service to Settlers (MSS), as well as federal nurses working in Aboriginal communities. Some of the public health nurses in rural British Columbia also fit the criteria for outpost nurses.[7] Although these programs took

different organizational forms, they shared a common approach to delivering health care to isolated populations. Recognizing the difficulty in attracting physicians, who could not make a living in remote areas with scattered, poor populations, most jurisdictions hired nurses to staff their outposts. Less expensive than doctors, they were also presumed to be the most efficient and sympathetic carriers of the public health message to mothers in their homes.

The VON-inspired model of outpost programs, in which influential lay women allied with nursing professionals, evolved into a bureaucratic undertaking directed by male government administrators and physicians. Like the VON, NONIA got its start through the organizing efforts of political wives, and represents the last gasp of lay women's leadership. After visiting coastal communities in the early 1920s, Lady Harris, wife of Newfoundland's governor, organized the Outport Nursing Committee. With the help of the Overseas Nursing Association, the group recruited four nurses certified in midwifery from England. The Committee supplied them with dressings and drugs,

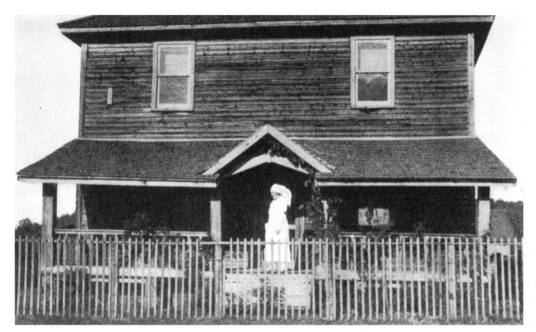

Figure 4
Wilberforce Outpost, opened in 1922
Hospitals in Ontario: a Short History, Toronto Department of Health, 1934

guaranteed a salary of $900 a year and sent them to four outport communities. When Sir William Allardyce replaced Governor Harris in 1922, his wife, Lady Elsie Allardyce, continued and expanded the program. As cash-poor outport communities could not afford the nurses' salaries, Lady Allardyce imported the innovative idea of "knitting circles," which had been used in the Shetland and Orkney Islands to service war needs.[8] In 1924, the organization became the Newfoundland Outport Nursing and Industrial Association. A total of 45 NONIA nurses served the residents of 29 outport communities from 1920 to 1934, treating over 83 000 patients and making over 232 000 home visits.[9]

In Alberta, the provincial government created the District Nursing Service in 1919 as the result of the lobbying of the United Farm Women of Alberta and other women's organizations. Anxious to keep the farm vote, the Liberal party passed the *Public Health Nurses Act* in April of that year. Government administrators and physicians, rather than lay women, sent nurses into remote areas with authority to practise midwifery where no doctors resided. Up until 1934, only eight nurses had been hired for the program, partly because communities were required to provide and maintain the nurses' homes, and partly because it was difficult to find nurses with the necessary obstet-

rical training. Expansion came during the Depression and then again as doctors left the province to serve in the Second World War. By 1945, the service maintained 36 nurses in the field.[10]

The CRCS created the largest of the interwar outpost nursing programs with the widest national coverage. Inspired by an international conference on health and social welfare following the First World War, and buoyed by its significant post-war prestige and financial resources, the CRCS launched a comprehensive public health plan. As one aspect of this program, the divisions of the Society combined with local community groups and provincial health departments to establish one-nurse outposts and small hospitals in the rural and remote districts of the country. A great deal of regional variation resulted, reflecting the autonomy of the divisions and varying levels of support from the provincial governments. The Ontario Division administered the most complex outpost program, opening the first of its 43 outposts in Wilberforce in 1922. The support of Adelaide Plumptre, as an accomplished lay woman organizer, was critical to the initiation of the outpost program, but a professional group of male physicians and elite nursing personnel guided its development at the national and provincial levels.[11]

In contrast, the MSS was created in response to

pressure from the clergy and was only officially formed after a ten-year period of testing. The Depression had motivated the provincial government to give land to indigent people wishing to settle outside the urban centres, and this movement had given rise to colonies or settlements comprised of very poor populations. Many of these poor communities, however, were unable to attract a physician. The clergy ministering to these communities suggested what came to be characterized as "the most reasonable solution": allowing nurses to perform interventions normally restricted to physicians (assisting with childbirth, diagnosing illnesses, prescribing drugs, and performing minor surgery). The first of such nurses, Eveline Bignell, came to settle on the North Shore on 26 August 1926 to assist birthing women and to provide medical assistance to people with "ordinary ailments." For the following ten years, Dr Alphonse Lessard, director of both the Provincial Bureau of Health (PBH) and the Bureau of Public Charities (BPC) from 1921 to 1936, used his discretionary powers, against vigorous opposition from the physicians, to hire nurses for poor communities instead of subsidizing doctors. Aurore Bégin in Abitibi, Anita Dionne-Ott in the Saguenay, and Gabrielle Blais in Témiscouata were also hired in the early 1930s by Dr Lessard as a temporary, urgent, and exceptional solution to the lack of medical services in settlements. There was still no administrative structure, and there were no facilities; the nurses often lived at the rectory, among the settlers, or at the village school.

As the Depression hit and government funded settlements in remote areas continued to multiply, a more structured solution was clearly needed. On 24 December 1935, representatives of the Department of Colonization, the BPC, and the PBH, under the prodding of Lessard, finally managed to agree to set up a service to systematically hire nurses to provide indigent settlers with minimum health assistance and to establish these nurses in residential dispensaries. Thus was created the Medical Service to Settlers in 1936, with Dr Émile Martel as its first director. Out of this structure emerged a network of outposts served exclusively by nurses working in collaboration with regional physicians. This "temporary" service proved

to be a fixture for 36 years. By 1953 there were 119 outposts, most with a residential dispensary, and even after the service was abolished in 1962, some residential dispensaries were maintained.[12] In Abitibi and on the Lower North Shore traces still persist today of the 174 outposts created, 122 of which had a residential dispensary financed by the government of Quebec.[13]

As far as the northern regions of the country were concerned, the federal government took reluctant responsibility for Aboriginal people at Confederation, but it was not until 1904 that the Department of Indian Affairs began to place a limited number of nurses in outposts throughout the Arctic and Subarctic regions of the country. In the words of one physician administrator, a health service was necessary both for "humanitarian reasons ... and to prevent the spread of disease to the White population."[14] By 1946, 24 nurses were in the field, although the Inuit people did not receive their first nursing station until 1947. The policies implemented by the federal department attempted to impose southern medical practices on the northern indigenous cultures. The nurses were usually culturally unprepared for their work, and some perceived their posting as a chance to expand their autonomy and authority. Nevertheless, many of them came to respect community traditions and were able to work congenially with the local midwives and other people.

Outpost Nursing: The Challenges of Nursing Practice in the Wilderness

As nurses and as supporters of the outposts at the local level, women played a significant role. A great deal of autonomy, albeit little support, was afforded outpost nurses by the distance to physicians and hospitals, which forced them to draw on all elements of their education, including public health teaching, district bedside nursing, emergency treatment, and, for some, in-hospital patient care. Alberta District Nurse Mary Conlin Sterritt, for example, managed difficult deliveries, sutured the victims of farm accidents, battled epidemics of flu and diphtheria, and held makeshift clinics at local dances because the people realized it was a "convenient opportunity" to consult the nurse on "the itch, the stitch, the gout and the

Gertrude Duchemin (1910–1990)

Brigitte Violette, Parks Canada

Gertrude Duchemin was born in Sainte-Thècle (Champlain County) on 20 May 1910, and grew up in Saint-Tite, in Mauricie. She trained at the nursing school of the Sisters of Providence in the hospital in Lachine, graduating as a nurse in Montreal in 1932. At first, she was in private practice in Montreal, and then she took a position at the dispensary of the Hôpital Notre-Dame de Montréal. An accident put an end to this employment in 1934. During her convalescence, she went to stay with her two brothers in Amos, in the Abitibi region, and on 15 December 1936 she was hired as a nurse to "work in hygiene and provide certain medical services to indigent settlers in the cantons of La Corne et Varsan [Vassan]."

Like all outpost nurses, Duchemin was called upon to attend childbirths. Over the years, she developed such an expertise in obstetrics that women in neighbouring counties came to ask for her services. Her fellow nurses stated that her excellent knowledge of pathologies and their treatment enabled her to practise with ease and without risk.

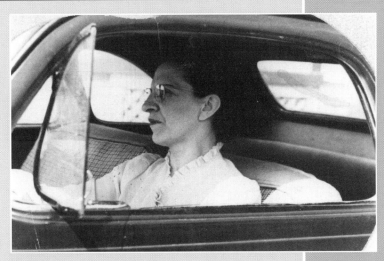

Figure 5
Gertude Duchemin in her car
La Corne, Abitibi, Quebec
ca. 1945
Photographer: Desparois
Collection of 'Le Dispensaire de la garde' Corporation

Like her colleagues practising in isolated regions, Duchemin crossed gender barriers on both the professional and personal levels. She had a brush with the second parish priest when he reminded her that it was forbidden for women to wear trousers. As she was the only one in the village to defy the curé's ban, all eyes in the community were upon her. Determined to have the ban lifted, Duchemin addressed the bishop of Amos, who stood behind her, confirming that the way she dressed was dictated by her functions.

Duchemin retired on 1 January 1976 after 40 years of service. Two years later, she became the owner of the dispensary-residence in which she had lived since 1940. She lived there until 1990, when she succumbed to cancer at the age of 80.

Sources: Claire Martin, outpost nurse [*infirmière de colonie*] in Abitibi-Témiscamingue, autumn 1992. Historical account presented by Le dispensaire de la garde Corporation, La Corne, Abitibi, as part of the Programme d'aide aux organismes en matière de patrimoine administered by the Ministère des Affaires culturelles du Québec, Direction de l'Abitibi-Témiscamingue; Société historique d'Amos, Fonds P63, Fonds Gertrude Duchemin, ANQ M.1-711, dossier P63/T-2-23.

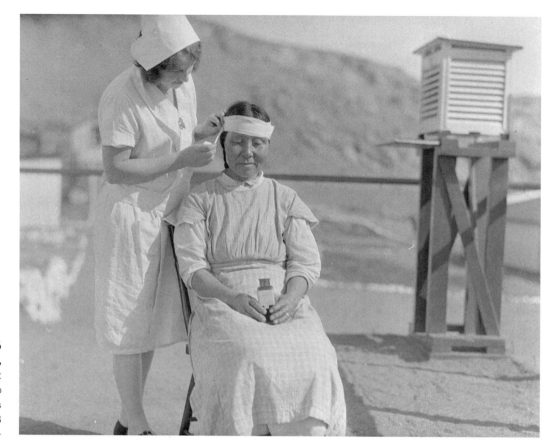

Figure 6
**Baffin Island,
Nunavut**
1930
Library and Archives
Canada, PA-1014458

palsy."[15] Remaining available on a 24-hour basis
for consultation, advice, and treatment, the nurses
directed much of the work on their own or with the
advice of a distant physician. School inspections
formed a large part of their public health work, where
they examined, immunized, and gave health talks to
thousands of school children. Outpost nurses also
organized tonsil, eye, and dental clinics for travelling
teams of doctors and dentists, and, in the case of the
Red Cross nurses working in the small outpost hospitals, helped local and visiting physicians to perform
hundreds of operations. Within certain limits, outpost
nurses could organize their time as they saw fit, an
aspect of professional nursing not possible for those
employed in hospitals or in private duty nursing.
Setting up new public health programs and finding
creative ways to adapt their nursing training to work
in an isolated environment was for some a welcome
challenge. On Gertrude LeRoy Miller's first tour of the
Wilberforce Red Cross outpost in 1930, she declared
that although "it wasn't much like a hospital ... I could
see the possibilities, and it was mine."[16] On the other

hand, the nurses were sometimes frightened of the
responsibility required of them. For Conlin Sterritt,"
[t]he idea of working on one's own, sometimes at
a distance of from 40 to 60 miles from a doctor,
appealed to me while it filled me with apprehension."[17]

Maternity care was the primary motivation
behind the establishment of nursing outposts and
remained one of the nurses' most important functions. As with this and many of the other tasks that
they performed, outpost nurses usually lacked the
necessary training. Although most authorities tended
to ignore these expanded nursing responsibilities
in the isolated areas, midwifery was illegal in every
jurisdiction except Newfoundland, which followed
the European model of regulating rather than eliminating midwifery. The 1919 *Public Health Nurses' Act*
in Alberta, however, did give nurse-midwives permission to practise midwifery in areas with no physicians. The federal government preferred to hire
nurses with midwifery experience for the northern
nursing stations. Nervous about the "alegal" status
of midwifery, based on the presumption that deliver-

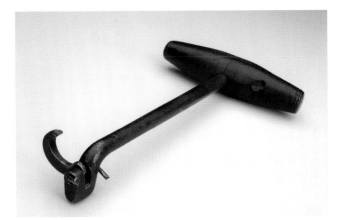

Figure 7 (left)
Tooth Extractor
early 20th century
Photographer: Doug Millar
Canadian Museum of Civilization, D-2289
Gift of Dr. Frederick Lowry

Figure 8 (below)
**Nurse Miller and patient discharged home
on toboggan from Red Cross Outpost**
Wilberforce, Ontario
Wilberforce Guild Heritage Collection

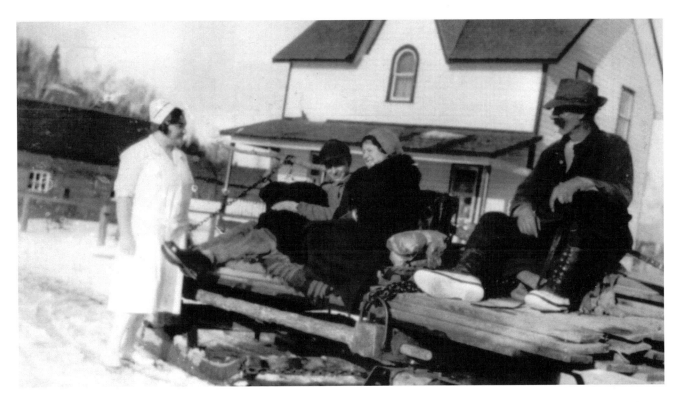

ing babies was the province of physicians, it refused financial recognition comparable to that given to nurses with public health education. Few outpost nurses received advanced education in obstetrics; most tried to remember what they had learned during their regular nurses' training and acquired their skills through experience. After the promised help of a nurse-midwife never materialized, nurse Jean Goodwill delivered 50 babies in her first year with the Department of National Health and Welfare in the Arctic with no special midwifery training. From 1932 to 1938, nurse Anita Dionne-Ott delivered 350 babies in northern Quebec, including five sets of twins. She also handled numerous abnormal presentations, and lost only one baby. Like physicians, she used forceps, performed episiotomies and often collaborated with local *sage-femmes*. Not all nurses were comfortable in their role as midwife, at least initially. Louise de Kiriline at the Bonfield Red Cross outpost "breathed thanks to God" after her first delivery, "[and] I was a little relieved the mother thought I was reliable."[18]

Other aspects of outpost nurses' work also encroached on the role of physicians. Although LeRoy Miller stated, "nurses never, no never diagnose," in reality, the isolation of outpost nurses forced them to make treatment decisions, including decisions

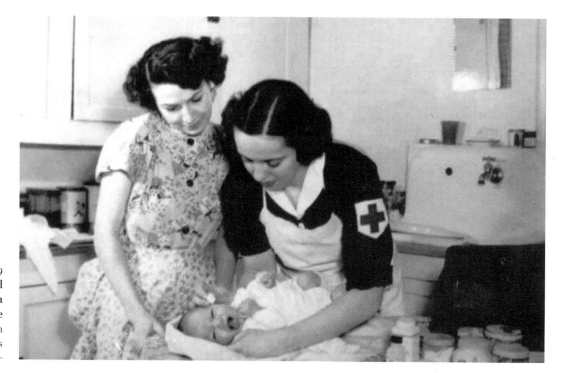

about whether or not patients needed to be sent to the nearest hospital. Nurses under the MSS in Quebec were instructed to first "make a summary diagnosis" — usually the jealously-guarded preserve of physicians — before hospitalizing a patient. As a result of being the only medical person in the district, nurses also found themselves regularly performing other non-nursing services: dispensing medications, dealing with dental emergencies, and even acting as the local veterinarian. In August 1942, Louisette Beaudoin took charge of the nursing station of Beaucanton, in Abitibi, where she was entitled to claim up to $5 for each child she delivered and was required to sell the drugs she bought herself for her little pharmacy. Several other Quebec nurses admitted that pulling teeth was a part of their practice that they heartily disliked.

Transportation for both nurses and patients in frontier areas was a constant challenge. By the late 1920s, some nurses had begun to use cars to visit their patients in areas with roads or well marked trails. This was limited to the summer and early fall when the roads were passable. Otherwise, nurses travelled by horseback or horse and buggy in summer, and horse- or dog-drawn sleigh in winter. Quebec nurses also used snowmobiles. Alberta district nurses sometimes used a stoneboat, a horse hitched to a flat piece of board used to convey stones from the fields. Those close to railway lines on the Prairies and in some parts of northern Ontario often used the railway jigger or speeder, sometimes with a trailer behind to transport a patient. Nurses in the Magdalen Islands travelled between the islands by lobster boat in all conditions of weather and sea.

Outpost Nursing and the Community

Most of the early outposts were located in pre-existing buildings, usually former homes, which allowed the various organizations to establish their nurses quickly and efficiently. Until a *dispensaire* could be built, some of the Quebec nurses lived in the homes of local residents, setting up their offices there. Precarious financing at the local level meant that living conditions for outpost nurses were often rudimentary. Alberta district nurse Janet Munroe Reynolds, who lived in a former granary, was forced to hack off a chunk of ice from an outdoor bin to obtain her water.[19] In the early years, only a handful of the nursing outposts were purpose-built. For example, the CNR, which also donated a travelling railway car/outpost station, financed two identical architect-

Figure 10

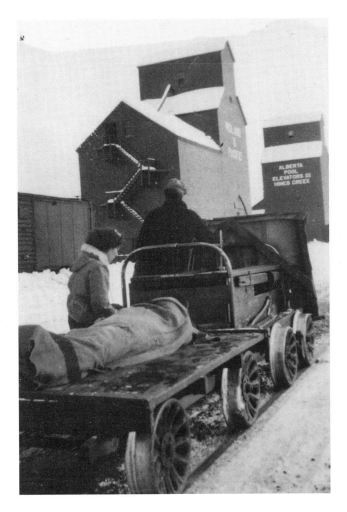

Alberta nurse and patient on a speeder
Glenbow Archives, Calgary, Alberta, NA 3953-5

nurse.[20] Other ways in which communities assisted were less formal. Many of the nurses, for example, received assistance from local men in transporting patients to hospitals or reaching isolated patients.

Not all outpost nurses were successful in integrating into the community. Some left after a short while, overwhelmed by the remote environment, loneliness, and lack of professional stimulation. Margaret Maclachlan noted that if she had remained with the Red Cross, she would have needed frequent breaks, "otherwise you are just bushed."[21] But those who made the transition were aided by taking part in local activities. Some played the organ at church and attended dances, card parties, and other events. Several Quebec nurses, one of whom won the Order of Canada, were active in such groups as *Cercle des fermières* and *Femmes chrétiennes* — one was even president of a local *Caisse populaire* (savings and credit cooperative). Federal government nurses working in the North who communicated respect for local midwives often gained their trust and confidence.[22] Quebec nurse Blanche Pronovost, whose life has been immortalized through the popular 1986 novel *Les filles de Caleb* (Arlette Cousture) and a subsequent television series, *Blanche*, donned breeches, cut her own firewood, and negotiated with local residents. Clearly their pioneering lifestyles allowed some nurses to step outside the bounds of traditional gender and professional roles.

Nation Building: Colonization and Building a Modern Health Care System

Outpost nursing ventures provided support to small communities by supplying much needed health care to settlers and resource workers, bolstering a sense of entitlement to health care, and increasing pressure for state funding. Community-based, women-led agitation for medical aid stimulated provincial governments in Alberta to institute the District Nursing Service, as well as the MSS in Quebec. The

designed buildings at Hornepayne and Nakina in 1925 for the Red Cross in Ontario.

The lives of the outpost nurses and the communities in which they lived and worked were often closely intertwined. Local committees formed in areas seeking an outpost nursing service, and were required to contribute both volunteer labour and financial support to the maintenance of the facility and the nurses. Although these activities were not exclusively undertaken by women, such groups as the Women's Institutes and the IODE figured prominently. Fundraising to support the outpost was an important task of the local group. Most of the outpost organizations paid the salaries of their nurses, but Newfoundland communities wanting NONIA nurses had to finance their salaries directly. Drawing on women's craft and organizational skills, each family was expected to provide the services of one volunteer knitter, part of whose profits contributed to the salary of the

Myra Grimsley Bennett, Newfoundland Outport Nurse

Dianne Dodd, Parks Canada

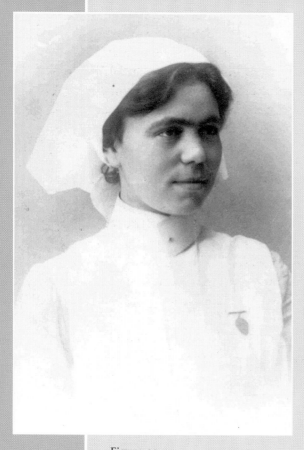

Figure 11
Myra Grimsley Bennett
England
1915
Myra Bennett House Foundation

Myra Grimsley Bennett (1890–1990), was one of several British nurses, all trained in midwifery, who came to outport Newfoundland in 1920 through the newly formed Outport Nursing Committee. The inspiration of Lady Constance Harris, wife of Newfoundland's governor, the committee was reorganized in 1924 as the Newfoundland Outport Nursing and Industrial Association (NONIA).

Grimsley was sent to Daniel's Harbour, Newfoundland, where she was responsible for 200 miles of coast, the nearest doctor being 120 miles away at Corner Brook and the nearest hospital, at St. Anthony, at the far north of the peninsula. Grimsley provided a wide range of health care services, from midwifery to minor surgery, in this poor and isolated outport community. She was fond of remarking that she was glad to have purchased a device called a "universal forceps" before her departure for Newfoundland. It proved handy for pulling teeth, another of her many tasks.

Grimsley married local resident Angus Bennett in 1922, and he proved to be her lifelong "para-medic." Her marriage and integration into the community helped ensure a good relationship with both patients and local lay healers. Myra continued to nurse on a voluntary basis even after her marriage forced her to "retire." When the Department of Health took over the nursing functions of NONIA in 1934, Bennett was paid a small salary as a part-time nurse, allowing her to refer patients to the hospital and to dispense drugs. Nurse Bennett later became a full-time employee, retiring at age 65. She has been honoured with a number of awards, including the Medal of the British Empire. Her former home in Daniel's Habour, the Nurse Myra Bennett Heritage House, is now a museum interpreting her outport nursing service.

CRS also fostered government participation in health care, attempting to "fill the gap" until both the people and various levels of government could take on the responsibility for the continuation of the outposts.

Outpost nursing programs significantly enhanced the available training facilities for public health nurses in Canada. In 1897, the VON established "Training Homes" in Ottawa, Montreal, Toronto, and Halifax, which offered the only opportunity for a trained nurse to follow a formal course in public health/visiting nursing in Canada. Immediately following the First World War, the Red Cross funded public health nursing courses in five universities across the country. The needs of the Alberta District Nursing Service in 1943 to boost the training of new district nurses encouraged the University of Alberta to institute a three-month course in Advanced Practical Obstetrics. Dalhousie University in 1967 initiated a midwifery course to supply more nurses to northern outpost communities.

In addition to formal training opportunities, the outpost nurses exchanged information with local lay midwives. In Quebec, Newfoundland, and the Arctic, for example, outpost nurses often included midwives in their rounds, and shared their knowledge of modern methods. One suspects that the nurses also learned a great deal from the midwives, whose experience in handling deliveries on their own was far greater. Federal nurses who served Aboriginal communities may well have helped to prolong traditional birthing practices even as they altered expectations for medical care, which fundamentally changed the delivery of health care in the North.[23]

Present Day Outpost Nursing

Few outpost nursing services remain, since most have been incorporated into the health care infrastructure. The first to be taken over by government was NONIA's nursing service, which became part of the Newfoundland cottage hospital system in 1934. The industrial side of the organization continues to provide outlets for women's entrepreneurial and artisanal talents. Following the Second World War, other outpost nursing services began to decline due to

improvements in transportation, the increasing use of hospitals for births, and the introduction of hospitalization and medical insurance. Renamed the Municipal Nursing Service, the Alberta District Nursing Service became, by the 1960s, virtually the same as that provided by public health nurses and the program was finally discontinued in 1976. After the introduction of hospitalization insurance in 1959, the Red Cross Divisions gradually relinquished their outposts; the Ontario Division finally transferred its last outpost hospital at Burks Falls in 1984. The Western Zone of the Red Cross, however, currently maintains six outposts in British Columbia. Federal nurses still staff outposts in the North, but most women are now flown out of their communities to have their babies, with the attendant social and emotional disruptions to family life that a prolonged absence brings.

In Quebec, the work of the nurses with the MSS agency underwent a profound transformation between 1961 and 1972. After the *Hospital Insurance Act* came into force in 1961, physicians refused to provide assistance to nurses delivering babies in the home. Nurses such as Louisette Beaudoin found themselves caught between the risks of prosecution in the event of complications and pressures from the women who still wanted to have home deliveries. In 1971, the *Act respecting health services and social services* completely restructured health and social services in Quebec, and the remaining staff were integrated into community health departments attached to the hospital centres and local community service centres (CLSCs). Physicians were still reluctant to practise in the remote areas, however. For this reason Thérèse Mercier, who had left the Montmagny CLSC in 1976, continued to offer weekend consultations for another two years at the request of the local population. A few nursing stations also lingered on in Abitibi, and as late as 1986 a new one was opened in Aylmer Sound on the Lower North Shore.

Conclusions

From the late nineteenth century, woman's organizations such as the VON had called attention to the high rate of maternal and infant mortality. When the military was forced to reject a high number of soldiers due to preventable childhood illnesses in the Great War, governments began to take the general state of health of its citizens seriously and gradually adopted and expanded work begun by women's voluntary groups. The administration of district nurses initially by lay women's groups such as the VON and NONIA, gave way to a professionally staffed program dominated by male physicians and bureaucrats. In search of a role in public health, the Red Cross established an outpost nursing network, utilizing and offering training to nurses, who were considered the ideal conduit through which public health education could be disseminated. The nurses brought health and medical care to neglected populations and shared many of the same difficulties with the isolated people they served. Willing to work independently, they obtained a level of skill in areas far beyond their training. Doing what they could, learning on the job, and hoping for the best, they delivered babies, performed minor surgery and first aid, pulled teeth, dispensed drugs, and diagnosed illness — all tasks considered beyond the traditional role of the nurse. Pioneers in all senses of the term, outpost, outport, and district nurses supported the colonization and settlement of large parts of Canada. As well, they helped lay the foundation for formal government involvement in health and medical care, aiding in the construction of a major component of the social welfare state.

Caregiving on the Front: The Experience of Canadian Military Nurses during World War I

Geneviève Allard

During the years leading up to World War I, the nursing profession in Canada had begun to be organized: among other things, schools were opened and associations were created, helping to establish the professional status of the caregiver's work in society. During this period, aware of the advantages that the presence of nurses would provide during military operations, the Canadian army invited groups of nurses to accompany the troops on various military expeditions, and these invitations were the prelude to the creation of a true military nurses' corps in 1908. However, in September 1914, even after ten years in existence, the Canadian Army Nursing Corps (CANC) comprised fewer than 30 reservists, only five of whom were permanent members. And its members were poorly prepared to handle the events that they were about to face. A few months before the war, Margaret MacDonald was appointed matron-in-chief of the CANC under the Canadian Expeditionary Force (CEF). Using her experience in the Boer War and in Canadian military hospitals, MacDonald had to mobilize a convoy of military nurses to serve overseas. An appeal was launched, and less than three weeks after Canada declared war, nurses with diplomas from all regions of the country offered their services for the duration of the war. Two thousand and three women enlisted in the CANC and were sent overseas. During the war, these nurses cared for almost 540 000 soldiers, working near the front lines, even risking their lives, as full members of the CEF; in fact, 53 of them lost their lives on active duty. They stirred the popular imagination and benefited from an aura of prestige.

At the turn of the twentieth century, the front was perceived as an exclusively male domain. In principle, women had neither the skills nor the qualities required to practise their profession there. The realities of the Great War, however, made the presence of women caregivers necessary, even indispensable, in proximity to the line of fire.

Acclaimed as war heroines at the time of demobilization, this group of caregivers had helped to provide the young profession of nursing and its training program with a stamp of legitimacy, and it saw its golden age in the years following World War I. Was this in part thanks to the visibility that the military nurses achieved? Although we know surprisingly little about the military experiences of these women — few historians have taken an interest and the nurses themselves have remained very discreet — the personal diaries, correspondence, and accounts of these women have begun to be gathered, analyzed, and studied. They demonstrate that on both the professional and personal levels, having been to war marked their lives. Nurses' presence in and

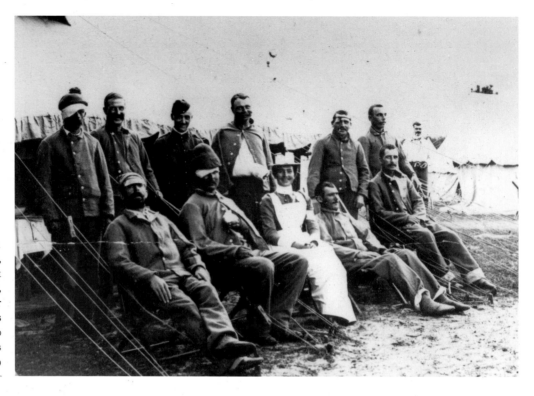

Figure 1
**Miss Minnie Affleck,
Nursing Sister, First
Canadian Contingent,
South African War
with wounded soldiers**
ca. 1900
Library and Archives
Canada, C-051799

contribution to the CEF improved the organization of medical care at the front and, as a consequence, had a noticeable effect on the physical and mental health of the soldiers under their care, just as, conversely, the conflict had an effect on the nurses' lives.

It is therefore of great interest to examine the origins and components of the CANC, as well as how nursing was practised at the front, in order to understand how military nursing during World War I fit within and had an impact on the development of the nursing profession in Canada.

The Canadian Army Nursing Corps

Brief History of the Military Nursing Service

The military nursing service is indebted, above all, to the volunteer efforts of nurses who, in various ways, made a difference during wartime by demonstrating the usefulness, and even the necessity, of their activity. Florence Nightingale is considered, rightly or wrongly, the pioneer of modern nursing, and in particular of military nursing. Her service tending to soldiers during the Crimean War (1854–56) and her constant efforts to improve the effectiveness of nurses' work convinced both the pub-

lic and the military authorities that it was essential to organize a more complete medical corps within the armed forces instead of offering the services of only one medical officer per regiment.

Nightingale's experiences[1] also showed that an effective nursing service had to be independent of the military authorities. As a consequence, the British nursing service began to establish its own structures in 1855. Although attached to the army, the nursing corps was autonomous on the administrative level. The British Nurse Corps borrowed some operating rules from the Armed Forces, notably the wearing of a uniform, respect for hierarchy, and adherence to a strict code of conduct. The CANC, created and placed under the charge of the Department of Militia and Defence, took inspiration from British traditions, but quickly went in its own direction.[2]

In 1870, military troops were sent to the Canadian Northwest to quell the Metis Rebellion, led by Louis Riel. Minister of Militia and Defence Adolphe Caron assigned Lieutenant-Colonel Darby Bergin the task of organizing the medical services to accompany the members of the RCMP. Bergin intended to hire women to be part of the medical service.

Georgina Fane Pope (1862–1938)

Cameron Pulsifer, Canadian War Museum

Georgina Fane Pope was the first full-time matron of the Canadian Army Medical Corps. Daughter of the prominent Prince Edward Island lawyer, politician, and "Father of Confederation," William Pope, she grew up in an environment of comfort and gentility. But in 1884 she entered the nursing program at the Bellevue Hospital in New York. After occupying a number of prestigious nursing appointments in the United States, in 1899 she returned to her native land to volunteer her services for the Canadian contingent that was due to leave for the South African War. Pope became the head of an initial party of four nurses, which was increased to eight in February 1900. Later she headed another group of eight Canadian nurses that served in South Africa for six months in 1902.

Pope possessed what her colleague Margaret Macdonald described as "splendid organizing ability," and under her "charming" but "stern" guidance the Canadian nurses did outstanding work under trying conditions caring for the wounded and helping to fight the ravages of the greatest killer in South Africa, enteric fever. A direct result of their work was the decision of the Department of Militia in August 1901 to create a cadre of part-time nurses. When, in 1906, the departure of the British garrison from Halifax increased the Canadian Medical Corps' responsibilities there, Pope and Macdonald were appointed to full-time positions, with Nurse Pope becoming matron in 1908. In August 1917, Pope left Halifax to join the staff of No. 2 Stationary Hospital at Outreau on the Western Front. But her health broke under the strain and she was repatriated to Canada, suffering from what was termed "shell shock." She died and was buried at Charlottetown in June 1938, a talented and energetic pioneer who stretched herself to and perhaps beyond the limits.

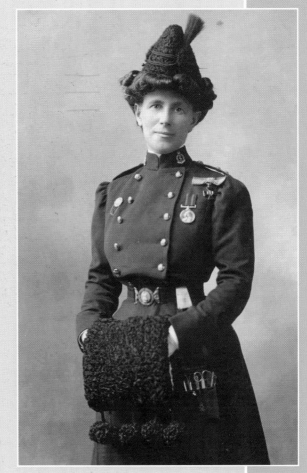

Figure 2
Georgina Fane Pope
Canadian War Museum, 19830041-182

Source: G W L Nicholson, *Canada's Nursing Sisters* (Toronto: Hakkert, 1975), 43.

Four volunteer civilian nurses were selected to care for the wounded for a period of several months. Having quickly proved how useful they were, these nurses were followed, at the end of their tour of service, by successive groups of volunteer nurses until the hostilities ended. The nurses were warmly applauded for their courage and endurance, and they received — rare for women at the time — a military decoration, the Northwest Medal,[3] as a reward for their efforts.

Given the success of the organization of medical care during the Northwest Rebellion, Lieutenant-Colonel Bergin planned to create a permanent army medical corps composed of doctors and nurses, which would be independent of the other army corps. Once peace was re-established, the project was more or less shelved, but the idea of maintaining a regular group of nurses to care for soldiers began to be considered.

In 1898, the federal government sent 200 volunteer soldiers to the Yukon to support the RCMP, which was dealing with problems caused by the gold rush. No medical officer accompanied the contingent, but four nurses from the Victorian Order of Nurses (VON) made the trip and bore the main responsibility for medical care of the soldiers on the long journey to Dawson City. They also tended to the residents of the various mining villages located on the route northward.

The trip took three months, and when they arrived in Dawson City, the four nurses remained there to tend to the region's population. Their work, performed under difficult conditions — inadequate facilities, lack of equipment, inclement weather — earned them praise and the respect of the Canadian military authorities.

However, the Canadian Armed Forces (CAF) had not yet integrated nurses into its permanent structures. When the Boer War was declared in 1899, the medical services of the Canadian Army, created when hostilities began between the British and South Africans, did not include a military nursing service. Nevertheless, the Canadian military authorities made the decision to attach a group of nurses to the convoy of soldiers sent to the front, and eight nurses were selected to accompany the several thousand Canadian volunteers.[4] The nurses sent to South Africa, unlike those who went to the Yukon under the VON banner, wore uniforms supplied by the Canadian army.

Following this war, in 1899, the general director of the CAF's medical services recommended that an official military nursing corps be formed. With the support of the commander of the Canadian militia, who had been impressed once more by the nurses' work in emergency situations, the recommendation was accepted, and the Canadian Army Nursing Corps began to be built in 1901. Even before the corps' administrative structure was established, Great Britain found itself embroiled in renewed hostilities in South Africa. Eight nurses, four of whom had served in the first episode of the war, went to South Africa, this time as full members of the new Canadian military nursing service.[5]

In 1904, the CAF completely reformed its medical services. As part of the administrative restructuring, it was decided that the nursing corps would become part of the Reserves, a section of the Armed Forces composed of semi-permanent members who, as the name implies, would supplement regular sections if armed conflict arose. Twenty-five nurses were selected to form the corps.

However, it was not until 1908, when Georgina Fane Pope became the first matron-in-chief of the CANC — and, as a consequence, the first permanent member of the unit — that the corps began its official existence. Among this pioneer's accomplishments was her contribution to the establishment of operating and recruitment rules for the corps' members. During her mandate, Fane Pope was concerned mainly with the management of military hospitals and recruitment of nurses. In addition, she had the nurses' uniform changed from khaki to navy blue and military insignia added.[6]

The Canadian Army Nurses: Who Were They?

At the dawn of World War I, the nursing profession was a sector of female professional employment that was expanding and becoming structured. Nurses represented only 2 percent of the female workforce as a whole — a negligible proportion.[7] But the profession was burgeoning, and training schools were being

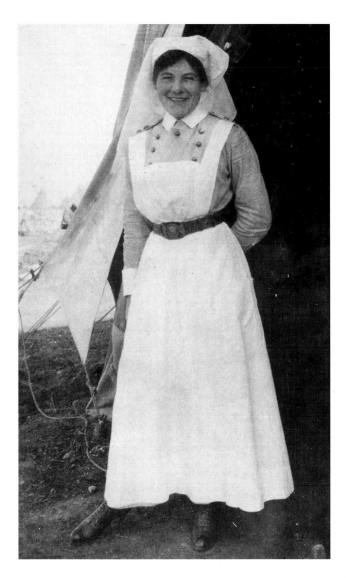

Figure 3
Nursing Sister Ruby Gordon Peterkin standing at the entrance of a tent
ca. 1916
Library and Archives Canada, ISN- 576261

centres. Most of them grew up in middle class milieus; their fathers were clergymen, physicians, accountants, or businessmen. They were generally better educated than the average among women at the time. Most had gone to high school, and some had even gone to university. A number had had paid work as governesses, teachers, or clerks before going to nursing school, which accepted applicants only aged 21 and over.

Some of the nurses in the CEF were trained in Canadian nursing schools; others, in Great Britain; a few had gone to the United States to study. Most joined the CANC soon after completing their training. In 1914, they were on average 24 years old.

At the beginning of the conflict, most nurses were sent to Europe, where convoys of nurses were posted until 1917. Many stayed until the hostilities ended. All were demobilized at the end of the war, and many got married and had children. However, a good number stayed single, not a common occurrence among women in general at the time. Among the single women, most returned to the labour market and worked in the health care sector, if not always as nurses.

Before the war, nurses recruited to serve in the Nurses Corps were chosen from among civilian nurses. They had to be single and in good health, and have a diploma in nursing from a recognized school. Once selected, the applicants went for four to six weeks of training at the Halifax military hospital to learn the rudiments of military nursing. They then took an oral and written examination, after which they were officially admitted to the CANC and received the rank of lieutenant, along with all the advantages of the rank: salary, leaves, retirement plan. However, their authority as officers was limited to the functions that they executed in the hospitals. They had no decision-making power at the military

opened at a brisk pace. By 1921, the number of nurses had quadrupled. World War I seems to have played some role in the expansion of the profession through, among other things, the creation of the CANC.

Few official statistics exist on the subject. However, although the analysis of the various sources available on the careers of Canadian army nurses does not allow us to make hasty generalizations on the military nurses who served in World War I, it is possible to draw out some interesting information and discern trends characteristic of the group.[8]

Most Canadian military nurses were born in Canada or the British Isles; the majority had been brought up in cities, and they therefore had easier access to training than did their rural counterparts, as nursing schools were concentrated in urban

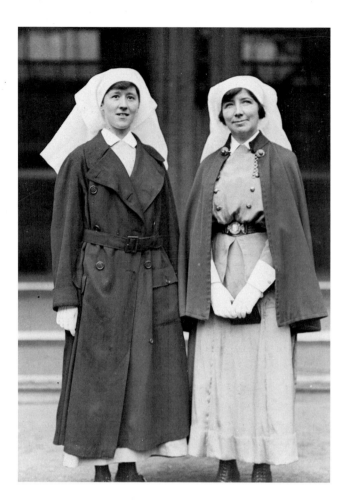

Figure 4
**Nursing Sister Guilbride, RRC (right)
and Nursing Sister E McLeod, RRC
in their dress uniforms**
ca.1914–1919
Library and Archives Canada, PA-007351

level, unlike medical officers. In addition, although they were lieutenants, they were known simply as "nursing sisters," a title reminiscent of the religious vocation with which caregiving tasks were often associated.

Of all the nurses on active duty during World War I, only the Canadian nurses were under the direct control of the army and held a military rank. In comparison, the British nursing services were affiliated with the army, but not integrated into it. The higher status accorded to the nursing profession in Canada than in Great Britain may explain, at least in part, this breach of tradition by the Canadian military authorities. Most Canadian nurses with diplomas had gone to high school, and in Canada, training in a nursing school was seen as a sign of prestige.[9]

Margaret MacDonald, who succeeded Fane Pope as matron-in-chief of the CANC, was quite critical of how members were recruited. The selection process, she felt, was an impediment to the rapid establishment of a large corps of nurses. To solve this problem, she suggested that the military nursing courses be given in various hospitals across Canada and that nurses be allowed to go to the soldiers' training camps to put into practice the military training that they had acquired, which differed, in her opinion, from training for civilian nursing. In addition, after applying pressure on the minister of defence, MacDonald went to Great Britain in 1911 to study the administration and organization of the British military nurses' corps, on which the Canadian corps was based. The goal of the trip was to learn the methods of British military nurses, who were more numerous and better organized, and import these methods to the Canadian corps so that it would operate more smoothly during armed conflicts.[10]

In spite of these efforts, in 1914, the CANC, like the rest of the CEF, was ill-prepared for the challenges that awaited it. Nevertheless, the lack of organization did not mean a lack of human resources. Throughout the war, enlistment applications by nurses always surpassed the number of places available in the corps.

Enlistment

It is not surprising that the Department of Defence received so many applications from nurses wishing to join the CEF, in spite of the danger inherent in the war context. The reasons for wanting to enlist in the CANC were many and diverse. The job prospects for nurses were still quite dim and salaries were low, so the possibility of regular and higher pay and the advantageous conditions associated with military work made it attractive. The CEF also offered adventure, an exciting life, and new professional challenges. In addition, the economic and political context of the time lent itself to an emerging desire for a military career. Propaganda in favour of the war encouraged young women, like young men, to take part in the war effort. The idea of enlisting was imbued with

Laura Holland (1883–1956)

**Glennis Zilm, Retired RN, freelance writer and editor and
Ethel Warbinek, University of British Columbia**

Laura Holland was a nurse and a social worker — a dual qualification that was highly unusual at the time; most nurses were not university educated, and social work was just being introduced into post-secondary education as a fledgling profession. She maintained active participation and held leadership roles in both professions at national and provincial levels and was one of Canada's first nurse advisors to government.

After graduating from the School of Nursing, Montreal General Hospital in 1914, Holland served as a nursing sister in World War I, and was awarded the Royal Red Cross. She then earned a social work diploma from Simmons College and became Director of Nursing Services for the Ontario Red Cross, establishing its first four outpost hospitals. For this, she was made a Commander of the British Empire. She was appointed Director of the Division of Social Welfare, Toronto Department of Public Health in 1923, and in 1927 moved to Vancouver to become manager of the Children's Aid Society. She then held several key government positions, including Deputy Superintendent of Neglected Children for the Province of BC, supervisor of the Provincial Welfare Field Service, Superintendent of Social Welfare for the BC government, and advisor to the Minister on Matters of Social Welfare Policy.

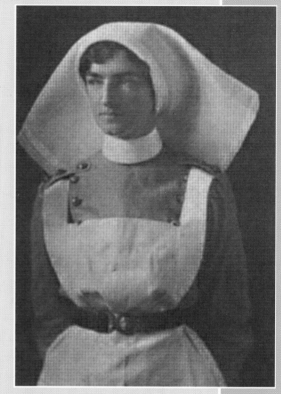

Figure 5
**Laura Holland, Nursing Sister in
the Canadian Army Medical Corps**
1914–1918
Courtesy of Mrs Kathleen Cooke

Her nursing accomplishments included an active role in the development of the Registered Nurses Association of BC, founding its job placement service and developing its functioning districts and chapters. She was noted for her professional achievements but, more importantly, for her warmth, kindness, and understanding. An article in *The Canadian Nurse* in 1934 said, "Miss Holland's great gifts of knowledge, technical competence, and administrative skill have brought her public recognition. These would all have been barren if it had not been for her warmth of personality, her personal kindliness and understanding, her spirit of altruism and her devotion. Her example will continue to shed a glow across both nursing and social work in the years to come."

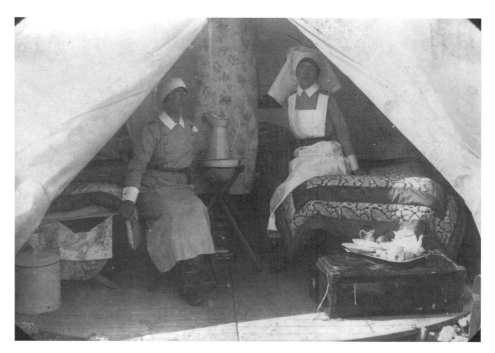

Figure 6
Nursing sisters Pugh and Parker sitting in their tent at the No. 2 Canadian General Hospital
Le Tréport, France
ca. 1915
Library and Archives Canada,
ISN 579194

romanticism, represented by the elegance of the uniform, it seems, and its draw as a symbol of courage and patriotism.

To mobilize rapidly the convoy of nurses required by the Department of Militia and Defence, the overly long selection process was considerably shortened. Top priority was given to reservist nurses who had already received the training dispensed in the military hospitals. The other nurses were chosen from among the hundreds of applications received. The young women were selected rapidly, all according to the same criteria: in good health, unmarried, with nursing training. However, the examination and six weeks of training were abandoned. Although morality was not one of the official selection criteria, a letter of recommendation from a religious leader was not without a certain influence in an application. Similarly, a young woman supported by a politician or wealthy person might see her application progress more quickly. No military experience was required, and military training was given quickly, as time permitted, often shipboard on the way to Europe. The first contingent, composed of 100 nurses, embarked for Great Britain in September 1914. A number of other convoys succeeded them in the following months.

The Work of Military Nurses

Living Conditions

Nothing in the conflicts that had gone before World War I foretold the breadth of that conflict. New weapons, new combat tactics, and the number of countries and soldiers involved were all factors that radically changed the ways that war was waged. As a consequence, the pace at which patients entered and left the various hospitals and dressing stations, the nature and seriousness of the wounds, and the care required meant that certain aspects of their job diverged greatly from what nurses had experienced as students or in civilian practice. It was not the administration of care itself that was transformed, but the conditions under which caregiving took place on the front.

The state of war, the reality of which the nurses really became aware on their ocean voyage to Europe on ships escorted by armed vessels, was even more striking when they arrived in England. While some rationing and conscription had been instituted in Canada, such measures, and others, such as the curfew, were naturally more severe in the United Kingdom and on the other war fronts.

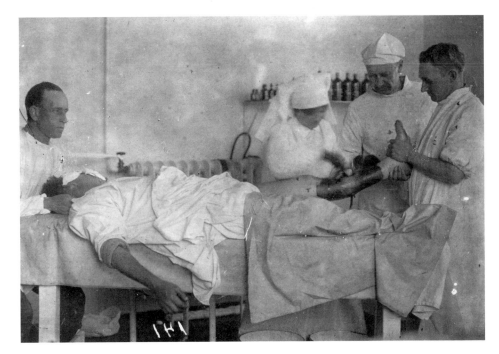

Figure 7
Doctor, Nursing Sister and two orderlies draining an infected leg
No.7 Canadian General Hospital
ca. 1917
Library and Archives Canada,
ISN 575652

The first war measures to which nurses were subjected concerned food and lodging. In each combat zone, whether England, the Continent, or the Mediterranean, specific difficulties arose. Provisions were reduced: sugar, butter, coffee, chocolate, and meat were rare foods. On the Mediterranean, the lack of potable water represented an even more severe health risk. Moreover, the poisoning of water reserves, a war tactic frequently employed by the enemy, made work and daily life even more difficult to manage; because the limited supply of potable water was reserved for drinking, the personal hygiene of the nurses, their patients, and their workplace quickly came to be considered secondary.

In terms of housing, some nurses had a better time than did others. In England and France, the nurses serving in towns or villages often had the chance to live in buildings, sometimes even villas or castles. Closer to the lines of combat, the nurses had to content themselves with canvas tents or wooden shelters. Whether or not their lodgings had walls, all nurses had to deal with a very real problem: vermin. Fleas, insects of all sorts, and rats infested all types of care units. The rats, in particular, seemed to be afraid of nothing. At night, they threw themselves on any trace of food and even attacked patients. Finally, frequent trips between dressing stations — an inconvenience, aggravated by the lack of communications, which resulted in wasted time, equipment, and personal objects — attacks, and bombings were all part of daily life on the front. Although they were accepted as inevitable in a war situation, bombardments were still a terrifying, and life threatening, reality.

Working Conditions

Within the army's medical services, doctors and nurses were assigned to four types of patient-care units: field ambulances, evacuation posts, stationary hospitals, and general hospitals. Wounded soldiers were first taken to the field ambulances, infirmaries located close to the front, staffed by soldiers who gave only first aid. Patients were immediately transported to medical evacuation posts for a more complete examination by a physician. In theory, no nurse was supposed to work so close to the hostilities, although some did so under specific circumstances — for example, to accompany a surgeon posted to one of these facilities. It should be noted that field ambulances and evacuation posts were not equipped to hold patients for more than a few hours.

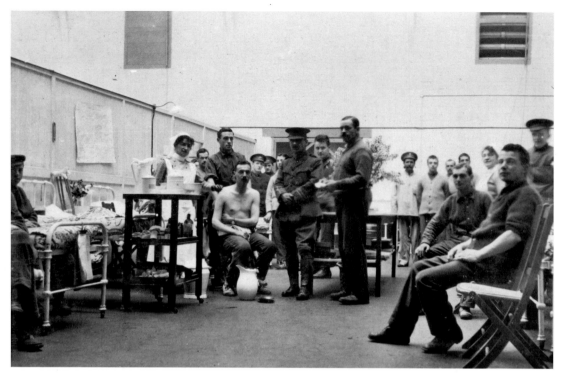

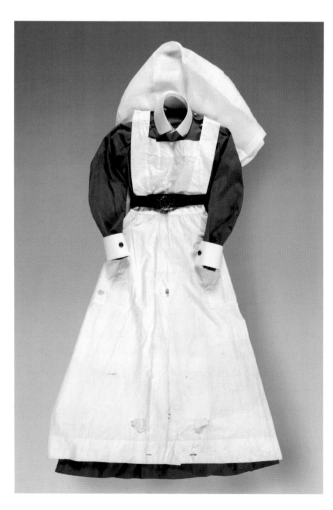

Patients were then transported to the stationary hospital, located relatively close to the front, managed by a matron-in-chief in charge of 16 nurses. These hospitals had about 250 beds. Those with serious injuries requiring a long convalescence or suffering from various diseases were sent to general hospitals, permanent buildings located in Great Britain that could house more than 500 patients. The nursing staff in these hospitals was composed of a matron-in-chief and 72 nurses. The nursing units rotated between various stationary and general hospitals; a nurse might change posts several times during her military service. In addition, a nursing unit might be broken up and its members allocated to various hospitals depending on personnel needs determined by the circumstances of the war.

With regard to the nursing work itself, it was the conditions surrounding administration of care, rather than nursing techniques in themselves, that were different from those in civilian society. Working conditions were considerably more rigorous because of the irregular pace of often massive admissions, a normal consequence of the advance or withdrawal of troops, which added to the already heavy load of care for those with diseases and accidental injuries. Nurses

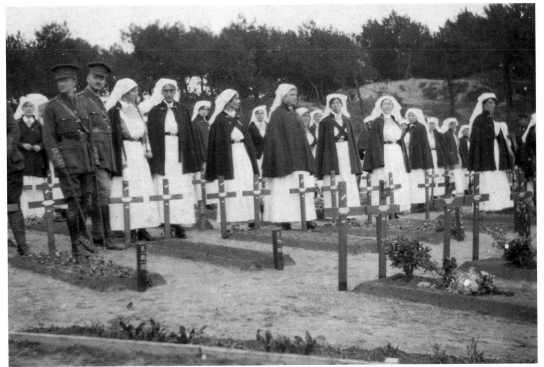

Figure 10
Nursing sisters and officers standing in graveyard
ca. 1916
Library and Archives
Canada, PA-134992

also had to deal with a lack of hygiene and insufficient equipment and personnel, but this shortfall was explained mainly by the irregular influx of injured soldiers, which made it impossible to know how many patients to be prepared for at any given time.

During an offensive, a dressing station close to the line of fire might be completely overwhelmed. Under cover of night, trucks filled with muddy wounded soldiers would be unloaded and handed over to the nurses, who, between stretchers crammed together or beside soldiers lying on the ground, had to try to staunch hemorrhages, set bones, and ensure the survival of their patients until they were transported farther behind the lines to receive appropriate care. The daily work of the nurses in units farther from the front was just as laborious. Climatic conditions and life in the trenches favoured the outbreak of epidemics, so many beds were occupied by soldiers suffering from infectious diseases, which in fact accounted for almost 70 percent of cases admitted to hospital.[11]

In this context, we cannot conclude that World War I was synonymous with a medical revolution in terms of practical nursing work and administration of care. Of course, certain techniques — blood screen-

ing, blood transfusions, and urinary screening for certain diseases — were developed and began to be widely used during this period, and some specialized disciplines — psychotherapy, physiotherapy, orthopedics, and dietetics — were in their infancy. But the fact remains that nurses were performing the same actions as in civilian hospitals: administering treatment for known diseases such as tuberculosis, influenza, and dysentery; changing dressings and disinfecting wounds; and, of course, seeing to the well-being of patients by providing food and tending to the body, and dispensing various ministrations and comforting words.

Another element had a considerable impact on military nursing: modernization of warfare techniques. The means used during military operations, such as poison gas, shrapnel, and bombardment, often caused injuries that represented medical challenges previously unknown to nurses. Along the same lines, the new combat tactics, the duration of the war, and the dropping morale of the troops were responsible for a constantly growing number of mental illnesses that manifested themselves in night terrors, insomnia, bed-wetting, and other symptoms. At the time, physicians did not have medications to prescribe for

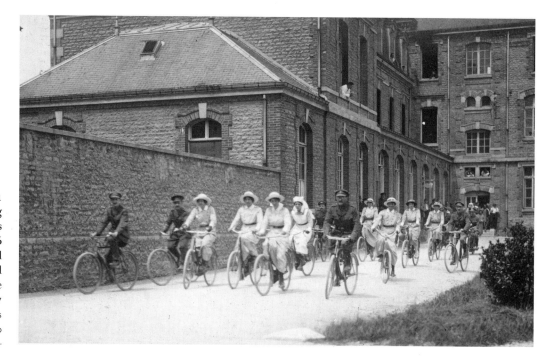

Figure 11
A Group of nursing sisters and officers cycling at No. 6 Canadian General Hospital
Le Tréport, France
ca. 1917
Library and Archives
Canada, ISN 576440

such conditions, and nurses had to call on their specific strengths to do what they do best in administering treatment: applying compresses, washing eyes, and applying balms for gas burns, providing comfort and a receptive ear, creating a warm and familial environment, and prescribing rest and diet for the most disturbed patients.

For the nurses, care provision at the front represented a major professional challenge at the technical, personal, and moral levels. Working in such unsanitary conditions, and at such a feverish pace, went counter to what they had learned in their professional training, with its emphasis on extreme cleanliness and personal attention accorded to each patient, and this at a time when hospital stays were very long. As a consequence, nurses often found themselves facing moral dilemmas for which they were not prepared, such as deciding to leave a dying patient alone to see to the pressing needs of those who had a chance to survive.

The high mortality rate of patients was another reality that military nurses had to face. Although they had dealt with death before, they had never been confronted with the loss of so many patients, especially ones so young, at once. Isolation — being far their families and friends — was another difficult aspect of

life at the front. On top of this was exhaustion, which also affected the nurses' health.

Professional Relations and Social Life

The isolation and sadness that were the realities of the front — along with the omnipresent danger, the constant work, and the forced proximity in which doctors, nurses, and patients had to live — encouraged a sense of friendship, solidarity, and loyalty. The members of the Nursing Corps were young, single, far from home, and often scared; social conventions tended to melt away in a time of war. All of this made it easy to form deep friendships. Military nurses remember a working atmosphere in which the rules of the game were based on co-operation and respect. Respect for authority and exemplary behaviour were top priorities on the front, and nurses had been indoctrinated into this comportment through their professional training. However, it seems that in the context of war, the perception of absolute authority was attenuated in favour of the collaboration needed to pursue a central objective: care of the ill and wounded.

But intimacy was the flip side of overcrowding. Groups of friends might form on the basis of the rep-

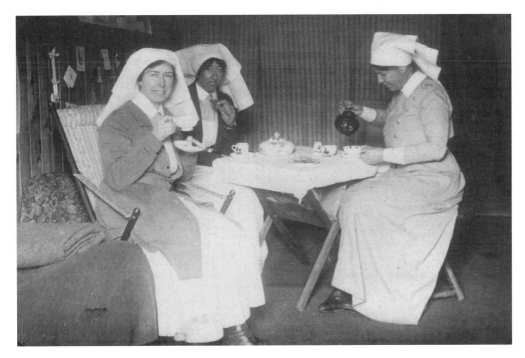

Figure 12
Nursing Sisters Thomson, Beers, and Isaacson having tea in the Sisters' Quarters
No. 2 Canadian General Hospital,
Le Tréport, France
ca. 1915
Library and Archives Canada,
ISN 579195

utation of their school, the size of the hospital where they had studied, where they had come from, or for other reasons. These distinctions might also provoke jealousy since they marked, symbolically, the professional status of the nurses, a status not yet secure in society at the time. Promotions and greater responsibilities could also be a source of envy, an indication that nurses were not without professional ambitions given the possibilities of advancement offered by military service.

More tense, it seems, were the relations between Canadian and foreign nurses, particularly the British ones. These tensions were due to the more advantageous conditions that Canadian nurses enjoyed. Their higher salaries, more distinctive uniforms, and apparent popularity with the officers seem to have inspired jealousy among their foreign colleagues. However, the greatest source of frustration with regard to the Canadian nurses had to do with their military rank. Indeed, their officer status gave them greater freedom of movement and a higher level of prestige, two elements that their foreign counterparts did not enjoy. The rules of the Canadian and British armies required that officers, female or male, communicate only with their peers unless they were in civilian clothing, so the British military nurses, without a military rank, could not spend time with their own officers or with

those of the CAF if they were in uniform. On the other hand, the Canadian military nurses could spend time only with other officers because of their rank as lieutenants. It is thus understandable that the British nurses perceived the arrival of the Canadians with some apprehension. What is more, the Canadians' rapidly acquired reputation for compassion, gentleness, and hospitality made them formidable rivals.

The military nurses also formed relationships with soldiers. At the time, hospital stays, even in the context of war, were quite long. Nurses therefore had the time to get to know the soldiers in their care and to enjoy their presence. They got to know patients and their families, and they often became attached to them. These relationships, formed over time, did, however, have certain disadvantages. Because they came to care for their patients, the nurses might worry about their futures and mourn their deaths — not to mention the pernicious effect of having to see them suffer.

Paradoxically, according to the testimonies, correspondence, and interviews that military nurses have left to us, the counterpart to the chaotic and dark world of war was the great importance accorded to social life on the front. Between enemy attacks and work shifts, nurses wanted to have fun, and they often went out with medical officers or other avail-

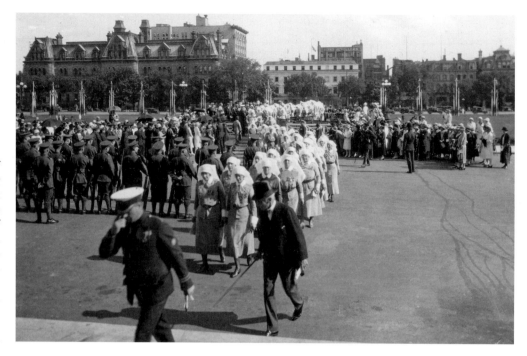

Figure 13
'The Last Parade' of
Canadian Nursing
Sisters on Parliament
Hill during the
unveiling ceremony of
the War Memorial
dedicated to
the Nursing Sisters
August 24, 1926
Library and
Archives Canada,
ISN 576343

able officers. Diversions included dances, eating together, and sports. The favourite British game, tennis, proved quite popular among the nurses, as did other sporting activities.

The most popular English ritual was afternoon tea. Having tea meant visiting friends in nearby hospitals, meeting officers or soldiers in an environment outside of the hospital, and a change in routine. Often, English families living near the care units invited nurses to tea in a gesture of welcome and hospitality.

The best-attended social events were evenings of dancing and music. During calm periods, any excuse served to get together, organize concerts, and have dances. Often, the patients took the initiative for these parties, or they took part, performing to entertain their friends. Professional orchestras, some of them very famous at the time, sometimes came to play. The possibility of meeting a suitor during these outings was on the minds of some nurses; such encounters might lead to marriage proposals, which, in the opinion of many young women, represented the best possible outcome to their career.

Travel was also an important aspect of military nurses' social life. They used their leaves to visit Europe, taking trips that were not easily available to civilian nurses. They enjoyed great freedom because of the distance and the circumstances of the war, which led to a degree of flexibility in the observation of conventions that normally applied to respectable young women.

Outings, encounters, and entertainment of all sorts might give the impression that life at the front was life as usual for these young, single nurses, especially because the context of the war meant that most of them led a much freer existence than their civilian colleagues. Nevertheless, the war and its consequences were a reality that bore its share of daily difficulties.

Conclusion

The participation of military nurses in the war seems to have been so highly valued that they enjoyed unequalled respect when they returned home. In the years following World War I, their contribution to the Canadian war effort and to the nursing profession was publicly commemorated by the erection of a monument in Parliament in honour of all Canadian nurses. This prestige reflected on the profession as a whole; from the time of the war to the 1930s was the golden age of professionalization of nursing in Canada. The recognition that nurses acquired is due, among other things, to the fact that military nurses, through their training, ingenuity, and resourcefulness, carved themselves a significant and respected place in a typically male bastion.

World War I thus represents an important time in the evolution of the nursing profession in Canada. The CANC, formed at the beginning of the twentieth century, provided an interesting opportunity for more than 2000 graduates from nursing schools, offering them stable employment (at least for the duration of hostilities) that was well paid and filled with professional challenges and adventure. Over the four years of the war, military nurses risked their lives, worked non-stop, overcame difficult living conditions, and went through emotional times watching patients and friends perish, but they also forged friendships and a sense of solidarity that transcended their military service and had fun. Above all, they made use of their training and their personal and professional experience to improve and even save the lives of their patients.

World War I did not change how nursing was practised in as notable a way as medical developments in the twentieth century would do during other wars. However, given the new combat tactics and weapons being used, along with the size of the conflict, the importance of the nurses' role as caregivers within the medical services of the CEF was convincingly demonstrated. In a context in which the power of medicine was limited and diseases abounded, nurses offered specific health care skills that were utterly indispensable.

In addition, the presence of nurses under such exceptional circumstances brought a feminine, almost maternal touch, expressed in all sorts of ways. It is in fact reasonable to think that the nurses helped to make the caregiving units warm places, providing soldiers with a home-like atmosphere.

This was the key to the success of the Canadian military nurses who served in Europe during World War I: by doing what they had learned to do, doing it well, effectively, and with dedication, they joined the other figures in the pantheon of World War I heroes. In the words of Marion Wylie, a nurse from Sutton, Ontario who served in England and France from 1916 until demobilization, "It was very necessary and very important, on the whole, I think, very well done. I am not boasting about that, but I think the nurses worked very hard and did good work."[12]

"Ready, Aye Ready": Canadian Military Nurses as an Expandable and Expendable Workforce (1920–2000)

Cynthia Toman

The majority of Canadian military nurses, known by rank and title as Nursing Sisters and later as Nursing Officers, served in the armed forces "for the duration" only. With few exceptions, military nursing has been primarily a temporary role. Although the need for nurses in the Armed Forces increased dramatically during times of war and crisis, there were very few permanent positions between wars and few opportunities for military nurses to maintain the full range of professional skills associated with civilian nursing. The episodic nature of military nursing practice was problematic for the civilian profession since the Armed Forces relied on the profession as an expandable workforce to "fill the ranks" whenever nurses were needed.

The civilian nursing profession was responsible for training and accrediting nurses who could and would fill both civilian and military needs, while guarding against an overproduction of nurses and the resulting severe unemployment when wars and crises ended. The episodic demand for increased numbers of nurses led to considerable anxiety and tension within the profession, especially during the Second World War when the largest number of nurses enlisted and served overseas. This chapter examines the Canadian military nursing experience since 1920 as nurses built upon the strong traditions inherited from the Nursing Sisters who served during the First World War, negotiated their own positions within the highly gendered military establishment, and made difficult choices about the return to civilian practice environments when their military service ended.

Active recruitment of military nurses was never necessary in Canada — unlike the situation in the United States, Great Britain, and South Africa. Even before Canada declared war in August 1939, the Executive Secretary of the Canadian Nurses Association, Jean Wilson, confidently assured the government that "there would be an immediate rush by nurses to answer 'The Call' for their professional services." Nurses would answer, "…'Ready, aye ready' to any emergency call."[1] And they did. Canadian nurses volunteered in numbers that far exceeded all available positions, in all Armed Forces branches, throughout the six years of war. Indeed, a moratorium was placed on their enlistment and the waiting list grew to an estimated 8000 names. As Nursing Sister (NS) Mary Bower explained, "We all were trying to get in the Army or Air Force or anything. We tried to go to Africa! Anything to get in the armed forces."[2] Other nurses chose to serve with the American, British, or South African forces rather than risk "missing the war." Nursing Officer (NO) Lee Anne Quinn echoed similar enthusiasm for military nursing more than 50 years later, calling her deployment to Somalia in 1994 "the high point in my nursing career."[3]

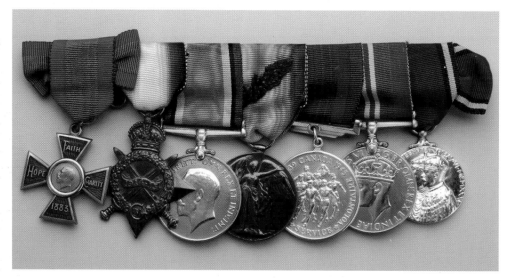

Filling the Ranks

At the end of the First World War, official plans called for an establishment of 25 permanent force nursing positions and a reserve force of 1110 nurses. But due to economic recessions and the Great Depression, there were only 12 permanent force nursing positions during the interwar years, and a mere 363 nurses' names on the reserve list at the end of the 1930s. These 12 interwar Nursing Sisters worked as supervisors and administrators within district military hospitals. They taught first aid to non-commissioned soldiers, known as "other ranks," who became medical assistants and stretcher bearers in field ambulance units. During the 1930s, a few Nursing Sisters served in converted military camps that became labour camps for unemployed men on relief. NS Elizabeth Pense claimed there was a ratio of "five Army patients to fifty unemployed patients" in these camps, and described "lots of pneumonia among the men arriving right off the trains."[4]

Reserve Nursing Sisters were "called out" on short notice for emergencies, such as a 1924 influenza outbreak at the Royal Military College in Kingston, Ontario. They could be posted for summer training camp duty, but military training was greatly curtailed due to the recessions. The only field training for medical units was held at Camp Borden on the eve of the Second World War in 1938. Meanwhile, reserve nurses depended on private duty nursing income while hoping for a vacancy within the permanent force.

Led by retired Nursing Sisters in Edmonton during 1920, military nurses who served overseas during the First World War organized local Overseas Nursing Sisters Clubs across Canada. These local units formed a national organization in 1929 for the purposes of mutual support, fostering a memory of military nursing service, and shaping a vision for military nursing. The Overseas Nursing Sisters Association provided continuity for the second generation of Nursing Sisters to whom they passed the torch in 1939. Indeed, five First World War Nursing Sisters were among the first persons to enlist for the Second World War.

As Matron-in-Chief of the Royal Canadian Army Medical Corps (RCAMC) during the Second World War, Elizabeth Smellie spoke about the special relationship between these two generations of Nursing Sisters in a 1940 CBC interview. She said, "[Y]our predecessors offer you greetings and good wishes. I suppose you will have your own distinctions, as we did.... Don't be resentful if, as we veterans pass you by, we reveal extraordinary interest in your uniform and tell you we wish we were going again, because we do so, scarcely realizing how much water has run under the bridge since 1918."[5] And NS Jessie Morrison put it this way: "We knew we had big shoes to fill."[6]

Nurses enlisted as officers with the relative rank of Second Lieutenant and became First Lieutenants at the end of their qualification period. They were

Elizabeth L Smellie (1884–1968)

Cynthia Toman, University of Ottawa School of Nursing

The career of Matron-in-Chief Elizabeth Laurie Smellie — the first woman in the world to become a full colonel — epitomized continuity between the two world wars and bridged civilian and military nursing practice settings. Always referred to as Miss Smellie, she worked her way up through the ranks, earning significant leadership positions in the military, with the Victorian Order of Nurses (VON), and with the Canadian Nurses Association (CNA).

After graduating from Johns Hopkins Hospital Training School in 1909, Miss Smellie worked briefly in hospital and private duty nursing at Fort William (Ontario) and Detroit. In 1914 she joined the Canadian Army Medical Corps (CAMC) with postings to Taplow, Le Tréport (France), and on North Atlantic hospital ship transport duty. Miss Smellie became Assistant Matron-in-Chief (1918–1920) after which she retired from the CAMC to pursue training in public health at Boston. She taught public health at the School for Graduate Nurses at McGill University (1921–1923), leaving to become Chief Superintendent of the VON for Canada. During the 1930s, Miss Smellie was also first Vice-President of the CNA.

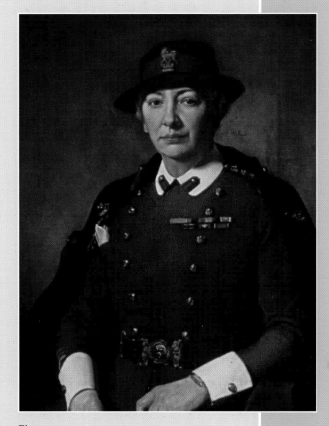

Figure 2
Colonel Elizabeth Laurie Smellie
Artist: Captain Kenneth Keith Forbes
1944
Canadian War Museum, 20000105-054

With this varied and knowledgeable background, she was reappointed as RCAMC Matron-in-Chief (Canada) in 1940, where she served for most of the Second World War. She played key roles in the formation of the Canadian Women's Army Corps (1941), and both the RCN and RCAF nursing services (1940–1941). Miss Smellie retired from the military in 1944 and returned to the VON until 1947, when she became the western supervisor of nursing for the Department of Veterans' Affairs, retiring again in 1948. With characteristic good humour, she called herself the "most retired nurse" in Canada. She was widely-known as "always a lady" who combined culture, wisdom, and practicality.

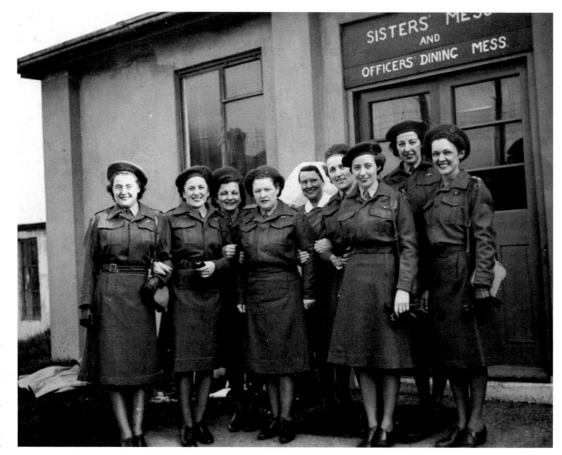

Figure 3
Nursing Sisters outside Sisters' and Officers' Mess
No. 13 Canadian General Hospital, England
1945
Library and Archives Canada, e002414889

further eligible to "progress through the ranks" with increased responsibility. Under relative rank, they were accountable to the Director of Medical Services through a parallel, female line of authority consisting of Matrons, Principal Matrons, and Matrons-in-Chief. From May 1942, nurses' commissions included the power of command over women but not until 1949 did nurses achieve full powers of command and rank parity.

At least 4079 military nurses served during the Second World War, comprising the largest group of nurses in Canadian military history. Whereas previous Nursing Sisters had been members of the Canadian Expeditionary Force attached to the British Army, Second World War Nursing Sisters served as fully-integrated members of the RCAMC, the Royal Canadian Air Force (RCAF), and the Royal Canadian Navy (RCN). Initially, the RCAMC supplied Nursing Sisters for both the RCAF and RCN until their respective nursing services were organized during 1940–1941. Matron-in-Chief Smellie guided the for-

mation of both new services, thus facilitating continuity in policies, uniforms, pay, and benefits across the three branches.

With few exceptions, Nursing Sisters served within Canadian medical units and wherever Canadian troops went: throughout Canada, Newfoundland, England, France, Holland, Belgium, Germany, North Africa, Sicily, Italy, and Hong Kong. NS Kay Christie and NS May Waters were posted to Hong Kong when it fell to the Japanese in December 1941. They are the only Canadian women to serve as prisoners of war, interned for 21 months under conditions of extreme privation and intimidation. An additional 302 Canadian nurses volunteered to serve with the South African Military Nursing Service while an unknown number enlisted with the British and American nursing services.

The title Nursing Sister was not restricted to nurses, however. Until the Armed Forces established Women's Divisions (1941–1942), all enlisted women were designated as Nursing Sisters regardless of their

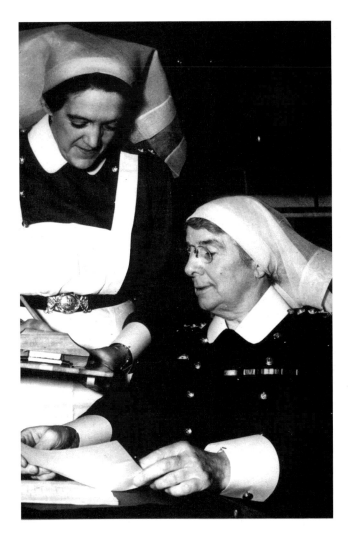

Figure 4
**Nursing Sister MN DeVere and Captain/
Matron Charlotte Nixon on the Lady Nelson**
1943
Alberta Association of Registered Nurses Museum and Archives
Marion C (Story) McLeod Scrapbook

service branch while a Nursing Sister stands alone at the top of the medal — belonging to all three.

Twelve RCAMC nurses re-mustered to the RCAF (November 1940) where NS/Flight Lieutenant Jessie E C Porteous became Matron in 1943. At the end of 1944, there were at least 100 RCAF air training stations with hospital facilities or infirmaries across Canada, Newfoundland, and Labrador. These units varied in size from several beds to 700 beds at the St. Thomas Technical Training School in Ontario. Nursing care primarily involved patients with infectious diseases and minor surgical procedures, since relatively few men survived air training crashes or bombing missions. Those who did survive sustained extensive burns requiring months or years of reconstructive surgery and rehabilitation. A small number of RCAF nurses served in England with No. 6 Bomber Group (Northallerton), No. 3 Personnel Reception Centre (Bournemouth), the Repatriation Depot (Warrington), and the specialized Canadian plastic surgery unit for burn patients at East Grinstead. Six RCAF nurses completed the American air evacuation course in 1943, and four of them became the first Allied women to land in Europe only 13 days after D-Day (6 June 1944) with No. 52 RCAF Mobile Field Hospital. Flight nurses were also posted to No. 6 Casualty Air Evacuation Unit, flying casualties between Europe and England. Nursing Sisters posted in Newfoundland and Labrador also evacuated civilian patients during emergencies.

Similarly, three RCAMC nurses re-mustered to the new RCN nursing service (1941) where Marjorie Russell became Matron-in-Chief in 1943. RCN nurses served primarily at nine land-based naval hospitals in Canada and two overseas postings at St. John's, Newfoundland (RCNH *Avalon*) and Grennock, Scotland (RCNH *Niobe*). RCN hospitals were strategically situated in relation to German submarine and U-boat activity off the east coast where the majority

professional or occupational category. Professional nurses made up only 91.8 percent of the rank during the Second World War. For example, RCAMC Nursing Sisters included physiotherapist aides, occupational therapists, dieticians, and Home Sisters (house-mothers) while RCN Nursing Sisters also included female laboratory technicians. The RCAF, however, used civilian services as long as possible, then enlisting dieticians and physiotherapist aides into their Women's Division. Nursing Sisters were never members of the Women's Divisions. Their rank remained a separate, unique classification of professional women subsumed within the medical services. This unique relationship within the military establishment is represented symbolically on the Voluntary Service medal, 1939–1945 (See Figure 1). Of the seven figures on the medal, a man and a woman represent each

of casualties were merchant seamen and survivors of the Battle of the Atlantic. They did not serve at sea because the navy had no hospital ships, and as NS Betty Surgenor explained, there were seldom survivors when ships sank. Most of the required first aid or medical care on naval vessels could be provided by enlisted men trained as sick berth attendants.[7] Although Nursing Sisters typically received an introductory cruise to better understand naval serving conditions, they were invited aboard ship more frequently as dinner guests when ships docked. The two Canadian hospital ships, the *Lady Nelson* and the *Letitia,* actually belonged to the RCAMC, and were staffed by RCAMC Nursing Sisters who transported wounded and recovering troops from the Mediterranean to England and back to Canada. Veteran Charlotte Nixon had served on a British hospital ship during the first war, and she came out of retirement at the age of fifty-four to serve as Matron of the *Lady Nelson,* which crossed the Atlantic 37 times during World War II (See Figure 4).

Like the RCAF nurses, RCN Nursing Sisters provided a much needed resource for local communities. In December 1942, they cared for 77 survivors suffering from burns, inhalation trauma, and fractures resulting from a fire at St. John's, Newfoundland. RCN nurses also staffed an innovative well baby clinic in Halifax, trained naval ratings as sick berth attendants, and dealt with an explosion at the Bedford Magazine Ammunition Depot in Halifax harbor.

A fourth group of Canadian nurses served in South Africa, on main evacuation routes between England and the Middle Eastern, North African, and Far Eastern theatres of war. The South African government received special permission to recruit 300 nurses for their military hospitals. The RCAMC selected them and verified their credentials. And while they wore RCAMC uniforms, the South African Military Nursing Service (SAMNS) was responsible for their transportation, pay, and postings. With Matron Gladys J Sharpe as liaison officer, SAMNS nurses signed one-year renewable contracts. At the 1000-bed hospital in Baragwanath near Johannesburg, Canadian Nursing Sisters comprised the major portion of the staff. They were also posted to Durban,

Pretoria, and Pietermaritzburg. Two-thirds of them extended their one-year commitment, and were subsequently posted to Egypt, North Africa, and Italy. More than 60 of these nurses also served with one of the three Canadian forces after initial contracts expired.

The Second World War extended well beyond the May 1945 European armistice for nurses as they continued to care for recovering casualties, civilians, and concentration camp survivors through 1946. Nurses served with the Army of Occupation (1946–1947) as medical units gradually downsized throughout Europe and England. The last overseas medical unit closed in May 1946 — six years and nine months after war was declared. Military hospitals across Canada also closed as soldiers transferred to Department of Veterans' Affairs hospitals, along with several hundred Nursing Sisters who accepted civilian nursing positions there. The Army of Occupation was replaced by the Canadian Army Active Force (Interim) with 79 Nursing Sisters at the end of 1947.

The post-war quota included 30 RCAMC, 30 RCAF, and 20 RCN Nursing Sisters, who received short service commissions of three to seven years, as medical units expanded services to military dependents and civilian personnel working for the Department of National Defence during the 1950s and 1960s. For example, RCAF nurses cared for both military personnel and civilians along the DEW (Distance Early Warning) Line and the Alaska Highway. And Nursing Sisters constituted highly valued mobile resources during the Manitoba polio epidemic (1953–1954) when posted to Winnipeg to care for entire wards of patients in iron lungs.

Fewer nurses served during the Korean War (1950–1953) and with North Atlantic Treaty Organization (NATO) forces in Europe during the Cold War era. Eight RCAMC nurses were posted to the British hospital unit at Kure, Japan, while two nurses served at the Commonwealth Hospital in Seoul, Korea. Three Nursing Sisters under Matron Elizabeth Pense served at Tokchong with No. 25 Field Dressing Stations, which later enlarged as a general base hospital. RCAF nurses continued to train in air evacuation and para-rescue with the American forces and 13 flight nurses were attached to the United States Air Force for the transport of Canadian

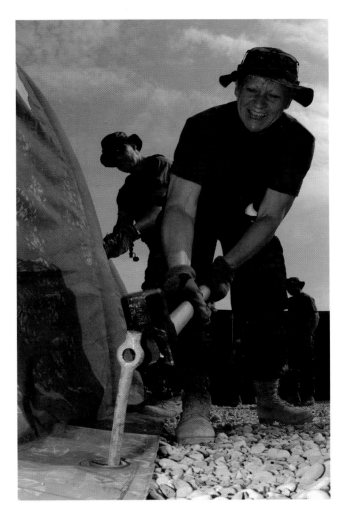

Figure 5
**Captain France Bergeron, a Nursing Officer
and second in command of the Advanced
Surgical Team, sets up the medical unit**
Port au Prince, Haiti
June 2004, Operation *Halo*
Photo: Department of National Defence

personnel. By the end of the 1990s, men comprised approximately 14 percent of the military nurse workforce.

The nursing service underwent further downsizing as Canadian military involvements shifted toward peacekeeping activities. Canadian Forces Nursing Officers participated in the Persian Gulf War (1991) when 32 nurses staffed a Canadian field hospital to support British land forces, four Nursing Officers deployed with the HMCS *Protecteur* and six deployed with the USN *Mercy*. Flight nurses participated in the air evacuation of casualties from war zones in the former Yugoslavia, Somalia, and Rwanda as part of deployment with the United Nations High Commission for Refugees (UNHCR) during 1993 and 1994. Captain Michelle Gagné described nurses' experiences, including advanced cardiac life support under adverse conditions such as weapon fire, with only minimal time on the ground for evacuation procedures. Since patients included both military personnel and civilian refugees, these nurses managed a wide range of equipment from volume ventilators to infant transport incubators. One flight nurse was deployed to Somalia for three months with United Nations Operation Somalia, while air evacuation crews with the UNHCR went to Rwanda where four Nursing Officers were posted to refugee camps. Yet another reorganization (1997) resulted in 244 Nursing Officer positions and introduced a rotation through civilian health care facilities to supplement practice experience.

Negotiating a Place in the Military

Overall, English-Canadian nurses responded enthusiastically to military nursing opportunities. The majority of them had strong British roots, either as immigrants or as first-generation Canadians born of British parents, for whom the war offered

casualties between Japan, San Francisco, and Canada. Flying Officer/NS Joan Fitzgerald was the first flight nurse to serve in this capacity.

The three nursing services integrated, along with the rest of the Canadian Forces Medical Services, in January 1959. There were 60 medical units on average, staffed by approximately 370 Nursing Officers during the period from the 1970s to the 1990s. A significant change took place in 1967 with the commissioning of the first male nurse, Lt. Roy D Field. Men, who were fully qualified registered nurses, were previously required to serve as non-commissioned officers, X-ray technicians, medics, in allied health care positions, or in the Medical Administration Branch where they could hold officer status but not as practising nurses. As more men enlisted in the nursing service, Nursing Officer replaced Nursing Sister as appropriate title designation for military nurses, although that title had been in use earlier by RCAF

opportunities to re-establish family connections. Their enthusiasm was partially based on the experiences of previous Nursing Sisters, whose officer status and overseas service had resulted in enhanced prestige and status following the First World War. As NS Helen Ross wrote, "I was influenced to choose a military career because I wished to emulate nursing sisters of the First World War who were close friends."[8]

The CNA clearly supported and promoted military nursing as a patriotic professional duty through its official voice, *The Canadian Nurse Journal*. As editor Ethel Johns wrote in 1940, "Although we Canadian nurses have distinct and vigorous characteristics of our own, our roots go deep into the rich soil of British tradition. The simplicity, the thoroughness, the devotion of the nurses in the Old Country are a continuing inspiration to us. This is the shining armour with which we may clothe ourselves in the day of battle."[9]

French-Canadians had generally opposed conscription during the First World War, and participation in this war was considered acceptable only to an extent necessary for home defence. French-Canadian nurses did serve, however, although they were much fewer in number and early plans for completely francophone medical units did not materialize. They were typically posted to Kingston for military and language training soon after enlistment. NS Gaëtane LaBonté described how difficult this transition was for her: "It was very hard for us who spoke English in a limited way.... The [English-speaking] nurses would give the lectures and they would stop. And then one of us would translate to make sure." When her unit moved to England as she wrote, "we thought the worst was over, as we had been transplanted very suddenly from our cosy French milieu to a completely different world in English."[10]

There were additional aspects of military nursing that made it extremely attractive to civilian nurses. Like their foremothers of the First World War, the second generation of Nursing Sisters was eager for travel and proximity to the men serving overseas. Still others were clearly looking for adventure and change. NS Edna Waugh wrote, "I joined the Army for better salary and a change of lifestyle." NS Joan Gore thought the Army offered a good chance to travel, while NS Marion Nichols "needed a change in my life and joining the Army was a spur of the moment decision." Some nurses considered enlistment "the thing to do" like NS Margaret Middleton who wrote, "I joined the Army because all the boys from school and relatives were joining up; it seemed the correct thing to do, go over and nurse them."[11]

Nurses had yet another important reason to welcome the opportunity for enlistment. The 1930s had been extremely lean years for graduate nurses who typically worked in private duty after completing their training. When the public became increasingly unable to afford the costs of private duty nursing, many nurses waited on registry lists for weeks before receiving a case that might provide several days of work at $5.00 per day. According to the 1932 Weir Report, approximately 40 percent of the private duty nurses in Canada were almost continuously unemployed and another 20 percent were only employed intermittently. Private duty nurses' wages were grossly inadequate to meet their costs of living.[12] But military nursing offered full-time employment, a salary triple the average civilian nurses' salary, accommodation, food, medical benefits, travel, proximity to men, and officer's rank.

All Second World War Nursing Sisters were women, and gender strongly influenced their experiences within the predominantly male Armed Forces. Although the 1941 Canadian Census reported several hundred men as nurses and student nurses, the military refused to grant them professional status as nurses — especially as a manpower shortage developed and the government implemented national conscription. Men were needed as non-commissioned combatants.

Nursing Sisters were not only a feminine workforce but they had to be either single or widowed without dependent children on enlistment. They had to sign an "undertaking" (contract) promising to resign their commission on marriage. But the Armed Forces revised this policy when a significant number of experienced military nurses resigned just as plans were developing for major offensives in the Mediterranean and Northwest Europe. Thus, Matron-in-Chief Smellie announced in 1943 that although

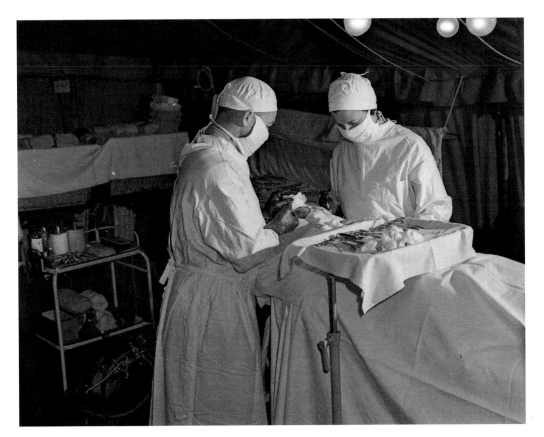

Figure 6
Surgery in Royal Canadian Army Medical Corps tent hospital
El Arrouch, Algeria 1943
Library and Archives Canada, PA-213783

married nurses were still not being *admitted* to the Forces, they could remain in the military if they married after enlistment — as long as they were "medically fit," which was code for "not pregnant."[13] Only 15 percent of the nurses married during the war, however, partially because married nurses were denied the opportunity to serve in active theatres, and many viewed this restriction as a career limitation. Most marriages took place during 1945 with the end of war in sight, or shortly after return to Canada.

Nursing Sisters were fully qualified professionals on enlistment, and while they already knew how to nurse, they had to learn how to be soldiers. Military training varied greatly but by 1943, the RCAMC provided an official "Qualifying Course for the Nursing Service," described as a four-week course and required for promotion. Some nurses described their orientation as focused on recognizing ranks and titles, and understanding military organization. Others described drilling, experiences in a gas chamber to become familiar with the proper use of gas masks, and several weeks or months of probationary work

at a military hospital within Canada. These activities served as a qualification period prior to promotion as well as screening devices for much-coveted overseas postings. Several nurses described additional field training, route marches, and field maneuvers that lasted up to ten days duration. As NS Evelyn Pepper wrote, "Learning how to march, salute, read a map, pitch a tent, take it down, put it up again, live in it and like it, eat out of a billy-can, drive anything from a motorcycle to an ambulance, fire revolvers and 303s, practice Judo techniques on our fellow-officers, plus a general orientation to army terminology and procedure, bulged our training days and hardened our muscles."[14]

Still other nurses received little or no formal military training. SAMNS NS Jean Keays explained that she did not have any "army training" because she was "just going to nurse after all."[15] NS Frances Oakes was one of the first four RCAF nurses in November 1940. She was posted overseas before the RCAF developed their three-week training program at Havergal College in Toronto, known as the "School of Aviation

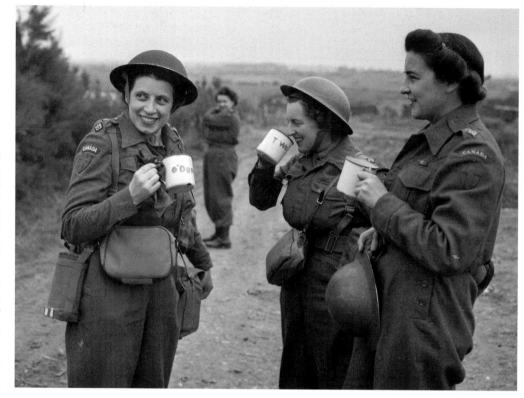

Figure 7
**Nursing Sisters
Hazel O'Donnell,
Teresa Woolsey, and
J MacKenzie with
No. 10 Canadian
General Hospital**
Arromanches
Beach, France
1944
Photographer:
Harold G. Aikman
Department of
National Defense
Library and Archives
Canada,
PA 132851

Medicine Course in Aviation Nursing." But most RCAF nurses who enlisted after December 1942 attended one of the twelve courses based on this program.[16] RCN NS Dorothy Surgenor portrayed the tenuous position of navy nurses who were considered as "support" personnel only. She said:

> I didn't even have a basic training. I just went from nursing to nursing. And this stood up very sharply because one day, [six] of us were supposed ...to be a colour party for launching of the corvette. And we didn't know anything about marching much less saluting or anything else. So for two days, the patients on the floors instructed us on how to do this because nobody really knew.... We weren't really part of the Navy.... We were not given any pre-instructions so we had to learn all about "galley" (and most of that was learned from the patients on the floor) because they *loved* teaching the Nursing Sisters.... We were in the Navy but not part of it.[17]

Later RCN nurses reported a "bewildering" introduction to barracks routine, the art of saluting, and the "significance and importance of all the different stripes and gold braid."[18]

The Armed Forces carefully regulated the selection of Nursing Sisters based on gender, age, marital status, educational preparation, and British citizenship. Once enlisted, the military proceeded to shape nurses into officers, and to constrain their activities and behaviours. Expectations as officers permeated all aspects of nurses' experience: the hospital, the military unit, and civilian settings. As NS Betty Nicolson said, "When you [were] in the Army, and especially overseas, you were in the Army all the time."[19] NS Doris Carter was reprimanded for having liquor. NS Mary Bower struggled with rank throughout her Army career and was "paraded" by her Matron for inciting soldiers to riot. NS Kathleen Rowntree liked to spend her evenings in a "neat little pub" with a dance hall while posted in England. However, as she wrote, "One morning I got called into the matron's office and told that 'jitterbugging' was not becoming to an officer." [20]

The military was ambivalent about the presence of women, especially in theatres of war. There were logistical issues to resolve, related to two sexes living and working together in close proximity 24 hours a day. There was the issue of nurses' rank and status as

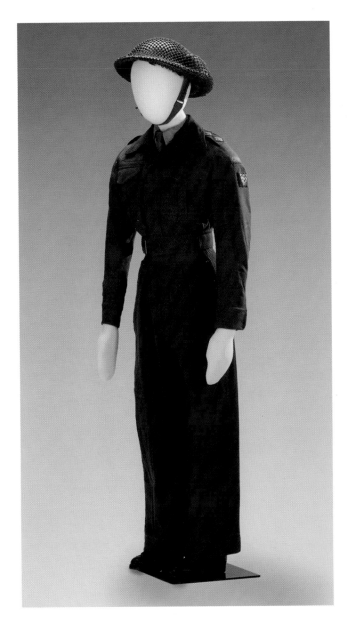

Figure 8
Battle Dress Uniform
Second World War
Canadian War Museum, 19900213, 19760457, 20020107

worth five to ten bottles of blood or plasma in the eventual outcome of a case."[21]

While the Armed Forces readily acknowledged the value of nurses to medical units, they avoided posting them to active theatres of war whenever possible. But effective medical and surgical care partially depended on the availability of nursing care on the frontlines because many of these casualties could not survive long evacuations to safer settings. The large number of surgical procedures, massive use of transfusion and fluid resuscitation, and introduction of injectable penicillin were only three wartime medical innovations that required the skills of nurses.

Nursing Sisters were supposed to train medical orderlies who could then be posted to front line field units — ostensibly to reduce the risk and danger for women. These orderlies provided valuable assistance but they were unable to substitute for highly skilled nurses. One Italian Field Surgical Unit clearly attributed their declining mortality rate of under 10 percent to "better nursing" as policies changed and nurses moved forward. As medical services historian and physician W R Feasby wrote, "It is emphasized that without the excellent post-operative care provided [by nurses], the work of the surgeons would have been of little avail however far forward they might have been positioned."[22]

The majority of nurses served in multiple theatres — up to four different theatres outside Canada. Almost all of them began their service in district military hospitals and troop training camps across Canada. One-fourth of them served entirely within Canada, either by choice or because there were no overseas vacancies. At least two-thirds of them served in England, slightly less than one-third in Europe, approximately one-fifth in the Mediterranean, 7 percent in the North Atlantic theatre, 4.3 percent in South Africa, and two nurses in Hong Kong.

The type and size of medical unit varied according to changing needs during the war. Canadian

officers that could potentially position these women in command over lower-ranking men, including lower-ranking physicians. And there was concern that public support for the war would be lost if women were injured, killed, or raped by the enemy — referred to euphemistically by several Nursing Sisters, as the "fate worse than death."

But the military expressed little doubt regarding nurses' value as professionals. Medical officer T S Wilson quantified their value this way: "Of especial importance in a surgical centre are the attached nursing sisters, whose services like that of a Thomas Splint in compound fractures of the femur, are often

General Hospital units in England were typically large 600- to 1200-bed facilities housed in borrowed spaces. They converted into field hospitals prior to moving to the Mediterranean during 1943 and 1944 and to Europe during 1944 — often doubling in size to accommodate casualties. Medical officers and nurses were added to units while regular personnel worked extended hours to complete surgical procedures and evacuate patients, and prepare for the next round of admissions.

Nurses also served in smaller 200- to 600-bed Casualty Clearing Stations (CCS), whose purpose was to stabilize and evacuate critical patients. Matron Agnes MacLeod described her CCS in England as consisting of an orderly room tent, an admission and discharge tent, a medical service tent, a surgical service tent, support services, and patient tents — in all, "well over fifty" tents. She noted rapid patient turnover because they kept only short-term cases that did not need a general hospital.[23] Size became cumbersome, and with the need for increased mobility, the CCS shifted toward the provision of immediate post-operative care of patients in addition to stabilizing casualties for evacuation. The RCAMC reduced the size of CCS further in 1943, often linking them to a small, 200-bed Stationary General Hospital for lower priority casualties and sick troops while also providing a pool of nurse reinforcements for the forward units. But as NS Jean Dorgan wrote, "The fact that we had 200 beds meant nothing. When we ran out of beds we used stretchers."[24]

Field Surgical Units and Field Dressing Stations were smaller yet, typically with two nurses plus medical and support staff. They operated in assembly-line fashion (sometimes receiving patients within 20 minutes of their being wounded), and left the follow-up care for larger units that moved in behind them. These small mobile units moved with the troops and adapted to available facilities: schools, convents, barns, bombed-out factories, chateaux, or canvas tents. Casualties requiring more than two weeks' convalescence were evacuated to England by hospital ships, trains, and air ambulance where general hospital and special units continued their care.

As nurses moved closer to the front lines, they were exposed to greater risk and danger. At least 12 nurses and an occupational therapist died on active duty, and one nurse died from enemy action. Ten RCAMC Nursing Sisters died from medical illnesses, septicemia, and motor vehicle/bicycle accidents. Two RCAF Nursing Sisters died in a training accident and one from disease. And one RCN Nursing Sister died from direct enemy action, drowning off the coast of Labrador in 1941. NS Agnes Wilkie was returning from Sydney, Nova Scotia to St. John's on the Newfoundland ferry SS *Caribou* when a German submarine torpedoed and sank it. Wilkie and her companion, NS/dietician Margaret Brooke, hung onto a capsized lifeboat for over two hours in the cold and rough waters of the Atlantic before Wilkie lost consciousness. Brooke was later rescued, and Wilkie's body was recovered for burial with full naval honors. According to Brooke,

> There was [*sic*] about a dozen of us. We clung to ropes. The waves kept washing us off, one by one, and eventually Agnes said she was getting cramped. She let go, but I managed to catch hold of her with one hand. I held to her as best I could until daybreak. Finally, a wave took her. When I called to her, she didn't answer. She must have been unconscious. The men left tried to reach her, but she floated away.[25]

While the military was extremely ambivalent concerning exposing nurses to danger, Nursing Sisters expressed far less concern. Typically, they felt their place was wherever wounded or ill soldiers were.

Making Post-war Decisions

When their skills were no longer required by the military, few Nursing Sisters returned to civilian hospitals in spite of a rapidly increasing nursing shortage across Canada. There were far more post-war nursing positions than nurses who wanted them. Military nurses were under pressure from the civilian profession to help solve this shortage but the majority of them were not interested in returning to "Civvy Street," as they called the civilian practice world. More than two-thirds indicated that they did not plan to return to civilian hospital nursing at the end of the war.[26]

Several groups of Nursing Sisters left the civilian profession immediately upon discharge. Almost

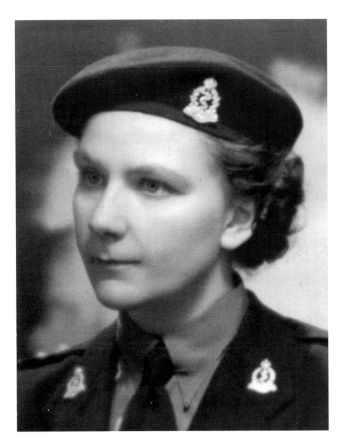

Figure 9
Nursing Sister Pauline Cox Walker
Italy
1944
Courtesy of Cynthia Toman

ent scene. And the very thought of working in civilian hospital didn't attract me at that point."[28]

Nurses indicated a wide variety of plans for their return to civilian life. Some planned to use their veteran credits to start small businesses, either independently or with a partner, such as grocery stores, a hardware store, a tea room or a bar, a ski lodge, a leather goods store, a beauty shop, a restaurant, hotel management, and a tourist camp. Others wanted to try advertising, farming, interior decorating, or handicrafts. Several planned to study art or music.[29] NS Margaret Roe considered going to California or Costa Rica but, as she said, "I wasn't ready at that time, mentally.... I had a chance to go back to university but I just wasn't ready for it."[30] During the 1945–46 academic year, 160 Nursing Sisters registered in universities across Canada and there were more applicants than could be accommodated. NS Mussallem recalled that, "You even had to sit on the steps — they were just overflowing, and a lot of them went back. [T]hat was a tremendous boost for Canada, wasn't it — all those nurses? It should have ultimately ended in better health care."[31] But the fields of public health and community nursing were the primary beneficiaries of post-war educational opportunities for many military nurses, instead of hospitals, which were experiencing the greatest shortages.

one-third married and planned to retire from nursing and raise children. As one Department of Veterans' Affairs (DVA) councillor wrote regarding a recently married nurse, she was already "happily rehabilitated." A second group of nurses remained connected to the military through permanent appointments, or to veterans as DVA nurses. Very few were able to build long-term military careers, as did NS Harriett Sloan who progressed through the ranks and became Lt. Col. Matron-in-Chief of the CFMS (1964–1968). A third group planned to work, but not in nursing. As NS Estelle Tritt said, "They wanted something different.... They would not have been happy at a civilian hospital — having the doctors try to order them around."[27]

Many Nursing Sisters were unsettled and restless when the war ended. NS Pauline Cox recalled that, "It took us awhile to adjust to civilian [settings].... [I]n the Army, you have your meals, you have your work, and everything is pretty much uniform and taken care of. And you were suddenly out doing it all on your own when you come back. It's an entirely differ-

Summary

For most of the twentieth century, military nursing remained a temporary role with the civilian profession successfully filling the ranks as needed. Relatively few nurses built long-term careers in the Armed Forces. Their roles and opportunities for professional advancement typically expanded during times of war but returned to status quo afterwards. They were motivated to enlist by multiple factors arising from the larger socio-economic and political contexts in which they lived and worked. Gender had a great deal of influence on their roles and expectations, particularly in relation to risk and danger. The composition of military nursing services gradually changed to include men, First Nations peoples, and people with multiple differences related to language, race, ethnicity, and sexual orientation. On one hand, military nurses have continued to value their experiences highly. On the other hand, they have also struggled with ongoing issues regarding gender, practice autonomy, building and maintaining core nursing competencies, and how to maintain clear identities as professional nurses within the military hierarchy.

Enough but Not Too Much: Nursing Education in English Language Canada (1874–2000)

Lynn Kirkwood

Training schools for nurses emerged as a means of improving hospital organization and increasing the quality of service to patients. They were just a practical means to an end, and were not intended to further the cause of higher learning or contribute to the overall development of human knowledge. Medical administrators, and today government officials, wanted a cheap, well-disciplined labour force; physicians wanted a nurse of pleasing personality and good character — that is, someone who would be pleasant to work with and would not challenge their authority. Nurses and nursing educators lacked the power to shape the future of nursing training and the emerging profession of nursing themselves. To begin with, the independent financial and administrative base from which Florence Nightingale launched modern nursing at St. Thomas's in Britain was not present in North America. Nor did leaders of the profession in North America have the necessary social standing and political clout to persuade a male dominated world to share the power and decision making. Thus the emphasis for nursing candidates in the early nursing schools in Canada and the US — and even in Britain where nursing leaders had a little more influence — was primarily on service, rather than on the academic or professional development of the individual. In addition it was felt that the tarnished reputation of the untrained nurse from earlier times was

something that had to be overcome, so social respectability was a primary requirement: Nursing candidates were expected to have "a minimum of educational attainment and a maximum of moral stature"[1] Even the nurse's uniform reflected bourgeois values. The high collar, long sleeves, and ankle length dress served to remind patients and nurses themselves of the womanly profession they had chosen to serve.

Arguments against nurses' educational aspirations, as against the education of women generally, have included claims of intellectual inferiority and of women's seemingly "natural" propensity to domestic service. To gain respect and recognition in nineteenth century society, nurses had to assume middle class values. Attempts to reform hospitals were to be conducted as an extension of women's role in the home. According to Adelaide Nutting, a Canadian who became the first professor of nursing at Columbia University, "hospital management consisted of expert housekeeping on an enlarged scale."[2] The mandate for nursing was not to disturb traditional male–female relationships. This stance did not threaten the professionalizing aspirations of physicians or their domination of health services. According to physicians, nurses were better off with a little education offered by physicians but not too much to make them bored with the mundane tasks of caring for the sick. The practical, domestic skills of

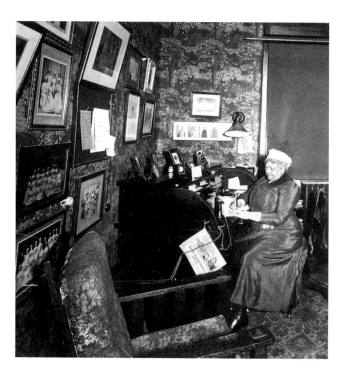

nurses were to complement the intellectual, scientific skills of medicine. The image of the nurse thus became that of the "good woman," nurturing, passive, self-denying, morally superior to men, but subordinate to physicians.

Histories of nursing education are primarily celebratory accounts of schools of nursing, usually written by graduates of the school for a particular anniversary. They focus on the fellowship, laughter, and tears of residence living and recount with humour, in song and verse, their relationships with patients and their hardships on the wards. A number of biographies about leaders in nursing education have been published in an attempt to underline the progress that nurses have made in gaining professional status. In the past twenty years, however, there have also been doctoral dissertations and numerous articles which provide a more analytic and critical analysis. More recently nursing has been discovered by historians interested in women's, labour, and social issues. These histories have added a different lens through which to view nursing's past. This chapter draws on published and unpublished work and also on the recollections of nurses who have "plied their trade" in the service of patient care. It does not cover the many and varied informal, certificate and lifelong learning courses that nurses have always been engaged in, or graduate education, nor does it address the growing number of men entering the profession and how they might influence nursing education.

Establishing Nurse Training Programs

In 1874 Theophilus Mack, MD, opened a school of nursing at the St. Catharines General and Marine Hospital in Ontario. As the three schools of nursing established in the United States a year before had done, Mack wanted to attract philanthropic funds by reorganizing the hospital while at the same time improving its sanitation and post-surgical mortality rates. He believed this could be done by replacing the untrained nurses already employed in the hospital with trained nurses. To accomplish this change, he brought two nurses who had trained in the Nightingale system to St. Catharines to set up a training program. According to Gibbon and Mathewson, the bylaws indicate that Mack was influenced by Nightingale's ideas; the motto of the school, "I See and I Am Silent," either chosen by him or paraphrased by another to clarify his meaning, was a strong indication of what hospital administrators really wanted: a saint, not a woman. He wrote:

> The nurses in the daily discharge of their duties must observe strictest secrecy, carefully avoid gossip, their demeanor should be kind and respectful on all occasions.... To evince no bias to any favorite medical practitioner. To attend scrupulously to the special duties to the patient with the gentleness and exactitude taught by their superiors, and never to interfere with or criticize the treatment.[3]

Other schools of nursing across Canada quickly proliferated. In 1881 a training school was opened at the Toronto General Hospital. Mary Agnes Snively, a former school teacher from St. Catharines, Ontario,

"We Have Played While We Worked and Worked While We Played"

James Wishart, Carleton University and Queen's University

The history of hospital training schools is enlivened by nurses' stories of their extracurricular exploits. In defiance of the strict rules of feminine decorum and the soul-crushing work regimen that characterized hospital training, nursing students had their own rituals of fun and fantasy that perhaps helped alleviate the harsher aspects of apprenticeship and strengthened the camaraderie that sustained them through their training and later careers. Breaking the rules was the rule, whether by racing laundry hampers through the underground tunnels of the hospital, stealing roast chickens from the Dietary Kitchen, or climbing in or out of residence windows after curfew. At Kingston General Hospital, student nurses from the 1920s to the 60s chronicled their escapades in a journal hidden in the splint room. On a water-stained page dated November 1933, for instance, we read of the practice of "sinking," a symbolic baptism that initiated new students to the surgery unit:

> Miss Freeman being away at the game, we the staff decided it would be an excellent time to put S—— in the sink.... L—— and P—— [two interns] assisted us in giving her a good ducking, in fact two to make sure she was wet. Then one by one all the new O.R. arrivals were lowered into the white enamel basins filled with nice icy water. One by one drowned maidens ran for the W.C. coming out dry but pantless. Very swiftly the flood was mopped up before our assistant supe arrived back...and we are back to work little worse for our party.

In the same clandestine journal, a 1928 graduate summed up her experiences of hospital training: "Three years ago to this day 23 shy bashful but willing girls [sic] entered the KGH to join the working class. Little did we know what was ahead because had we — well I wonder where some of us would be today. However, not one of us is sorry because we have played while we worked and worked while we played."

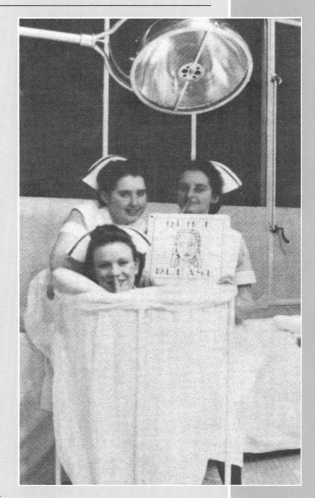

Figure 2
Fooling around in the O.R.
Royal Jubilee Hospital School
of Nursing, Victoria, BC
1960
Alumnae Association of the Royal Jubliee
Hospital School of Nursing

Source: Queen's University Archives (QUA) Kingston General Hospital Fonds (KGH) R500, Nurses' "Comment," 4 Nov. 1933, 18 Sept. 1928.

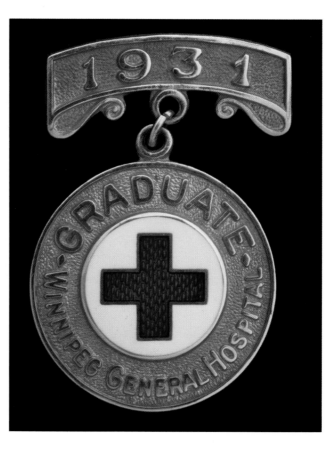

who had just graduated from the Bellevue Hospital Training School in New York, took over the school in 1884 and succeeded in making it one of the most successful schools of nursing in Canada. She ultimately became the leading advocate for the professionalization of nursing, both in her role as an educator and also as founder of the Canadian Nurses Association. In 1890, after two abortive attempts by others, Nora Livingston, a recent graduate of the New York Hospital's Training School, was successful in establishing a training school at the Montreal General Hospital, over which she reigned for twenty years. Training schools were established in the Maritimes in the 1890s, influenced primarily by the successful programs on the eastern seaboard of the United States. They also spread to the West along with the settlers and the railway. The Winnipeg General Hospital School of Nursing claims to be the first in western Canada (1887). The Sisters of Charity of Montreal (the Grey Nuns) established the first French-speaking school of nursing at Notre-Dame Hospital in Montreal in 1898. The Grey Nuns were quintessential educators, later establishing other religious schools in Quebec and throughout the country.

Throughout the early development of nursing training, however, no mechanism was ever put into place to identify a formal knowledge base called "nursing." The skill of nursing was linked to duty (the good woman), obligation (altruistic care of the good mother), and order (the self-discipline of a good soldier). And these qualities together became the expertise of nurses. Little is known about the untrained nurses who staffed hospitals before the shift to a formal training system. There is no evidence to suggest any were accepted into, or allowed to participate in, the new trained nurse movement, nor anything to suggest their knowledge and experience were recognized in the new training schools. The first genera-

tion of nursing education reformers tended to be teachers or even university graduates, many of whom had some association with Teacher's College, Columbia University, which established a course for nursing educators in 1899. They wanted an education similar to that of their brothers, so a liberal education became the basis for nursing training. Elizabeth Logan, who had a double degree in psychology and biology from Acadia University and a masters in nursing from Yale, explained: "... We were encouraged to be creative, we could do a few more things perhaps a little differently because of it [liberal education]. And I found this very stimulating. ... And so this sort of set my sights on what I thought nursing could and should do."[4]

By 1902 there were 70 training schools in Canada with courses of two or three years in length offering young women training in nursing in exchange for service to patients. By 1930, at the time of the *Survey of Nursing Education in Canada* (The Weir Report), there were 212 training schools in the 886 hospitals across Canada. Data at the time did not separate students from graduate nurses or untrained nurses. The census for 1901 identified 280 nurses. By 1921, following the First World War, there was a dramatic increase to 21 163, of which 223 were male. According to Kathryn McPherson,[5] mental hospitals relied on male nurses and did accept them into training. These programs were two years in length with students often completing two more years in a general hospital program. However, these male students were more frequently disciplined, and hospital administrators preferred the deference and docility of female students. By 1960, at the time of the *Royal Commission on Health Services* there were as many students in training as there were students and nurses combined in 1921 — 21 297 students in 188 hospitals across Canada. Interestingly, these numbers have changed very little. In 2000 there were 21 390 nursing students enrolled in nursing programs. Nursing was one of the few occupations open to women in 1900 and offered them skills, respectability, and financial security. By the 1960s, however, it was competing with numerous other occupations many of which offered better employment opportunities, working conditions, and remuneration.

In the early days, the reasons for going into nursing were many and varied. While nursing provided a cheap labour force for the development of hospitals, the new schools also offered independence and freedom, much needed employment for those no longer needed on the family farm, and safe and respectable work opportunities that stayed within the bounds of women's expected role in society. Certainly conditions were harsh, the hours of work long, and education and training sparse. New recruits were often sent into the wards with no preparation for the work they were supposed to do. Some have argued that the training was not really apprenticeship but something less, with students learning from one another or on their own.[6] Kathryn McPherson has argued that, although conditions in early hospitals were severe, hospitals offered women a passage out of the harsh economies of rural Canada and a relatively privileged occupation compared with women in other sectors of the economy. Some women who really wanted to go to university went into training because the family finances were earmarked for the sons' education. But social

limitations on women's opportunities also drew women into nursing. Rae Chittick, who taught school on the Prairies during the First World War and later became Director of Nursing at McGill School for Graduate Nurses, said:

> There was so little one could undertake in those days. I thought at first I wanted to be a doctor. I didn't have the money. My father discouraged me. He said, "you'd never get a practice"... I was trying to do some nursing during the flu epidemic. There was a nurse who worked in the Royal Bank as a secretary, she had given up nursing. She came back to organize it.... She was so efficient. I thought nurse training would help me become more efficient. So I went to [Johns] Hopkins.[7]

In the 1930s schools were flooded with applicants whose families were financially stricken by the Depression. Nurse training provided free lodging and plenty of good food, making nurse trainees better off than many of their friends. One student recounts: "The crash of 1929...affected many of our parents.... Skilled people could not find jobs in their chosen profession. We in training were lucky; we worked hard and studied hard, but the sisters fed us well."[8]

There were very few students from visible minority groups in nursing before the 1970s. Many schools refused to admit these students, and job opportunities were scarce. For example, in 1932 the Vancouver General Hospital admitted a Japanese-Canadian student, and in 1936 a Chinese-Canadian student (Louise Lore [later Yuen]) graduated and immediately entered the public health certificate course at University of British Columbia. But her career options were restricted, since she was expected to work in the Vancouver Metropolitan Board of Heath with her own people. And to work for less pay than white nurses.[19]

Nurses had no control over the development of nursing in the clinical area; that remained the domain of physicians. And administrative control of educational programs belonged solely to hospital administrators, whose primary aim was to acquire a cheap and docile labour force. Nurse superintendents, therefore, were assigned the task of character building and the discipline of students. Although there were some attempts to improve educational standards,

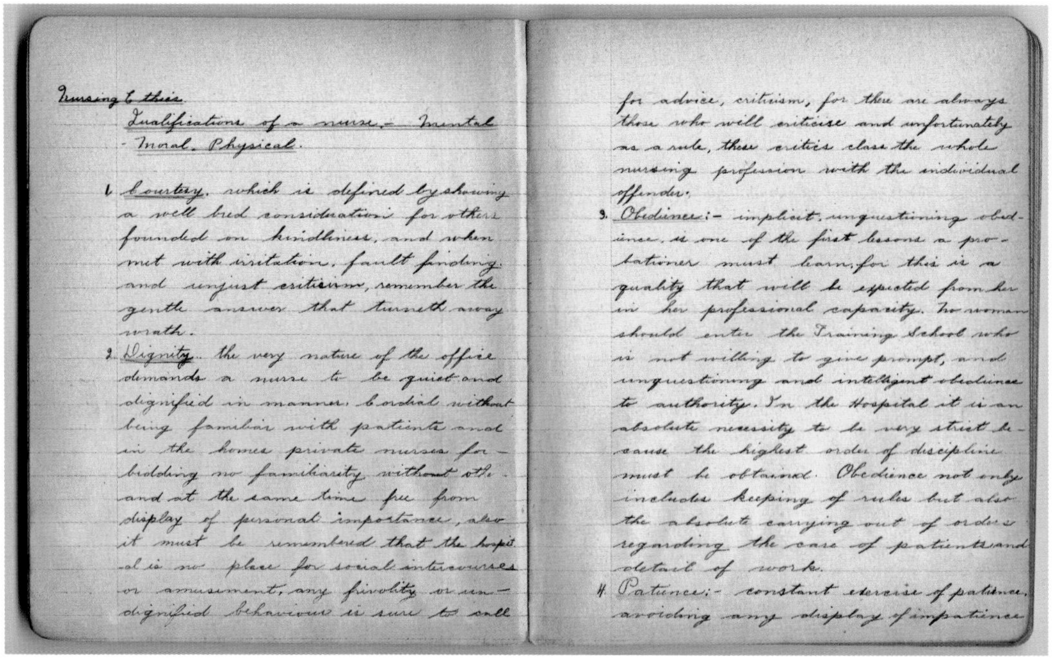
Nursing Ethics.
Qualifications of a nurse. - Mental - Moral. Physical.

1. Courtesy. which is defined by showing a well bred consideration for others founded on kindliness, and when met with irritation, fault finding and unjust criticism, remember the gentle answer that turneth away wrath.
2. Dignity. the very nature of the office demands a nurse to be quiet and dignified in manner. Cordial without being familiar with patients and in the homes private nurses forbidding no familiarity without oth- and at the same time free from display of personal importance, also it must be remembered that the hospital is no place for social intercourses or amusement, any frivolity or undignified behaviour is sure to call

for advice, criticism, for there are always those who will criticise and unfortunately as a rule, these critics class the whole nursing profession with the individual offender.

3. Obedience:- implicit, unquestioning obedience, is one of the first lessons a probationer must learn, for this is a quality that will be expected from her in her professional capacity. No woman should enter the Training School who is not willing to give prompt, and unquestioning and intelligent obedience to authority. In the Hospital it is an absolute necessity to be very strict because the highest order of discipline must be obtained. Obedience not only includes keeping of rules but also the absolute carrying out of orders regarding the care of patients and detail of work.
4. Patience:- constant exercise of patience, avoiding any display of impatience

Figure 4
Page of nursing student's notebook, "Nursing Ethics: Qualifications of a Nurse, Mental, Moral and Physical"
Grace Hospital
Windsor, Ontario
1920
Canadian Museum of Civilization Archives
Gift of Lynn Kirkwood

generally speaking lectures — usually given by doctors — were held after long days of clinical service. Only students who had "free time" from the wards attended. During the early years, superintendents of nursing, with very little collegial or professional support, struggled to maintain a delicate balance between meeting the demands of patient service and those of student education — while, of course, trying at the same time to meet the expectations of parents and society at large. To avoid compromising her position, the superintendent had to set an example of socially acceptable womanhood at all times.

Reforming Nursing Education

By the 1920s nursing educators were unhappy about their loss of control of nursing education. Physicians, on the other hand, were mistrustful of nurses moving outside the hospital, where doctors controlled nurses' practice, into the new domain of public health, which had not yet come under full medical jurisdiction. Nurses wanted to develop areas of nursing expertise beyond what was considered medicine — the prevention of illness and the maintenance of health — while still acknowledging medical dominance in areas that overlapped both professions. In 1927 members of the Canadian Nurses Association (CNA) and Canadian Medical Association (CMA) agreed to work together to determine the educational needs of nurses. *The Survey of Nursing Education in Canada,* commonly known as The Weir Report, was funded two-thirds by the CNA and one-third by the CMA. In order to address all the issues on the table, George Weir, Professor of Education at the University of British Columbia, was given sweeping powers to study all aspects of nursing and nursing education. There was so much opposition to nurses' desire to improve their education that Weir felt compelled to address the question directly in a chapter entitled "Does the Nurse Need to Be Educated?" He wrote: "A little reasoning is not a dangerous thing if it is sound; but unsound reasoning that tends, intentionally or otherwise, to deprive the nurse of the advantages of a sound education is not only dangerous but indefensible."

And quoting from an address of a university president, he wrote: "Nursing education is something more than the scraps of a hospital's spare time or a source of cheap labour."[10]

In order to improve education and raise standards, Weir recommended the removal of education from hospital control, that small schools be closed, and that entrance standards and working conditions be improved. He also warned universities that sooner or later they, along with the well-equipped hospital, would be called upon to educate nurses, since university education was an essential part of professional progress.

Following his report, some new measures were put into place: Some small schools were closed and common standards of education were set forth by the CNA. However, the standards were not compulsory, so many hospitals did nothing to improve conditions. Thirty years after this report Helen Mussallem found that very little had changed.[11] Although the number of schools had decreased from 218 in 1936 to 171 in 1959, only 16 percent met the standards set by the CNA.

It is too easy to use the Depression of the 1930s to justify non-action. In hindsight, the Depression offered great opportunities for change. Many nurses were out of work and could easily have replaced student labour at very little cost — and to some extent this did happen. However, the apprenticeship system had become firmly entrenched and was economically satisfactory for hospital administrators. They feared that replacing students with graduate nurses would undermine their authority and present discipline problems. The public, parents in particular, were generally pleased with the supervision, discipline, and training that schools offered their daughters, at little expense to themselves. As Helen Carpenter suggested:

> Many Schools of Nursing had achieved recognized standing in the community and were the pride of hospital boards, administrators and doctors, as well as graduates of the school and their families. To suggest change was to imply criticism. Universities and governments hesitated to interfere with a system acceptable to the public and one that required minimal financial support.[12]

The twenty-year period following the Second World War saw drastic changes in nursing education. The advances in medical science after the war, the hospital insurance act of 1957, and increased government funding to health care and education in the 1960s helped to finally bring about the major recommendation of The Weir Report — the transfer of nursing education to educational institutions. In the 1950s, hospitals began to question the feasibility of funding nursing education programs. In a study done at Toronto Western Hospital in 1950, it was found that "the net loss to the hospital [of running a training school] was $230.46 per student." The author concluded, therefore, that "exploitation of students did not exist."[13] At the same time, a study to demonstrate that nurses could be trained successfully in less time if they did not have to provide service was conducted by the CNA at the Metropolitan Hospital in Windsor, Ontario. This program was two years in length, and during that two years the students concentrated only on their own training and were not responsible for service to the hospital. The program was conducted between January 1949 and September 1952. At the end of the study, it was determined that the 87 graduates of the program were as well prepared for basic bedside nursing as were graduates of the three-year hospital training program "control" group.[14] But a similar study done at the Regina Grey Nuns Hospital in the 1960s did not produce as positive results.[15]

Without giving up training schools altogether, hospitals found a way to recoup costs in what was called the nurse intern program. As patient care became more acute, it was apparent that junior students did not have enough experience to be put in charge of very sick patients. But more senior students could take over much of this responsibility. During the 1960s, courses consisting of two years' training plus a one-year internship were introduced across the country. In these programs student nurses spent more time than previously in the classroom during the first two years, with the third year devoted primarily to full bedside service. Almost every province adopted some form of this system. Later during the 1960s, when the shortage of nurses became more acute, these programs were reduced to two years.

It is interesting to speculate about why nurse educators bought into the idea of a reduced training period when length of training is directly associated with professional status. In accepting shorter training periods, did nurses lose an opportunity to provide a sounder scientific foundation and strengthen nursing courses? And did they miss a chance to completely transfer nursing education into the university, at a time when other professions, such as teaching, were doing just that? In answer, however, it is important to remember that hospital administrators and physicians still wielded considerable power, and the notion that the educated nurse might not want to do the dull, menial, and boring tasks of bedside care was still an obstacle to be overcome. Even though the CNA was involved in the Metropolitan Hospital Project, they were only an advisory body. With few nurses having the qualifications to teach, nurses were satisfied to settle for the best deal they could get: that is, some control of the education process.

By the 1960s, after just about every jurisdiction had debated nursing education, the system of apprenticeship had finally outlived its usefulness. With the cost of training students rising and more government money available to hire graduate nurses, hospital superintendents were willing to turn over the training of nurses to others. Although many graduates of these early hospital programs extol the benefits of residence living, young women of the new feminist era did not view the petty rules and discipline of residence living with much amusement. As well, the profile of nursing applicants was changing to include older students with previous experience, males, and visible minorities. Gradually, during the late 1960s and early 1970s, hospital training programs were transferred into the developing colleges of applied arts and technology or regional nursing centres. With this transfer, the major philosophical underpinnings of nursing education — service to the hospital and the lifelong friendships and support of residence living — came to an end.

Significantly, the shift of nursing education to the educational system eroded physicians' hold over nursing education at the diploma level. Moyra Allen and Marie Reidy also found that as nursing education programs moved into educational institutions, students focused more on the care of their patients than they did on the policies and practices of their hospitals.[16] Although there have been no studies done to determine how nursing fared in the technical education institutions, anecdotal evidence suggested that faculty and students were highly regarded and were seen as a positive contribution to the academic and political development of the institutions.

Professional Nursing Education

The establishment of nursing programs within five Canadian universities in 1919–1920 provided an educational foundation for nursing from which nursing leadership could achieve their goal of professionalization. At this time, university education was seen as a means of providing a small group of nurses who would become teachers, supervisors, and public health nurses with the leadership skills to reform nursing.[17] Instead of moving all of nursing education into the university, nursing educational reformers justified university education for a few nurses, thus creating a two-tiered system of entry into the profession and two cultures for nursing — the professional culture, rooted in education and science, and a craft culture, rooted in domestic skills. Although there were physicians who supported the programs, there were also many critics. Nurses knew better than to promote university education for all nurses at this time. Instead they chose to "tread softly" and be satisfied with university education for a small group of nurses. Ethel Johns, the first director of the UBC program, assured the many critics that: "[T]he number of women who will choose or who are fit for the higher reaches will be necessarily small. It is not intended for one moment to recommend that all pupils be compelled to take the combined course."[18]

University programs in nursing began in Canada in 1918 with a short two-month course for public health nurses at the University of Alberta. In 1919 the University of British Columbia (UBC) established a five-year program for nurses. It was the first baccalaureate program in nursing in the British Empire. This program and other university programs of that time were closely tied to two key social reform issues of the time: scientific management and public health. The program at UBC was established through the efforts of an influential hospital superintendent, Dr Malcolm MacEachern at the Vancouver General Hospital, and Henry Esson Young, the provincial medical officer of health. These men, as other physicians throughout our history have done, promoted the expansion of nursing education when it served the purpose in which they were interested. MacEachern believed that better educated nurses (in contrast to

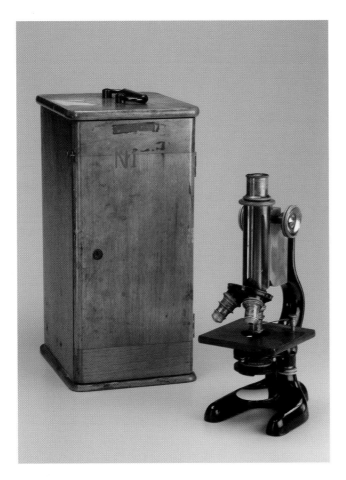

Figure 5
Microscope
Faculty of Nursing, University of Western Ontario
ca. 1930
Canadian Museum of Civilization, 2004.62.1.2
Gift of Marion McGee

Normal Schools for teachers, would not have been publicly supported. But most importantly, nursing reformers were aware that affiliation in the modern university ensured professional status.

In 1920 the Red Cross Society, which was looking for a role in peacetime health efforts, agreed to fund university programs for public health nurses on a temporary basis. After much negotiation they convinced five universities to co-operate in the new endeavour. Courses of one-year duration started in September 1920 at Dalhousie University, McGill University, the University of Toronto, and UBC, all funded by provincial Red Cross Societies. The University of Western Ontario began a course the same year funded by the local branch. Each university received $5000 yearly for three years. The Ontario branch also provided ten yearly scholarships to students of $350 each. McGill included courses for teachers and supervisors as well as public health nurses, because physicians did not believe that there were enough nurses interested in university education to financially support a course solely in public health nursing. After the Red Cross funding was withdrawn in 1923, only Dalhousie closed its program. All other universities had enough students interested to warrant continuation without outside funding. But funding remained (and still remains) an acute problem. The only program that received outside funding after the Red Cross agreement expired was the French language Institute Marguerite d'Youville, sponsored by the Grey Nuns and associated with the University of Montreal. Between 1925 and 1930 the program received $34 000 in funding in order to deal with the high rate of tuberculosis in Quebec's rural areas.[20] And as important as this program was, its funding did not survive the Depression.

Within the university, nurses faced deep seated prejudices about female intellectual inferiority. While

the better trained nurses of Theophilus Mack's day) would be able to carry out hospital and community health reforms more efficiently, competently, and cost effectively than those who were then being trained. The initiatives in hospital and public health reform gave nurses the opportunity they had been looking for to use scientific advances in bacteriology and hygiene to develop a systematic knowledge base for nursing. However, nurses committed to independence in the developing profession of nursing feared that medicine would continue to interfere with their progress. In a letter to her colleague Isabel Stewart, Adelaide Nutting wrote: "…[I]t seems to be entirely clear that our efforts towards freedom in universities are going to be blocked by our medical friends. We get out from under the hospital only to pass under the hands of the medical school."[19]

Even so, in the early years of the twentieth century there were few options available. Colleges of applied arts and technology had not been established, and a system of independent schools, such as the

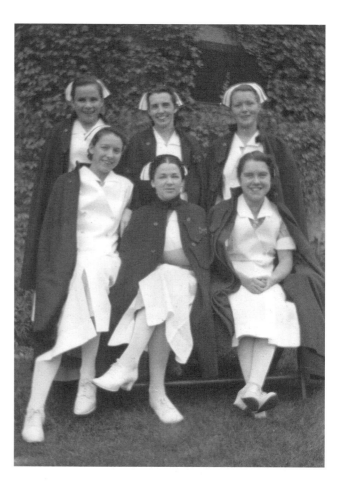

this plagued all women, nurses faced discrimination related to both their gender and their chosen discipline. Not only were nurses women, but they were perceived to be doing women's "natural" work, for which university education was not seen to be necessary. During the Depression, nursing programs met with both skepticism and open hostility from male faculty, who were themselves threatened with salary cuts. The School for Graduate Nurses at McGill had to be rescued from closure by nurses from all across Canada, whose pledges and support were enough to keep the school open until 1943, when the university saw fit to once again take over funding. Ironically, in that year the school received $12 000 from the Kellogg Foundation but was too bereft of resources to spend all of the money. The early diploma courses at the University of Toronto and McGill were weighted towards the new social sciences, which had not yet received university sanction. At McGill, like other women students, nurses were introduced to the great scholars of the day such as Stephen Leacock, whose fundamental opposition to higher education for women was certain to affect their self-esteem. In his essay "We Are Teaching Women All Wrong," he decried women's ability to do even elementary science. He wrote: "At McGill the girls of our first year have wept over their failures in elementary physics these twenty-five years. It is time that one dried their tears and took away the subject."[21]

In the 1950s when nursing students entered the university in greater numbers one professor at McGill coped with the influx by failing all the nurses. Elizabeth Logan recounts: "We introduced about 50 students to the English course. ... In order to deal with it the professor decided to fail all the nurses because she said that nurses could never learn English."[22]

University administrators were willing to offer nurses certificates or diplomas as part of the universities' contribution to the public health movement if, and only if, it was economically feasible.

However, in order to be awarded the sacrosanct university degree, nurses had to be tested in the traditional curriculum by which universities judged educational standards, liberal education. Nurse reformers were committed to both to higher education for nurses and to the development of the profession of nursing, so nursing educators had to figure out how to find an academic standard for nursing that compared to that of the traditional university courses. Kathleen Russell, director of the University of Toronto nursing program, came to realize that before they could reform nursing education, nursing educators had to prove themselves and their students academically worthy. She wrote:

> The nursing school of Canada must accommodate itself to the Canadian university if it wants to work with it.
>
> ... Later when we have become part of our country's universities we can hope to take our part (small though it may be) in the general development of the whole institution. At present, I must

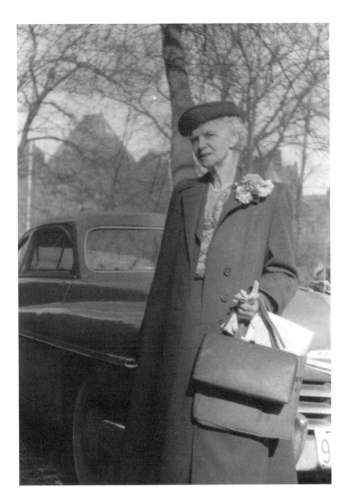

Figure 7
Kathleen Russell
Courtesy of Lynn Kirkwood

a full year of university courses to begin with. Students then went into training at the Vancouver General Hospital (later at St. Paul's Hospital) and then returned to the university for a year of courses in public health, teaching, or administration (the non-integrated or sandwich program). Students learned in two worlds — the world of the university, where education was highly valued, and the world of the hospital, where service was valued. Nursing faculty at the university had no control over student time and learning. Later some of these programs were increased to include three years of university, thereby giving students the equivalent of a general arts degree plus nursing training.

The second type of undergraduate program was called an integrated program. This program was pioneered in Canada by Kathleen Russell at the University of Toronto. After being refused degree status by the university in the 1920s, Kathleen Russell set about developing a nursing program that would meet all the standards of a university degree. She was determined to control all aspects of university nursing education — administrative, financial, and educational — within a school of nursing, "loosely connected to the university." In 1932, with funding from the Rockefeller Foundation ($17 500 yearly for five years), she established a diploma program in which university nursing faculty had full authority for the teaching of nursing practice in the wards of the Toronto General Hospital. In this radical departure from traditional nursing education, neither the faculty nor the students had any responsibility for service needs to the hospital. Over a ten-year period, Kathleen Russell and the faculty integrated nursing theory and practice with the academic courses of the university. By 1942 she was convinced that the program met all the criteria for degree status — sufficient academic courses for a general arts degree as well as high quality nursing education — and she successfully applied to have it made a degree-granting program. Several factors, apart from the readiness

repeat once more, we must know our university and use it *as it is*.[23]

The five-year basic degree programs grew very slowly until after the 1970s. These lengthy and demanding programs were not attractive to the majority of young women wanting to go into nursing or to their families. For example, ten students were registered at UBC in 1929 and 32 in 1958. By 1971 only one nurse in 14 held a university degree, and in 1989 12 percent of new graduates had completed university degree programs, far short of the 25 percent recommended in 1962 in the Royal Commission on Health Services.

These early nursing programs reflected the segregation of theory and practice. Universities were willing to offer nurses access to general university courses but refused to take on responsibility for practical learning in the hospital. The program justified by the university, like the one started at the University of British Columbia in 1919, provided

Northern Nursing Program

Pertice Moffitt, Instructor, Aurora College; PhD candidate, University of Calgary

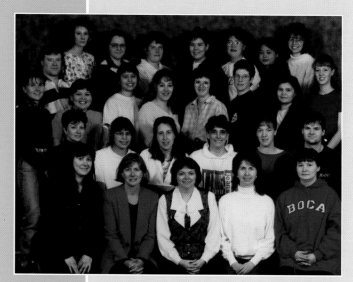

Figure 8
First group of nursing students and faculty of the Diploma Program
Aurora College, NWT
1995
Courtesy of Pertice Moffatt

In Canada's territories since the 1940s, nurses have been recruited from southern Canada to provide nursing care to the majority Aboriginal populations. With the onset of the Northern Nursing Program at College West (now Aurora College), nurses are now home-grown Northerners, many Aboriginal.

The establishment of the NWT Northern Nursing Program required many systemic transformations, however, and one of the most memorable of those changes was the legislation process that occurred to accommodate nursing education in the Northwest Territories.

At the time I was president of the Northwest Territories Registered Nurses Association. On 6 March 1995, *Bill 17*, an Act to amend the *Nursing Profession Act* to allow registration of nurses educated through the Northern Nursing Program, was scheduled for public hearings by the NWT Standing Committee on Legislation. Four nursing students went to the meeting of their own volition with personal stories about the significance of the legislation to them.

Tony Whitford, a highly respected territorial politician and the chairman of the Standing Committee, presided over this particular meeting. The students spoke from the heart and without rehearsal about their desire to become nurses. Although the setting was formal (the caucus room of the Legislative Assembly), the students' spontaneous presentations and the listeners' responses were laced with laughter and tears.

Karen Binder, an Inuvialuk from Inuvik, began the students' presentation, saying, "[W]e are presently in our second semester and we have been working very hard in our studies." Adele Tatti, a Dene from Deline, who was the next to speak, began her talk in South Slavey. The committee was not prepared for presentations in languages other than English and Tony apologized that there was not a translator in the room. Adele emphasized the importance of nurses being able to speak their own languages and told of the hopes and aspirations of her home community for her to become a nurse. Linda Panika, an Inuk from Rankin Inlet, spoke directly to the eastern Arctic MLA on the committee and told him, "[M]y granny will be so upset if I cannot become a nurse." Shannon Saunders, a Metis from Yellowknife, stated that since she was a little girl she had always wanted to be a nurse and if this Bill did not proceed her dreams would be unfulfilled. With that she broke into tears, and Tony got up from his chair with a box of tissues, walked over to Shannon, and consoled her.

There was not a dry eye in the room. The Bill was passed without a hitch. I have no doubt that the influencing force behind *Bill 17* was those four nursing students.

of the program, probably influenced her decision to apply for degree status at that time: Graduates of her program, believed to be the best undergraduate program in Canada, were not eligible for graduate education courses in the United States without a degree. And another predominantly female discipline — Health and Physical Education — had just been granted degree status.[24] Given the generally slow and reluctant acceptance of nursing within the academic world, one wonders whether the university would have acted on its own to offer degree status to the program without Kathleen Russell's advocacy.

A third type of university nursing training, the post-RN program, was introduced after the First World War to meet the need for nurses with specialized preparation to serve in the expansion of public health services. These programs provided two years of university education for previously qualified RNs, and for a time, were immensely popular. For the universities they were an inexpensive way to train nurses, because the institution only took responsibility for the relatively low cost academic component, leaving the costly clinical training to others; and for nurses it was a relatively inexpensive route to a degree — and better career opportunities. In practice, however, the separation of theory and practice was not very effective. Learning is said to be better if theory and practice are integrated or if theory comes first. As the academic revolution of the 1960s changed university dynamics and government funding increased, universities heeded the recommendations of the Royal Commission on Health Services to adopt the integrated model as pioneered by Kathleen Russell at the University of Toronto.

At the time when nursing programs were becoming fully integrated within the university and diploma programs were finding a new home in institutes of art and technology, the CNA made their last stand towards achieving professional status for all nurses. In the move from hospitals to educational institutions, nursing, for the first time, was able to establish and gain control of educational standards. Diploma programs were evaluated by a provincial association, and in 1986, the Canadian Association of University Schools of Nursing established an accreditation system, thus meeting one of the major criteria of professionalization. Following the American lead, the CNA, in 1982, adopted a policy making university level education the goal for entry into the practice of nursing. "Entry to Practice by the year 2000" became the rallying cry of the association. In 1995, with universities' reluctance and government doubts, Alberta established a unique program in which college and university programs formed a partnership to provide education and degree status. By 2005 all provinces offer full degree status, although there are still diploma programs in British Columbia, Alberta, and Quebec. In this move the two cultures of nursing education might be bridged. As university degrees become the only entry to nursing practice, questions of where to educate the nurse have been resolved for the time being. Now nursing educators can turn their full attention to how to educate the nurse.

Conclusions

With university education now accepted as entry to practice, nurses have met the demands of the university for professional education. However, nurses, as women generally, continue to struggle to have their experiences and knowledge validated within the university and society. Nurses' demands for equal access to education and professional autonomy were based on its complementary relationship with medicine. To date, nurses have not been able to shed the shackles of this role in any meaningful way. And they continue to profess reluctance to give up practice as both a learning and research model. Although faculty in all professional schools are committed to some form of practice, the concept of excellence promoted by the university suggests a hierarchical system, with knowledge gained through practice occupying a lower order than theoretical or scientific knowledge. To date universities have tended to devalue nurturance and caring. A coming issue in nurses' association with the university will be whether they accommodate themselves to the university and "use it as it is." Or will nurses as the largest group of women academics "take their part in the general development of the whole institution," challenging the dictates of traditional professional education and pushing the boundaries of science to include feminine values such as caring?

CHAPTER 13

Professionalism and Canadian Nursing

Diana Mansell and Dianne Dodd

Two distinct paths toward the development of nursing as a profession, the Anglo-Protestant "Nightingale" tradition and the French-Catholic tradition, will be dealt with in separate sections of this chapter. In English Canada, the campaign to gain professional recognition, enhanced by the Nightingale mystique, was very much a part of early nursing history. Drawing on various, often conflicting, definitions of what constitutes a profession, the chapter will assess whether the goals of nursing leaders were achieved. In Quebec, nursing developed within the French hospital system established in 1639 by skilled and devoted religious women, exemplified by the Augustines. Questions relating to professional status will be assessed in light of the impact of the Nightingale system on the French-Catholic model. Different responses emerged out of Montreal and Quebeco a nursing model that ill-suited the French-Catholic hospital tradition.

The Anglo-Protestant "Nightingale" Tradition

In a recent *Globe and Mail* obituary, nurse Dorothy Macham was described as "an efficient, thrifty administrator who exerted a spirit of gentleness and compassion." Macham was a leader in health care and professional advancement at home and abroad, attaining the military rank of Major, receiving the Associate Royal Red Cross medal for Second World War service, and heading Women's College Hospital for three decades. Yet, nowhere in the article is the word "professional" used. Can a nurse not be both compassionate and professional?[1] The term "professional" has had different meanings at different times, and each generation of nursing leaders had its own vision of what a professional nurse was. Underlying all their visions, however, lay one common thread: the desire to instil in nurses at all levels the belief that they were, or could become, professionals. And nursing leaders did achieve, over the course of the past century, the basic elements considered necessary to meet most definitions of professionalism,[2] although there were certainly disappointments and obstacles encountered along the way.

Critiques of Professionalism

The debate about professionalism among both nurses and historians centres on the question of whether or not nurses achieved professional autonomy and public confidence. We must also ask whether professionalism provides a satisfactory model for analyzing nursing work and nursing history and for assessing the effectiveness of the professionalization strategy.

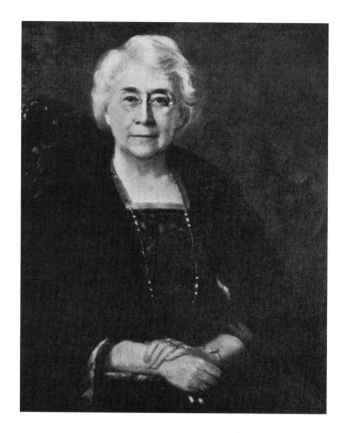

How did early nurse historians and nursing leaders define the components of a profession? Early leaders do not appear to have defined it at all. Rather, they assumed the nurse was a professional, more as a demand than a statement of fact. They asserted that the graduate or trained nurse was a full-time paid worker who had received formal training in a hospital school, and that she was not a woman religious or a domestic worker. She was still expected, however, to behave in a pious and respectable manner.

This model was accepted until the 1980s, when historians began to examine the components of professionalism. Feminist historians and academics have examined the way in which patriarchal society delegates nurturing to women, exploits their alleged capacity for compassion, and subordinates the nurse to medical authority. Some historians have wondered whether nurses are members of the "pink collar" ghetto of women workers. Yolande Cohen and others, for example, speak of nursing as a subordinate profession, citing the paradox of nurses having a legally recognized right to practise, yet having so much of their actual professional practice dependent on medical authority.[3]

Using the medical profession as her point of comparison, Margaret Levi defined the criteria for a professional as:

- the performance of full-time work
- the formation of a national professional association
- the development of a formal code of ethics by which to eliminate the incompetent and unscrupulous
- political activity in a state granted monopoly
- the requirement of an advanced degree, usually at a university.

Levi suggests that, although nurses achieved some of these criteria, they still fell short of the mark, concluding that a remaining obstacle is functional redundancy, that is, "there is very little, if anything that is defined as exclusively the province of the R.N."[4]

Kathryn McPherson has pointed out that the historical focus on professionalization ignores other hierarchies that sometimes pit nurses against other health care workers such as midwives, and neglects the rank and file nurse who may not have adopted the professional goals of her leaders. McPherson suggests that the professional image is complicated by an equally compelling image of the nurse as a worker, arguing that, in moving from self-employed private duty nursing to salaried positions in hospitals, nurses underwent a de-skilling process, or proletarianization. The latter is analogous to the nineteenth century craftsman who was reduced to a waged labourer when his skilled work was subdivided and brought under the control of professional managers. Similarly, nursing educator Shirley Stinson and historian David Wagner conclude that between the years 1920 and 1960, nursing experienced "deprofessionalization" characterized by "a diminution of independence, increasing stratification and division of labour, and growing revolt against assembly-line conditions."[5]

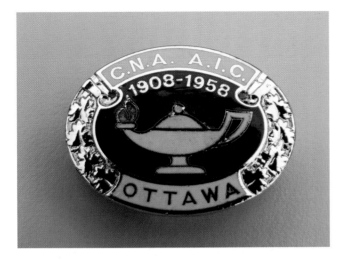

Figure 2
**Canadian Nurses Association
Meeting Pin**
1958
Photographer: Doug Millar
Canadian Nurses Association Collection
Canadian Museum of Civilization, 2000.111.18

Other historians have argued that nurses did attain some form of professional status. Cynthia Toman describes nursing as "one of several women's occupations that professionalized during the early 1900s."[6] Similarly, historian Mary Kinnear argues convincingly that, while acknowledging the gender inequities in the professional workplace, nurses did win the right to call themselves professionals and that their gains opened the door to professional employment and university education for other women. Kinnear rejects the stringent medical or legal model often used to assess professional status, as it allows no more than a small handful of self-employed practitioners to qualify. Kinnear also notes that the vast majority of twentieth century professionals are salaried employees and often members of professional unions. This paper will argue that nursing leaders were successful in attaining professional status, by showing that they met all of Kinnear's criteria for a professional which include: "Post-secondary education and training in a subject requiring scientific or esoteric skill and knowledge; a certification test;... a degree of self-regulation by practitioners...[and] service to the public."[7]

The Campaign for Professional Recognition

As professionalization promised a pathway to achieving legitimacy, power, and autonomy, Anglo-Protestant Canadian nursing leaders worked toward it by establishing professional associations; lobbying for registration legislation and exclusive use of the title RN; enhancing nurses' education; and improving their public image. The language of professionalism is identifiable throughout their writings. Even one hundred years after the opening of the first nursing school in English Canada in 1874, Margaret Street, nursing leader and biographer of Ethel Johns, continued the discourse:

> looking back over the past 100 years, one sees the gradual evolution of nursing as a profession from embryo to maturity...history records the vision, dedication, and courageous action of our predecessors, and their slow uphill climb interspersed with plateaux where dogged determination was required just to hold the ground that had been won.[8]

Formation of Professional Associations

The career of Mary Agnes Snively, who was at the centre of the push to form professional associations at the nursing school, provincial, and finally national levels, exemplified the professional trajectory. A former teacher and graduate of the Bellevue Hospital Training School for Nurses in New York, she became the nursing superintendent at Toronto General Hospital School of Nursing in 1884. In 1893 Snively was part of a group of nurses from the United States and Canada who attended the International Congress of Charities, Corrections and Philanthropy at the Chicago World's Fair. They addressed the need to establish separate, independent professional associations of nurses that could work to direct educational policies and standards. After her return, Snively organized an alumnae association at the Toronto General Hospital and by 1903 was instrumental in establishing other Ontario alumnae associations. She then brought these together to form the Graduate Nurses Association of Ontario. By 1914, all provinces but Prince Edward Island, had formed provincial associations. The alumnae associations remained the backbone of the professional movement, organizing social events, fostering school identity, and providing services such as registries to help private duty nurses find employment. From these beginnings, the Canadian Society for Superintendents of Training Schools of Nurses in 1907 was established, later renamed Canadian Association of Nursing Education (CANE). In 1908 CANE created the Canadian National Association of Trained Nurses (CNATN), which was affiliated with the International Council of Nurses (ICN). In 1905 the Toronto General Hospital School of Nursing Alumnae Association again took the lead and established its newsletter as a national nurses' journal, giving nurses a voice, facilitating exchange and serving as the mouthpiece for its leaders' professional aspirations. At first, the physician Dr Helen MacMurchy served as editor; however, when the CNATN purchased *The Canadian Nurse* in 1916, the organization felt confident enough to appoint a nurse editor.

In 1924 CNATN became the Canadian Nurses Association with Snively as its first president. Leaders of the three principal groups of nurses — private duty, public health, and hospital — as well as leaders in nursing education were represented in the organization's new committee structure. A determined and committed group of nurses emerged from the twenties with significant gains in terms of their collective self-confidence.

Registration Legislation

Nurses were mindful of the need to distinguish themselves from the untrained caregivers who often called themselves nurses. They lobbied for reforms that would lead to standardization of curriculum across all nursing schools, a standard accreditation test that all nurses would take, and the legal recognition of the title Registered Nurse. Between 1910 and 1922 nursing associations secured registration legislation in all provinces.

Education: From Hospital to University

Control over education is a key element in professionalism. For nurses, this began with the establishment of the first nurse training schools in the late nineteenth century. As the function of the hospital was

shifting from custodial care to curative medicine, the need for literate, trained nursing staff as well as improved hospital organization and sanitation arose. Often it was physicians, especially surgeons, who started these schools, appointing a graduate from one of the early Night-ingale-inspired British or American schools, as nursing superintendent. Snively, for example, was one of a number of nursing leaders who established training programs.[9] As early as 1895, she was looking at ways to upgrade educational standards through uniformity in school programs, to be achieved by establishing the three-year program and appropriate textbooks and lectures followed by formal examinations, as the norm. Superintendents felt the system of apprenticeship education served the hospital's staffing needs at the expense of the nurse's education and continually fought for both time and facilities to provide formal training for students, such as nurses' residences equipped with classroom space and libraries. Nursing leaders also built materials for a nursing curriculum independent of the physicians' sporadic lectures.

After registration was achieved, nursing leaders focused on improving existing hospital facilities through regular inspection. In 1922, the Ontario government appointed Alice Munn, Director of Nursing at Stratford General Hospital, to be director of the Department of Public Health and to investigate the schools of nursing. As a result of her study, 51 nursing schools were closed in the first year for a variety of reasons including the lack of a library and double occupancy of one bed in the nurses' residence.[10]

The Canadian Nurses Association (CNA) and the Canadian Medical Association (CMA) jointly sponsored a survey of nursing education in Canada. Dr George Weir issued his report in 1932, and supported the claims of nursing leaders that education be upgraded. He recommended a three-year program of study, and that small hospitals (under 50 beds) not be allowed to run a nurse training school.

As discussed in Lynn Kirkwood's chapter on education, nursing leaders focused their long-term sights on higher education. In 1914, the CNATN committee on nursing education recommended that nurse training schools be established in connection with the educational system of each province. A baccalaureate

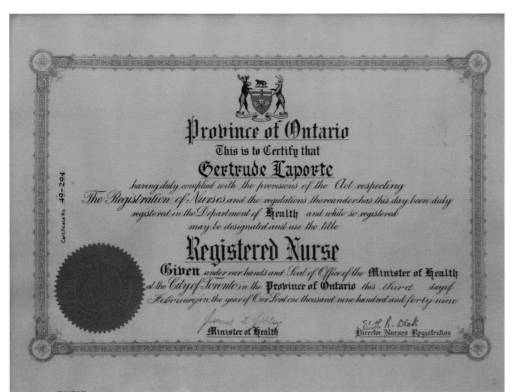

Figure 3
Registered Nurse certificate, Gertrude Laporte
1949
Photographer: Doug Millar
Canadian Museum of Civilization, 988.1.30
Gift of Charles Morin

degree course in nursing was established at the University of British Columbia in 1918 under the direction of Ethel Johns, followed by a McGill diploma course in teaching and supervision in 1920, five Red Cross-funded programs in public health nursing in the 1920s, and a University of Toronto program, established by Kathleen Russell in 1933. As will be discussed later in this chapter, the University of Montreal offered a program that developed into the first French language university program, the Marguerite d'Youville Institute, in 1934. Thus, by 1945, many nurses were enrolled in universities across Canada acquiring post-graduate education. A Master's program was established at the University of Western Ontario in 1959 and the first faculty of nursing, autonomous from the faculty of medicine, was established at the University of Montreal in 1962.

Public Image

Another important element of professionalism is service to the public. Prior to the Nightingale reforms, nursing in Anglo-Protestant Canada was regarded either as an unremarkable part of a woman's "natural"

domestic function, or something that working class charwomen did in dirty, disreputable hospitals. Nightingale changed all that with her dramatic and highly publicized campaign in the Crimean War and soon Nightingale-inspired nursing schools began to graduate neatly uniformed, respectable young nurses. Several well-publicized events served to highlight nurses' courage and service, including the Victorian Order of Nurses' journey to the Klondike during the Gold Rush, as well as the contribution of nurses during the First World War, the Halifax Explosion (see figure 4), and the Spanish flu epidemic of 1918–19. The outbreak of the Second World War gave nurses a superb opportunity to prove their worth and nearly 4000 nurses joined the Expeditionary Forces. When this caused a severe shortage of nurses at home, the CNA struggled to find new sources of nursing personnel, thus increasing the organization's political visibility.

Professionalism Achieved — Still, There were Disappointments

The post–Second World War period seemed to be the golden age of nursing, with hospital expansion and

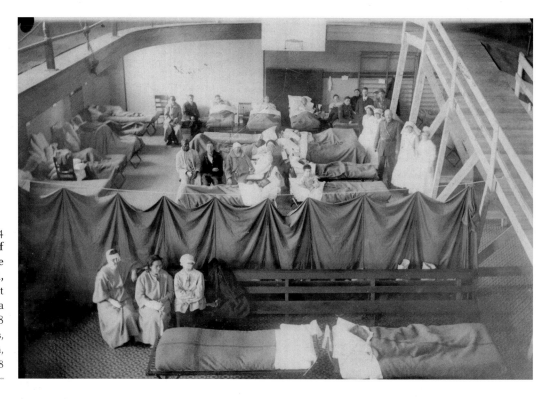

Figure 4
Emergency relief hospital in the YMCA,
Barrington Street
Halifax, Nova Scotia
1917–1918
Nova Scotia Archives,
Lola Henry Collection,
1979-237.8

thousands of new nursing positions being created. Private duty nurses, toiling in isolation in patients' homes, had largely been replaced by hospital staff nurses who joined the trend toward professional unions. They bargained successfully with hospital employers for better wages and conditions of work, the 8-hour shift and other long-standing demands. Education had become standardized and advanced programs were available in a number of post-secondary institutions. All provinces demanded a certification test, and there was a degree of self-regulation by nurses. All the components of Kinnear's criteria for professionalism were in place. As well, in 1955 the CNA adopted the Inter-national Council of Nurses' Code of Ethics, adding to the prestige surrounding the title Registered Nurse. Particularly from the perspective of the early twentieth century, when the very concept of a professional was strongly associated with men, the achievement of even an imperfect status in the professional world marked a significant symbolic victory for nurses, and for women. These achievements had been won due to strong women such as Mary Agnes Snively who led nurses toward her vision of professionalism. Not surprisingly nursing leaders such as Ethel Johns were also active in the early

women's suffrage movement that in turn supported the efforts of nurses to gain professional recognition.

Still there were disappointments. Although nurses achieved the right to use the title Registered Nurse, registration laws varied greatly from province to province, and all were weaker than nursing leaders had hoped for. In Ontario, for example, legislation was passed in 1912 as part of the *Hospitals Act*, and the Ontario Nurses' Association did not win the legal right to administer the process until 1951.[11] Nurses never gained power to police incompetent or unscrupulous practitioners in the manner that physicians could. Indeed, through both education and practice, nurses struggled for autonomy. Overshadowed by physicians' state-granted monopoly over diagnosis, a recognized area of exclusive authority and expertise eluded nursing. Even their major survey on education was conducted by a physician, and jointly sponsored by the CMA. Universities granted nurse education programs only a tenuous and insecure status, and their code of ethics was not as well known or prestigious as the medical profession's Hippocratic Oath, which dates back to antiquity. Clearly the picture of the professional nurse is complex and perhaps lends itself to McPherson's acknowledgement that components of all

Ethel Johns (1879–1968)

Glennis Zilm, Retired RN, freelance writer and editor, and Ethel Warbinek, University of British Columbia

Ethel Johns, head of the first baccalaureate nursing program in Canada, passionately believed in university education for nurses. Raised in rural northern Ontario, she lacked the means to attend university, but nevertheless was a well-educated, highly literate woman.

She graduated from the School for Nurses at Winnipeg General Hospital in 1902, one of its outstanding students. After graduation she became first editor of a nurses' alumnae journal and a regular contributor to the newly-founded *The Canadian Nurse*. After a few years as a private duty and staff nurse and a year at Columbia University, she was appointed superintendent of Winnipeg Children's Hospital.

When the University of British Columbia opened a nursing degree program in 1919, Johns was appointed head of the department as well as acting as superintendent of Vancouver General Hospital. During her time at UBC she firmly established the degree program and initiated a one-year public health diploma program.

In 1925 the Rockefeller Foundation of New York invited her to take on a series of major projects. Later on she assisted in developing university nursing education in Hungary, Romania, and other European countries.

From 1933 to 1944 Johns was editor and business manager of *The Canadian Nurse*, greatly increasing its international influence. She started columns on "Just Plain Nursing," which later were published as pamphlets and small books that were widely popular throughout North America. After retirement she was commissioned to write histories of the Winnipeg General Hospital School of Nursing and Johns Hopkins School of Nursing. As well, she was appointed to national and international committees, such as the United Nations Relief and Rehabilitation Administration.

Her distinguished contributions were recognized with many awards, including the CNA's Mary Agnes Snively Memorial Medal (1940) and an honorary doctorate from Mount Allison University (1948). She died in Vancouver in 1968 at age 89.

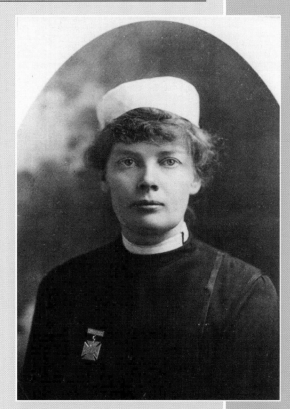

Figure 5
Ethel Johns
ca. 1920
University of British Columbia
Special Collections
UBC School of Nursing Historical
Collection

Jessie F MacKenzie 1867–1960: Reform Comes with a Price

Sheila J Rankin Zerr, University of British Columbia

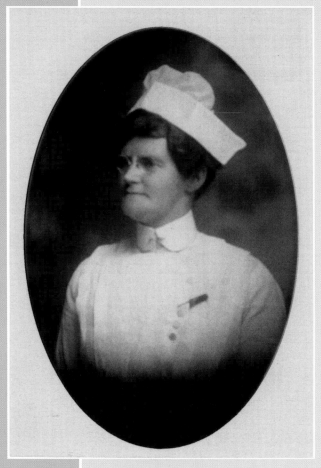

Figure 6
Jessie F MacKenzie, Matron and Superintendent of the Royal Jubilee Hospital School of Nursing
Alumnae Association of the Royal Jubilee Hospital School of Nursing

Jessie Ferguson MacKenzie was dismissed from her position at the Royal Jubilee Hospital (RJH) in Victoria, BC, in 1927. During her 14-year tenure as Matron and Superintendent of the hospital and school of nursing, she raised both the standards of patient care and the standards of nursing education. Her strong, outspoken advocacy for high standards, however, often placed her in conflict with others. Even her students, who held her in high esteem, found her intimidating. When told she often frightened them she quipped, "I only bark at those who benefit from it."

Jessie MacKenzie's campaign for improved hospital facilities at RJH resulted in the building of a new wing as well as the addition of a maternity unit. And despite opposition from medical men and the RJH board, she succeeded in making significant reforms at the hospital training school. Because of the many advances she introduced at the school, RJH had no difficulty attracting students — even during World War I and in the post-war period, when there was fierce competition for nursing personnel due to a countrywide nursing shortage. She was respected by her professional colleagues and took an active part in reforming the curriculum in schools of nursing across BC.

Miss MacKenzie was also not afraid to use her influence in matters ranging outside hospital walls. She encouraged her nurses to vote when women won the franchise and hired a car to take them to the polls. As one student recounts, she even told them how to vote: "Liberal so we took matters into our own hands and voted Conservative."

In January 1927 when the RJH hospital board asked Jessie MacKenzie to resign, the hospital was $13 000 in debt. There were board members and some hospital personnel who felt that her insistence on high standards, particularly for nursing training, were too costly, and that students would be better occupied on the wards. Nurses were outraged and felt she had been made a scapegoat for the hospital's financial problems. Reform comes with a price.

Source: Anne Pearson, *The Royal Jubilee Hospital School of Nursing 1891–1982* (Victoria, BC: Alumnae Association of the Royal Jubilee School of Nursing, 1984), 47.

three approaches to nursing history — the professional model, the proletarianization model, and the feminist analysis — are necessary to fully explain changes in nursing history.[12]

The Professional Nurse in the French-Catholic Tradition

If professionalization can be characterized in Anglo-Protestant nursing as almost a linear progression from the illiterate domestic to that of an educated, secular professional, no such assumptions can be made about nursing in Quebec. Some questions, such as nurse autonomy, the role of physicians in influencing the contours of nursing practice and the "what is a professional?" question are shared with the historiography of English-Protestant nursing. However, the historian must also assess the impact of the Nightingale model. Did it destroy an otherwise well-functioning Catholic hospital system, usurping the role of skilled women religious? Or did Nightingale reforms bring, despite some unwanted cultural baggage, real advances? The question has been divisive, with some Montreal-based nurses supporting a co-existence with the Nightingale model while most in the Quebec region resisted it. As well, the roles of church and state clearly add another dimension to the complexity of this historiography.

Debunking the Nightingale Myth

Promoters of modern nursing have invested much rhetoric in placing Florence Nightingale at the centre of its very creation and her Canadian disciples are no exception. Despite occasional concession to the pioneering Augustines and Jeanne Mance, who established the first hospitals and whose successors continued to competently manage them for over 300 years, Nightingale's supporters nonetheless cast aspersions on the apprenticeship training that nuns received and the emphasis they placed on religion in their role as nurses. Recently Sioban Nelson, an Australian nurse-historian who studied the international phenomenon of women's religious communities and nursing, has joined other voices in suggesting that Nightingale's fans might have had it backwards. It appears that Nightingale actually borrowed consider-

ably from Irish-Catholic orders in her work in the Crimea and that cross-fertilization between the two models of nursing occurred not only in Quebec, but in many Canadian communities where Catholic hospitals were often the first to be established. Far from unskilled, Catholic nuns had a well-established system of novice training using the time-honoured apprenticeship model, and kept up-to-date on medical and scientific advances. While most lay nurses worked for a few years until marriage, Catholic sisters made a life-long commitment to learning as a way of perfecting their level of service to God and community. Living in community with other women also allowed older sisters to act as mentors for the younger postulants.[13]

In truth, professionalization of nursing in Anglo-Protestant communities was suited to the haphazardly organized and poorly funded British/Canadian hospital. However, these reforms were less urgent in French-Catholic hospitals where, as Brigitte Violette outlines in chapter 4, religious orders, led by the Augustines, had achieved a high degree of excellence in nursing, pharmacy, and hospital administration. Thanks in part to the laissez-faire attitude of British authorities toward feminine orders following the Conquest, the longevity of this tradition may indeed be unique to Quebec, and its influence felt far beyond its borders. Between 1639 and 1939, more than 50 religious communities established and/or ran several hundred hospitals including the first hospitals in western Canada. Even as late as 1940, Catholic hospitals accounted for 34 percent of all hospital beds.[14]

Professionalization Campaign Led by Montreal Anglophone Nurses

In Quebec, the first nurse training schools were created at the anglophone hospitals, beginning with the Montreal General Hospital in 1875, although a school was not successfully established until 1890 under Canadian nursing leader, Nora Livingston. Women such as she established the first nursing organizations including the Canadian Nurses' Association of Montreal, a local group despite its name, which made efforts to include francophone nurses. At their first annual meeting in September 1918, they welcomed six lay nurses from L'École Jeanne Mance at

Hôtel-Dieu de Montréal and three nuns from Notre-Dame Hospital run by the Grey Nuns. The association drafted legislation for nurse registration, leading to passage of the *Loi constituant en corporation l'Association des gardes-malades enregistrées de la province de Québec* in 1920. It accorded the title Registered Nurse exclusively to members of l'Association des gardes-malade enregistrée de la province de Québec (AGMEPQ).

Sparked by an initial protest from nurses at l'hôpital Sainte-Justine, denied recognition under the Act, organized opposition arose particularly to the requirement for a three-year program and the 50-bed minimum for a hospital to run a training school. Due to the prevalence of religious nursing, nurse training schools in Quebec were established later and tended to be smaller. However, the real anger was not focused so much on specific stipulations governing what constituted a recognized hospital training school than on the prospect of ceding administrative control of Catholic hospitals to an anglophone movement. Led by an alliance of women religious and Catholic physicians, the protestors successfully gained an amendment in 1922, allowing recognition, with approval of one of the faculties of medicine at Université Laval or Université de Montréal, of nurses trained in a two-year training school program, and it eliminated the 50-bed minimum. This change meant that nurses registered in Quebec through AGMEPQ would not be recognized as RNs in other provinces. More ominous, however, was the power it gave the university faculties of medicine. Although not dissimilar to provisions negotiated in other provinces, the nursing association AGMEPQ had been relegated second place to physicians in the registration of graduate nurses.[15]

The Francophone Response to Nightingale

The Nightingale model of nursing was foreign to the Catholic religious tradition in which nursing was a religious mission or vocation, and nuns firmly controlled well-established French hospitals. Still, the response to it was not united: it reflected a divi-sion between Montreal nurses who worked in close proximity to anglophones, and those in the Quebec region, where Anglo-Protestant nursing had not made the same inroads. While the erudite Augustines, whose network of hospitals was confined to francophone regions, held out the longest against the Nightingale onslaught, the Grey Nuns, administrators of hospitals across North America, tried to gain concessions by adapting Nightingale to the French-Catholic system. Undermining any protest against Nightingale nursing was the increasing aggressiveness of physicians in Catholic hospitals, who were only too happy to adopt the more restrictive nursing model, if not the Anglo-Protestant aspects of Nightingale's system.

Beginning with the Hotel-Dieu de Quebec, the Augustines had implanted the French tradition of caring that was guided by the Catholic principle of "healing the body and saving the soul." Gifted healers, administrators, and nurses, they organized their hospitals around the key function of the learned apothecary who not only created and dispensed medicines, but contributed to medical knowledge. However, modernization was already undermining that role, beginning with the Hotel-Dieu's affiliation with Université de Laval in 1855. As was happening elsewhere throughout the nineteenth century, male physicians used university education to formalize, and indeed masculinize, medical knowledge, excluding women from its learned aspects. As well, physicians exerted pressure to expand hospital services to include surgery and other sophisticated medical treatments and to train a subordinate nursing workforce to support them. In response, the Augustines opened a training school for nurses in 1900, although it remained modest, not admitting lay students until the 1950s. Disrupting the Augustines' long-standing power over the hospital's direction, including professional and scientific matters, these changes meant that nuns retained only administrative functions and control over nurse education. They had to slowly relinquish medical and scientific roles.

Little wonder that the Augustines were lukewarm to Nightingale nursing. They joined a loosely allied group of women religious who rejected the idea of

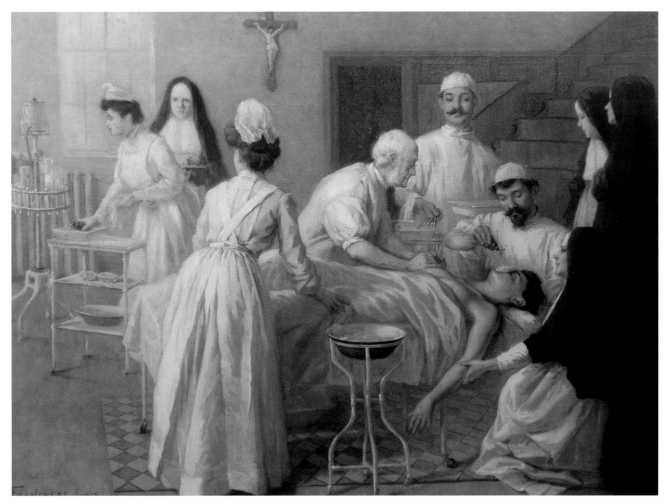

Figure 7
"Doctor Hingston and the Operating Room"
Artist: Joseph-Charles Franchère
Hotel-Dieu Hospital, Montreal
1905
Collection des Hospitalières de l'Hôtel-Dieu de Montréal

Both religious and lay nurses are assisting the doctors.

giving AGMEPQ, a "neutral" association — in fact controlled by anglophones — the authority to implement registration legislation. They made no effort to have their nursing school meet the AGMEPQ's requirements for recognition, and indeed it was not recognized until 1937.[16] Leading the protest were the Sisters of Charity of Quebec who didn't allow their nurses to register, and created a rival nurse organization, l'Association des gardes-malades catholiques licencées de la province de Québec (AGMCLPQ) in 1928. It remained active in the Quebec region, Gaspé, Trois-Rivières, and the North Shore areas and

offered a modest alternative for several decades. The religious congregations who resisted registration paid the consequences in not having their students recognized elsewhere in the province and outside of Quebec. However, until later in the century this would not have hurt them, as most did not need to train lay nurses. As members of a large international Catholic phenomenon and, after 1915, active participants in the Catholic Hospital Association, they had access to an impressive network of Catholic hospitals and other institutions throughout North America and the world.

The Grey Nuns and the Religious Hospitallers of St. Joseph

Among the orders that made accommodations to the Nightingale system were the Religious Hospitallers of St. Joseph who established the Hôtel-Dieu de Montréal, and an early French-language nursing school, l'École Jeanne Mance in 1897, accepting lay students from 1901 on. The acknowledged leaders, however, were the Grey Nuns, founded in 1747 by Mother Marguerite d'Youville. They took on the nursing function at Notre-Dame Hospital in Montreal in 1880, and by 1927, administered 22 hospitals. They were responsible for 30 percent of hospitals and health care facilities established by all women religious in Canada before 1939.[17] With an extensive chain of hospitals across Canada and the United States, the Grey Nuns clearly had an interest in having their nursing recognized anywhere in Canada.

Historian Yolande Cohen suggests the Grey Nuns took aspects of the Nightingale reforms they felt could be beneficial and tried to adapt them to fit the Catholic health care vision, which did not separate the body from the soul. Some even suggested that this represented an early manifestation of "total patient care" or holistic nursing.[18] Under the direction of Mother Élodie Mailloux, who had collaborated in the founding of a nursing school at Saint-Vincent Hospital in Toledo, Ohio, they established a French-language hospital nursing school at Notre-Dame in 1898, accepting lay students one year later. They were also the driving force behind the first university-level program to admit francophone women, which began as a summer course at the Université de Montréal in 1923, taught by Sister Fafard, then director of the Notre-Dame nursing school, and a Montreal-trained nun, Sister Duckett. Following the death of Sister Fafard, the course ended, but the congregation hired Mother Virginie Allaire, then superior at St. Boniface, to develop a program. She studied methods and curriculum, travelled to schools in Europe, and planned a university-level program for French-speaking nurses. The Institut Marguerite d'Youville (IMY) was established in 1934, in affiliation with the Université de Montréal, offering a baccalaureate in nursing. This allowed francophone women to gain a foothold in the

university, up to this point closed to them. In 1962 an autonomous faculty of nursing was established at the university. The creation of a nursing baccalaureate program that was not controlled by a faculty of medicine was clearly no mean accomplishment, one that Cohen attributes to the depth of hospital management experience acquired by the hospital orders.[19]

In support of their teaching programs, the Grey Nuns also published a French-language textbook of nursing, *Le soin des maladies: Principes et techniques,* in 1947.[20] This complemented the 1931 *Principes élémentaires concernant le soin des malades,* written by Sister Allard of L'École Jeanne Mance. These nursing manuals filled the pressing need for French-language nursing textbooks. Cohen posits that through their textbooks and courses, the Grey Nuns formalized the centuries-old knowledge and skill that women religious had acquired running hospitals, nursing the sick, preparing medicines, and administering hospital finances, thus giving greater legitimacy to women's knowledge.[21]

Under the direction of AGEMPQ, the first francophone professional nursing journal, *La Veilleuse,* was established in 1924. Influenced by the Grey Nuns and initially supported by Catholic physicians and clergy, the journal attempted to promote a French-Catholic vision of the modern nurse, one that melded the Nightingale nursing tradition with its Catholic counterpart. The effort was not entirely successful and *La Veilleuse* was replaced in 1928 by *La garde-malade canadienne-française (GMCF).* Continuing to promote a French-Catholic model of nursing until the Quiet Revolution, the GMCF also reflected the increasing influence of lay nurses in positions of authority in Quebec nursing. In 1956 it was discontinued, when the CNA decided to introduce a French-language version of *The Canadian Nurse, L'Infirmière canadienne.* It became in 1957 *Les Cahiers du nursing canadien,* its name signifying adoption of the professional model of nursing developed by anglophone nurses.[22]

Not always divided, francophone nurses did come together, for example, in defending themselves against The Weir Report on nursing education. Dr Weir did not speak French, and he included only one Quebec member on his committee, A T Bazin of the Montreal General Hospital, an anglophone institution. Despite visiting 145 nursing schools and travelling 35 000 miles, he produced a report that showed a complete lack of understanding of nursing in French-speaking Quebec, ignoring the contribution of women religious. Although he had conducted 2280 intelligence tests with English-language nursing students, he did none with French-language students, as "he was convinced that English tests could not be translated into another language and another environment." Weir's assertion that "the ecclesiastical tradition, however laudable in the abstract, has exerted and is exerting a somewhat prejudicial influence on the evolution of Canadian nursing" was met with outrage. The congregations, led by Mother Virginie Allaire of the Montreal Grey Nuns did not let such an insult — to a sector that had been active in the field for centuries! — go unchallenged. They created the Conférence provinciale des hôpitaux catholiques de la province de Québec whose purpose was to promote and maintain the progress of hospitals in the spirit of Christian charity.[23]

The existence of rival nursing associations in Quebec finally came to an end in 1946 when the *Loi concernant l'Association des infirmières de la province de Québec* was passed. It made the licensing of nurses obligatory, and required that all members of a new association, l'Association des infirmières de la Province de Quebec (AIPQ), be licensed nurses, restricting to them alone the right to practise.

Lay Nurses

The contours of nursing were changing rapidly by mid-century as an increase in the demand for nurses coincided with the growing predominance of lay nurses. While in 1931, 51 percent of all nurses in Montreal were women religious, by 1941 they constituted only 23.2 percent. The 1946 legislation recognizing collective bargaining by nurses reflected this. It also restricted the practice of nursing to women, a stipulation that was not rescinded until 1969.

Francophone lay nurses were not passive on the question of professional advancement, although they often employed different strategies than did anglo-

phone nurses. As women religious dominated administrative positions, lay nurses were initially congregated in bedside nursing where many found it difficult to earn a living. Unlike nuns, who worked for heavenly rather than earthly rewards, who were well educated and often came from the upper echelons of society, and who benefited from their congregations' support in sickness and old age, lay nurses worked in a climate of economic insecurity. The 1946 *Nurses' Act* providing for collective bargaining, led to the formation of l'Alliance des infirmières de Montréal, which was successful in gaining better wages and conditions for its members with a collective agreement signed in 1947. Earlier, the Quebec-based AGMCLPQ had offered some services such as an employment bureau, although historian Johanne Daigle disputes its status as a union because the nurses' employers had created it.[24]

With changes that culminated in the Quiet Revolution, the belief that the state, rather than the church, should be responsible for health care became widespread. Women religious lost control of their institutions and lay nurses assumed leadership of the nursing profession. Soon francophone lay nurses were taking their place in leadership positions, at home and in the world. Alice Girard's life story exemplifies some of the transitions Quebec nurses had to make in moving from the religious to the secular tradition. Alice Girard was born in 1907, the last of seven children in a French-Canadian family living in Connecticut. She returned to Quebec with her parents, and at the age of 11 resolved never to marry because "housework didn't interest her." She obtained her normal school diploma in 1925, and eventually trained at Saint Vincent de Paul Hospital in Sherbrooke. Deciding to devote her life to nursing, she observed, "Of course, nurses lived like nuns at that time, so our parents didn't have to worry about us." Following a varied public health career in Montreal, other parts of Canada and the United States, Girard went on to gain national and international recognition as the first francophone president of the CNA in 1958, and the first Canadian president of the ICN in 1965. As the first dean of the autonomous Faculty of Nursing at the Université de Montréal from its creation in 1962 until 1973, she

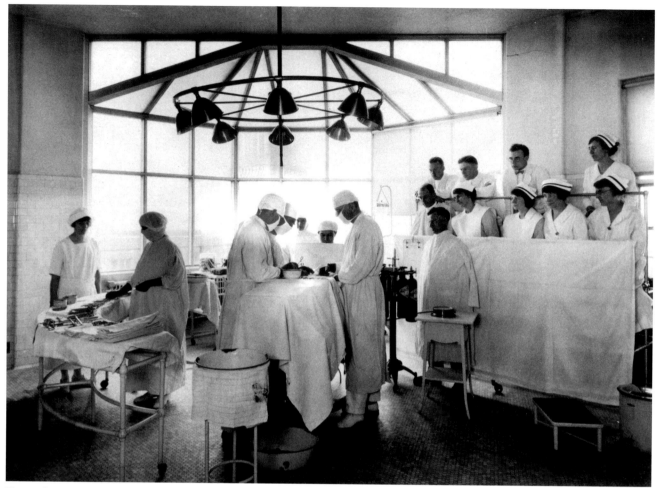

Figure 8
Nurses observing an operation
St. Michael's Hospital, Toronto
1924
St. Michael's Hospital Archives

had an enduring influence on nursing education and practice, an influence that could rival any of the religious nursing leaders who came before her. She died in 1999.[25]

A Forgotten Dimension: English Catholic Hospitals

The influence of the French hospital tradition in English-speaking communities has not been studied extensively; however, such a study might well illuminate some of the reciprocal influences of the two nursing models. The Religious Hospitallers of St. Joseph established well-respected Hotels-Dieu in Acadian areas of New Brunswick and in Kingston, where their nursing school was influential throughout eastern Ontario. In Toronto, the Sisters of Saint Joseph, who came to Canada in the 1840s from France via the United States, established St. Michael's Hospital in 1892, winning the community's trust through the courageous care of epidemic victims, and immediately opened the first Catholic nursing school in Canada, accepting lay students from the beginning.

Assessing the French-Catholic Model of Nursing

The decline of the tradition of Augustine nurses, apothecaries, and administrators was clearly a loss for women and for francophone society, one that parallels similar losses in women's access to knowledge that came with the nineteenth century professionalization of knowledge. Yet Nightingale's reforms would not have succeeded without the collusion of the male-dominated medical profession. And the early women religious for all their entrepreneurial and medical skills were, after all, products of an era in which the Catholic view of health care was paramount and the role of the church largely unquestioned. The pan-Canadian Grey Nuns led the effort to merge the anglophone Nightingale with the French-Catholic model of nursing, an effort that allowed them to operate across North America and helped open up superior educational programs to francophone women and provide opportunities for lay nurses.

Conclusions

This preliminary overview of the literature on professional formation leads to the view that the Nightingale, Protestant influence on the French-Catholic nursing model was not one-sided but, in fact, reciprocal. In English-Protestant Canada, nursing followed a course influenced by the degraded status of the pre-professional nurse, and the unclean and poorly organized charitable hospital. Anglo-Protestant nursing leaders, schooled in the Nightingale system, succeeded in gaining professional recognition for nurses through education, a recognized title, and improved public image, despite encountering some disappointments. The path to professional formation differed in Quebec where the long-established French Catholic hospital, presided over by skilled women religious, was the cornerstone of a well-developed health care system. Nursing leaders were initially divided in their response to the Nightingale system of nursing, a model that ill-suited their needs. Some sought to accommodate themselves to the Nightingale presence, while others opposed it as an anglophone import. A lay nursing leadership later emerged, establishing a secular profession similar to that of English-speaking Canada, yet one that inherited many strengths from the rich legacy of women religious.

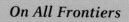

CHAPTER 14

Unionization of Canadian Nursing

Sharon Richardson

The sight of nurses walking the picket line — much less being involved in illegal strikes — is contrary to the public stereotype of nurses as self-sacrificing, caring professionals. Within recent years, however, there have been province-wide nursing strikes in Newfoundland and Labrador, Saskatchewan, Quebec, and more threatened in Saskatchewan, Alberta, and British Columbia. In today's climate of political uncertainty about health care, it is unlikely that labour unrest among the more than 75 percent of Canadian registered nurses who are unionized is over. This chapter outlines some of the significant events and factors in Canadian society that have contributed to the high rate of nursing unionization in the post–Second World War period, focusing on three eras: (1) professional nursing associations' support of collective bargaining; (2) creation of autonomous nursing unions; and (3) nurses' strikes.

Development of General Duty/ Staff Nurse

Hospital, general duty, or staff nurses have always comprised the significant majority of unionized nurses in Canada. Contrary to popular belief, however, it was only after the Second World War that the majority of Canadian nurses began to work in hospi-

tals. Before that, 60 percent of the graduates of hospital nurse training programs worked in private duty. As outlined in chapter 3, these nurses worked for patients in their homes and were paid directly by them, on a fee-for-service basis. Only a few graduate nurses worked in hospitals, supervising the student nursing workforce, which did most of the bedside nursing. Hospitals admitted as many nurse trainees as were required for work on the wards, resulting in an over supply of graduate nurses and their chronic underemployment. This stimulated some hospital nursing superintendents to offer work to their recent graduates at a reduced salary and these nurses, who provided patient care, were known as general duty or staff nurses. They stabilized the hospital's nursing service and facilitated clinical placement of nurses-in-training on the basis of their learning needs. One senior nurse administrator commented in 1942: "Experience has taught us that it is not possible to fulfil the highest standard of the Curriculum and at the same time give the best care to the sick if the hospital is obliged to depend entirely on the student body for its nursing service."[1]

The outbreak of the Second World War in 1939 dramatically lessened the unemployment of nurses. As outlined in chapter 11, approximately 4000 graduate nurses were absorbed into the Canadian and Allied nursing sisterhoods during the war, leaving vacancies to be filled by underemployed private duty nurses and recent graduates. Between 1930 and 1943, the proportion of nurses employed in private duty declined by one-half, while the proportion working in hospitals almost doubled.

Dissatisfaction with Hospital Working Conditions

Unfortunately, Canadian hospitals failed to adapt their employment policies and practices to meet the needs of the increasing number of registered nurses they hired as general duty or staff nurses. Throughout the Second World War, hospital staff nurses demonstrated their patriotism by continuing to work 12-hour shifts, six days a week, with mandatory call-back, for minimal remuneration. The Canadian Hospital Council (CHC) countered nurses' repeated requests for replacement of 12-hour shifts with 8-hour shifts by claiming that the long-awaited 8-hour day would go into effect, "if only nurses were available in sufficient numbers to make this possible."[2] The real issue for the CHC, of course, was the unavoidable increase in hospitals' overall expenditures for nurses' salaries that would result from 8-hour shifts, which required three, rather than two rotations of nursing staff.

Helen Saunders, a demobilized military nurse, stated in a 1946 issue of *The Canadian Nurse* that salaries of $100 a month or less, plus room and board, were inadequate payment for the level of responsibility demanded of registered nurses in Canadian hospitals. Not only that, but there was no standardization; an individual nurse's salary depended on her ability to persuade her employer of her worth rather than on her qualifications and cumulative nursing experience. Although hospitals claimed they had instituted 8-hour work days, many nurses were still required to work a "split eight-hour day" from 7:00 a.m. to 7:00 p.m. with three hours off some time during the day, rather than a continuous eight hours on duty. As a result, they were unable to engage in the usual recreational and social activities enjoyed by other single working women of comparable status. Because hospital boards refused to employ sufficient housekeeping and other staff, nurses did a significant amount of non-nursing

work such as cleaning furniture, sinks and equipment; making dressings and supplies; folding linen; washing and testing rubber gloves; and rinsing out soiled laundry items. As well, hospitals neither acknowledged the important contribution nurses made to improving patient care nor ensured for their professional development.[3]

Nursing Associations and Collective Bargaining

Despite ongoing discontent with their unsatisfactory salaries and working conditions, the growing cadre of hospital staff nurses was slow to accept unionization. Trained in a tradition of dedication to service and loyalty to the hospital, staff nurses initially perceived collective bargaining at the very least unladylike, if not down right unethical. The spectre of nurses putting their needs ahead of their patients', and possibly withholding services to enforce demands, unnerved many of them. The gendered nature of nursing also meant that hospital staff nurses espoused the values of womanhood held by society at large: patience, respect for authority, and above all, putting others' needs ahead of one's own. As late as 1960, only one in four practising nurses was married and conventional wisdom held that women were destined for marriage and motherhood. Most women perceived salaried employment as a temporary episode before being supported by a husband. Prior to the 1960s, approximately one-third of registered nurses left the work force within ten years of graduation, and only half of those remaining stayed employed until pensionable age.[4]

During the Second World War, federal government regulations proved a major stimulus to union formation. In an effort to gain the support of unionists for the war effort, in 1943, the Canadian government issued Order-in-Council PC 1003, which gave employees the right to freely choose a union to represent them, and compelled employers to "bargain in good faith." It also established a board to investigate "unfair labour practices" and regulate certification of unions as bargaining agents. Subsequent court decisions further protected unions by making payment of union dues compulsory.[5] As a result, some labour unions began to organize municipal and hospital employees. Many nurses, however, did not fully trust industrial unions, fearing the influence of outside groups with different motives and limited knowledge of nursing. These suspicions were particularly strong among leaders of provincial and national nursing associations who feared losing influence over their members.

During the Second World War, the Canadian Nurses Association (CNA) had been able to significantly expand its influence over nursing in Canada thanks to a large grant from the federal government. Adroitly capitalizing on the patriotic fervour of the early 1940s, the CNA obtained funding "for emergency nursing needs," to ameliorate the anticipated shortage of nurses during wartime. It administered $774 000 from 1942 to 1946 for teaching and public health nursing, and to fund a national Emergency Nursing Advisor. It disbursed funds through provincial nursing associations and used a portion to create a full-time salaried chief executive officer, paid secretary, and permanent office space, enabling the CNA to consolidate its national presence and increase its influence over provincial nursing associations.[6]

Notwithstanding the CNA's opposition to unions, in 1942 something happened that caused organized nursing to consider collective bargaining: Toronto public health nurses were being pressured, reportedly against their wishes, to join an American Federation of Labour City Hall workers' union. In response, the Registered Nurses Association of Ontario (RNAO) asked the CNA to consider collective bargaining for nurses and they in turn created a Labour Relations Committee to investigate its legal implications. In 1944, the CNA's Executive Committee approved the principle of collective bargaining for registered nurses through their provincial nursing associations, but not through trade unions. If provincial laws forbade certification of professional nursing associations as collective bargaining agents for their members, the CNA proposed that the provincial association should establish an advisory labour relations committee to assist local groups of nurses to become certified as independent bargaining units. Some provincial nurses' associations (Alberta, Saskatchewan, Manitoba, Ontario, Quebec, New Brunswick, and

Prince Edward Island) had members who were registered nurses holding managerial positions. Since they had members on both the labour and management sides of the table, these associations could not legally be ratified as bargaining agents for hospitals or public health nurses.[7]

To further dissuade nurses from joining trade unions, the CNA warned "that no nurse should become a member of an association or a trade union under conditions that might call for the stoppage of necessary nursing service, in other words, to strike."[8] This anti-strike stance enabled the CNA to persuade many rank and file nurses that membership in trade unions was unprofessional, and they were encouraged to support their professional nursing associations. A 1946 editorial in *The Canadian Nurse Journal* rhetorically asked:

> Should the nurses of Canada join unions? They already belong to a stronger body than any that could now be formed. It is up to the individual nurse to rally to the support of this emerging giantess — the Canadian Nurses' Association, the nine federated provincial associations, the local districts and chapters.[9]

The CNA's position led to the passage, at its 1946 Annual General Meeting, of a resolution opposing "any nurse going on strike at any time for any cause." This anti-strike position was not repealed until 1972.

A notable exception to provincial legislation forbidding the professional nursing associations from bargaining on behalf of their members existed in British Columbia. In 1946, the Registered Nurses Association of British Columbia (RNABC) received official recognition as the bargaining agent for its members below the level of assistant director of nursing. The RNABC negotiated a collective agreement covering salaries, hours of work, statutory holidays, annual vacations, credit for experience, and postgraduate training. In 1959, the RNABC agreed to a proposal by the BC Hospitals' Association for province-wide collective bargaining. This meant that all eligible nurses in the hospital bargaining unit were covered by one collective agreement. By 1967, in addition to 78 groups of nurses employed by 62 hospitals, the RNABC was certified as the bargaining agent for 13 public health agencies, several clinics

Figure 1
**Fédération des infirmières et
infirmiers du Québec poster**
2000
Courtesy of the Fédération des infirmières et infirmiers du Québec

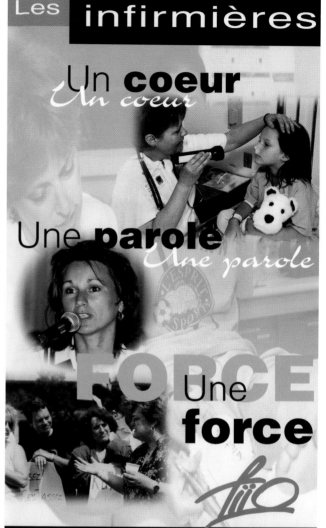

and a medical insurance company. Evelyn Hood, RNABC's director of personnel services, concluded that overall benefits included increased communication and understanding between nurses and their employers, and greater influence by nurses on their working conditions. Some specific gains made by the Association included doubling of nurses' salaries, increased vacation time, higher rates of pay for nurses with more experience and education, a reduced work week (40 hours), an end to discrimination against hiring married women, and a grievance procedure to process nurses' problems and complaints.[10]

In Quebec, as late as 1921, the *Quebec Public Charities Act* reaffirmed the historic importance of religious social service work where female religious orders provided a pool of skilled administrators for Catholic hospitals. Thus lay nurses enjoyed limited occupational advancement in Quebec's health care hierarchy until the 1960s and 1970s.[11] Quebec lay nurses advanced their professional position through collective action earlier than in other parts of Canada. For example, in 1939, with the support of their employers and the Catholic union movement, nurses in Quebec City formed Syndicat professionnel des infirmières catholiques (SPIC) to negotiate their collective interests with employers. In 1946, the *Quebec Nurses' Act*, providing for collective bargaining, was passed, and Montreal nurses turned to the Quebec Federation of Labour to establish the first independent nurses' union in the country, l'Alliance des infirmières de Montréal (AIM), an affiliate of the Confederation of National Trade Unions (CNTU). Other hospital-based nurses' unions formed under their guidance and in the next two decades became la Fédération québécoise des infirmières et infirmiers (FQII). A second federation of nurses' unions in the province was formed by Quebec City nurses and named the Fédération des syndicats professionnels d'infirmières et infirmiers

du Québec (FSPIIQ). In 1965, an anglophone nurses' union called the United Nurses of Montreal formed. Soon this new union became a bilingual organization, eventually transforming into the third Quebec nurses' federation, Fédération des infirmières et infirmiers unis, Inc. (FIIU). In 1987 a composite union was formed by the merging of the FQII, the FSPIIQ, and the FIIU. Together, they became Fédération des infirmières et infirmiers du Québec (FIIQ). The early assistance from organized labour to Quebec nurses and the greater stratification in Quebec nursing helps explain why nurses in that province have stronger ties with organized labour than elsewhere.[12]

Although unionized nurses in British Columbia and Quebec made significant gains in salaries and working conditions during the 1950s and 1960s, nurses in other provinces were slower to seek certification for collective bargaining. Instead, they attempted to improve their wages and working conditions through voluntary, non-certified agreements with employers. Their reluctance reflected the values associated with ladylike, "professional" behaviour, as well as the variability in trade union achievements across Canada. Both Quebec and British Columbia had a much longer tradition of successful trade unionism than did agrarian provinces such as Alberta and Saskatchewan and the economically depressed Atlantic provinces. This voluntary bargaining approach (as it was called by nurses) usually involved provincial nursing associations establishing advisory labour relations committees to prepare recommended salary schedules and standardized plans for hours of work, which they circulated to all employers. This non-confrontational strategy illustrated nurses' rather naive expectations, and by the mid-1960s, it became clear that voluntary bargaining was not being respected by many employers, who made decisions without consulting the nurses. Consequently, provincial nursing associations in Alberta, Manitoba, Ontario, New Brunswick, Nova Scotia, Prince Edward Island, Saskatchewan, Newfoundland, and Labrador increased their assistance to local staff nurse associations to help them become certified and negotiate contracts with individual hospitals and public health units. In Ontario and Saskatchewan, the RNAO and the SRNA sought legislative changes permitting them to act as bargaining agents for their members. In Alberta, although changes in the *Registered Nurses' Act* in 1966 made it legal for the Alberta Association of Registered Nurses (AARN) to act as a bargaining agent, a year later the AARN was certified as the collective bargaining agent for only four of 53 provincial staff nurse associations.[13] Nurses' reluctance to join the union movement faded during the late 1960s, when they saw the significant gains made by newly unionized public service sector workers in Canada.

Public Sector Unionization

The mid-1960s saw the sudden emergence of unionism amongst mainly white-collar workers in the Canadian public sector including teachers, health care, and government workers. Previously organized into professional associations and denied collective bargaining rights on the grounds that their services were "essential," they had been outside the mainstream union movement. During the 1960s, dissatisfaction among these workers escalated when their wages fell far behind those in the private sector, and they began to challenge the status quo. Newly militant public service employees in Quebec held illegal strikes in 1963 and 1964 that later forced the provincial government to grant collective bargaining, and even the right to strike, to all civil servants, teachers, and hospital workers, with the exception of police and firefighters. At the national level, the postal strike of 1965 was similarly effective. Two years later, the federal government passed legislation giving its employees the right to bargain collectively and to strike in the event of disputes. All other provincial governments soon extended bargaining rights, but not always the right to strike.[14] By 1975, almost all public employees in Canada belonged to union-like organizations.

By 1978, half of the ten largest Canadian unions were from the public sector and they made up 38 percent of total union membership, shifting the labour movement away from its male, blue-collar focus and allowing a more prominent role for female, white-collar and professional organizations. For example, Canadian unions appearing before the federal Royal Commission on the Status of Women in 1967 stressed married women's right to work, the need to accept two-income families, and women's right to better education.[15] The proportion of women joining unions rose from 17 percent to 31 percent between 1965 and 1980, and among this number were many nurses.[16]

The increasing unionization of women also reflected the ideals of the feminist movement and a new family ideal, no longer based on adult women confined to the home as wives and mothers. Young women were demanding equal access to post-secondary education, but they also continued to marry and have children. The new dual income, shared parenting family model was reflected in a conspicuous change in the Canadian nursing labour force. By 1990, married women comprised more than 70 percent of the nursing workforce, whereas 30 years earlier, only one in four practising nurses was married. Many married nurses also continued to work even after the birth of children, moving to part-time employment while their children were young and back to full-time employment as children reached adolescence and became more independent. The increasing number of nurses who continued as salaried employees for a significant proportion of their adult lives reinforced nurses' collective demands for working conditions in keeping with their needs, including maternity leave and other benefits that came at a time of escalating demand for nurses' services. In 1965, there were 104 349 registered nurses living and/or working in Canada, and by 1989, this number had increased by almost one-and-a-half times to 252 189. The most common field of employment was the hospital, as general duty or staff nurses.[17] Demands for adequate salaries and improved working conditions could not be ignored.

Separation of Nursing Unions

By the early 1970s, many Canadian nurses in all provinces but British Columbia and Quebec were members of local collective bargaining units, which negotiated with hospitals and public health units on their behalf. Many of these bargaining units were indirectly supported by provincial nursing associations. Two events in 1973 affected the course of nursing unionization: the RNAO's 1973 decision to support a separate, autonomous nursing union in Ontario, and a 1974 Supreme Court decision to disallow certification of an SRNA supported staff nurses' unit as a collective bargaining agent.

In Ontario, the RNAO supported local collective bargaining units in voluntary talks with employers. Through persistent bargaining, Ontario nurses were able to negotiate improved wages and working conditions during the late 1960s and early 1970s. Unable and unwilling to invoke strike action to resolve impasses with two rural health unit boards, the RNAO achieved success through "gray listing," which

involved advising all Ontario nurses of a bargaining impasse, and requesting they avoid employment with offending boards. So successful was the RNAO strategy that by 1972, the association was deluged with requests from nurses to establish collective bargaining units. Due, however, to a unique situation in Ontario, some of the nurses requesting assistance were not RNAO members. The Ontario government had removed regulatory functions from the RNAO in 1961 and created a second provincial nursing organization, the College of Nurses of Ontario, which was given responsibility for licensing both registered and practical nurses. The legislation also made membership in the RNAO voluntary and not all registered nurses chose to join. In all other Canadian jurisdictions but Ontario, the provincial professional nursing association is legislatively empowered to regulate nursing by licensing and disciplining registered nurses.

Faced with escalating costs of assisting a rapidly increasing number of local nursing collective bargaining units, not all of whose members were also RNAO members, the board recommended creation of a separate nursing union. The RNAO offered to provide services to this new union that would bargain province-wide for registered nurses. They hoped it would fulfil the RNAO's longstanding goal of standardized collective agreements for hospital staff nurses throughout the province. Thus was created a third province-wide nursing organization in Ontario, the Ontario Nurses Association (ONA), whose mandate, approved by the Ontario Labour Relations Board in 1974, was to bargain collectively for nurses. Approximately 100 local nursing collective bargaining units merged with the ONA.[18]

The creation of a separate nursing union independent of the provincial professional nursing association in Ontario, the province where one-third of all nurses worked, influenced other jurisdictions. Nurses in other provinces considered establishing separate nursing unions, although the cost of supporting a rapidly growing number of local nursing collective bargaining units was a consideration. In all Canadian provinces and territories (except Ontario), the professional nursing association was also legislatively responsible for protecting the public through the

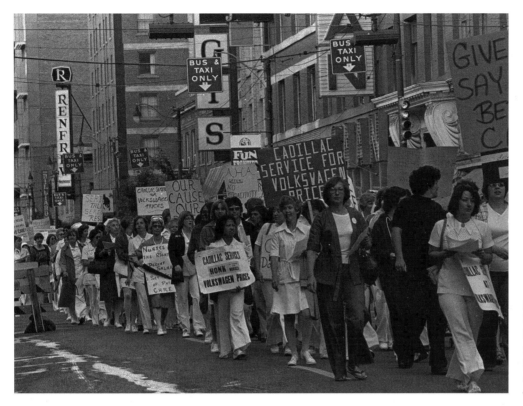

Figure 2
Nurses picketing
Calgary, Alberta
1977
Glenbow Archives, Calgary,
Alberta, NA-2864-16924

licensing and discipline of registered nurses to ensure that they provided safe, ethical care to patients. Most provincial nursing associations realized that they did not have the resources to support both their regulatory responsibilities and collective bargaining. Since not all members benefited from collective bargaining — nurses in management roles, for example — the elected boards of management of the various provincial nursing associations were unwilling to increase annual fees to support collective bargaining activities. The formation of a separate, independent organization to handle collective bargaining was a logical solution to the internal struggle to balance the various other roles faced by the provincial nursing associations.

Just as significant as the RNAO's creation of a separate nursing union was the SRNA's late 1973 decision to withdraw entirely from collective bargaining. This resulted from the 29 October 1973 Supreme Court of Canada ruling that upheld an earlier decision of the Saskatchewan Labour Relations Board (SLRB) to disallow certification of the Nipawin and District Staff Nurses' Association as a collective bargaining agent. According to the SLRB ruling, the staff nurses' association had been assisted by a "company-dominated organization," the SRNA, which had helped local groups to become certified. However, the SLRB accepted the argument put forward by a trade union interested in representing nurses: that because the SRNA included on its board nurses in managerial positions, it was ineligible to assist local nurses in this way. Rather than incur the additional costs and controversy associated with ongoing debate about its involvement in collective bargaining, the SRNA chose to withdraw completely from such activity. Early in 1974, Saskatchewan nurses established the Saskatchewan Union of Nurses (SUN) to bargain collectively for nurses in any Saskatchewan health care institution. It successfully negotiated a model province-wide contract that gave general duty staff nurses a 21 percent salary increase in their first year and 9 percent in the next year.[19]

Influenced by the Supreme Court's decision, other provincial nursing associations also withdrew from collective bargaining, helping their in-house advisory labour relations committees establish themselves as autonomous nursing unions. Within eight years, there were independent nursing unions in all provinces except Quebec and Prince Edward Island.[20]

Figure 3
Cartoon
Artist: Bob Kreiger,
1998
Simon Fraser University Editorial Cartoon Collection
MsC 25.KRI.140

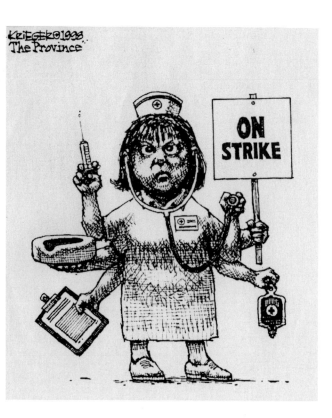

The heads of these fledgling nursing unions perceived a need for a national association to support provincial activities, and in 1981, six provincial nurses' unions came together to found the National Federation of Nurses' Unions, later renamed the Canadian Federation of Nurses Unions (CFNU). This model mirrored that of the provincial professional nursing associations, all of which, with the exception of Quebec, were members of the CNA. The nursing union presidents and their executive committees were rank and file hospital general duty or staff nurses rather than nursing administrators, educators, or public health nurses. Initially, their focus was collective bargaining; however, by the 1990s, with their phenomenal growth in membership and increased experience, they began to challenge provincial and national nursing associations in influencing the public policies affecting nursing. As Kathleen Connors, President of the CFNU from 1982 to 2002 asserted:

> My goal for CFNU was to make it truly national.
> Now we have nine of Canada's ten major nurses
> unions as members, from Newfoundland and
> Labrador to British Columbia. We are also seen
> by the Federal Health Minister and her deputies
> as a critically important constituency — one that
> must be consulted. And many in the national
> media regularly call for comments.[21]

Today, the CFNU represents 122 000 registered nurses, registered psychiatric nurses, and licensed practical nurses. It is the largest organization of nurses in Canada.[22]

Strikes and Nurses

Collective bargaining and the right to withhold services if an impasse in bargaining is reached — the "right to strike" — have been inextricably linked in Canadian trade unionism. They are less tightly linked in public sector unionism, since provincial governments have varied in their willingness to permit "essential service" workers access to the strike weapon.[23] Just what constitutes "essential services" in any province has been, and continues to be, hotly disputed. In Quebec, massive unionization of public employees transformed the union movement in the 1960s and the province had the highest rate of strikes in Canada, including those in the public sector.[24] However, rather than outlawing strikes, the Quebec government chose to permit them while requiring certain designated essential services be maintained during strike action.

More recently, Canadian nurses have demonstrated their acceptance of the strike tool. Between 1966 and 1982, there were 32 strikes by nurses in Canada. In 1991, nurses in Manitoba and Saskatchewan engaged in province-wide strikes. In 1999, there was a province-wide strike in Newfoundland and Labrador, although nurses were legislated back to work after nine days. The following month, Saskatchewan nurses went on strike. They were also legislated back to work, but this time they defied the legislation for 11 days. Then Quebec nurses staged a strike for most of the summer of 1999. In 2001, British Columbia nurses refused to

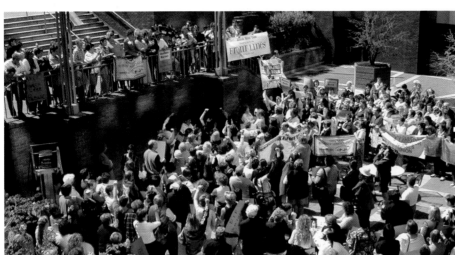

Figure 4 (above)
Canadian Federation of Nurses Unions Biennium
Edmonton, Alberta
June 2001
United Nurses of Alberta

Over 400 nurses descend on Canada Place to exert pressure on the Federal Government to improve the public health care system.

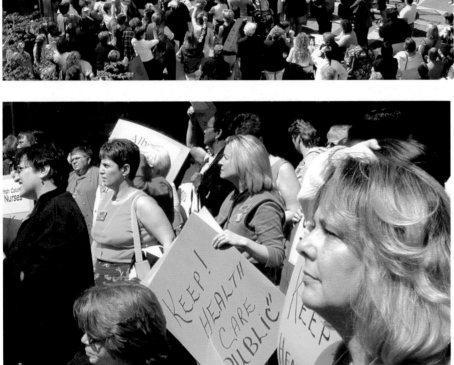

Figure 5 (left)
Canadian Federation of Nurses Unions Bienniun
Edmonton, Alberta
June 2001
United Nurses of Alberta

Delegates chant "We are the nurses, the mighty, mighty nurses" at a march to Canada Place in Edmonton.

work overtime until the provincial government legislated a settlement. Unquestionably, effective use of the strike has done much to advance the socio-economic status of nurses during the past 30 years. Not incidentally, strikes promoted nurses' sense of political efficacy and forced governments to deal with their complaints.[25] Strikes by nurses have also changed stereotypic images of them as passive female workers.

Legislative denial of the right to strike has not always prevented strikes. In Alberta, for example, in 1988, a 19-day illegal strike of 11 000 staff nurses from 96 hospitals led to fines totalling $450 000 against the United Nurses of Alberta (UNA). However, it also prevented employers from rolling back salary increases and contract provisions gained in previous collective bargaining. Strategically planned on the eve of the Calgary Winter Olympic games, the UNA strike showed that nurses would not tolerate unjust treatment. The illegal strike was supported by the public, despite disruption in hospital services throughout Alberta.[26] In 1989, a seven day illegal strike by 21 777 Quebec nurses in 300 hospitals led to improved salaries, but it also resulted in severe penalties levied against the FIIQ. The union underwrote all individual fines, precipitating a major financial crisis for the FIIQ.[27] Nevertheless, despite penalties, some Canadian nursing unions are unwilling to relinquish their right to strike. The success of

A Nurse on Strike

Margaret Gorrie, British Columbia Institute of Technology

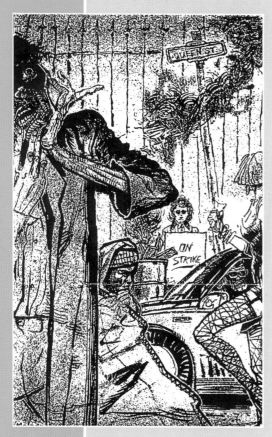

Figure 6
Cartoon
Artist: Molnar
Globe & Mail, Toronto
Winter 1996

My 20 years of nursing hasn't prepared me for this. I've never been on strike before and find the experience exciting — even frightening — while managing also to be tedious. I stand in front of the Queen Street Mental Health Centre from 3:00 to 11:00 p.m. wearing a sign urging passersby to help save public services from government cuts.

It is winter 1996 and the first strike of the Ontario Public Sector Employees Union. The union represents nursing and other staff in nine provincial psychiatric hospitals as well as staff in a myriad of other provincial agencies. The Conservative government of Mike Harris has plans to eliminate 13 000 jobs. Nurses make up the majority of the essential workers who continue to provide patient care during the five-week strike.

As I stand on the sidewalk, I think of the connections between my years of nursing and my new involvement in this direct political action. The specialty of psychiatric nursing, once defined solely by the setting in which it took place — psychiatric hospitals — is now more properly termed "psychiatric/mental health nursing," reflecting an increased emphasis on health promotion and community-based care:

> The psychiatric/mental health nurse understands how the psychiatric disease process, the illness experience, the recuperative powers and the perceived degree of mental health are affected by contextual factors.

In other words, recovery from mental illness is best achieved when patients are connected to society — when they have a place to live and work to do — things that most of us take for granted. But these are the very social programs threatened by the government's haste to shrink the public sector.

I find I am absorbed in learning about Queen Street West through my new stationary position on the sidewalk. While I am able to claim a temporary place at the curbside, I fear those with whom I share this space — the homeless, prostitutes, and mentally ill persons — will face a future of increased hardship and fewer supports.

"It's all closed up," said a dishevelled looking man, "you can't get in to get warm any more."

Source: Canadian Federation of Mental Health Nurses (CFMHN), "Beliefs about Psychiatric and Mental Health Nursing," in *Canadian Standards of Psychiatric and Mental Health Nursing Practice*, 2d ed. (CFMHN, 1998).

this strategy was demonstrated in March 1997 when the UNA threatened an illegal strike a few days before a provincial election. Because nurses had been the group most affected by massive cuts in health care system restructuring, which cost thousands of full time nursing positions, the Alberta public supported them. Within a few days, a government appointed mediator recommended an enhanced salary package over three years, as well as concessions on a number of patient care issues.[28]

Although nurses' salaries continue to be pivotal in negotiating collective agreements, quality of the work environment and its impact on patient care have recently surfaced as significant issues. The elimination of thousands of nursing positions, coupled with increases in the severity of patients' illnesses and the complexity of their care, have made patient safety a significant workplace issue. Additionally, as workloads increased and environments became more stressful, nurse absenteeism rose alarmingly. Many were forced to work significant numbers of overtime hours, including scheduled days off. In some instances, a minimum level of safe patient care has even replaced salary concerns as the focus of nursing unions' negotiations with employers.

Conclusion

Today, more than 75 percent of all Canadian registered nurses are unionized and the significant majority are members of nursing unions. Beginning soon after the end of the Second World War, collective bargaining for nurses, by nurses, heralded a significant change in Canadian nursing. Capitalizing on the advances of public sector unions during the 1960s, nursing associations in all provinces except Quebec were instrumental in dramatically improving the salaries and working conditions of their members. Quebec nurses had already advanced in that respect, having begun unionizing in the 1930s. This phenomenon can be explained by the hierarchical structure of nursing in the French-Catholic tradition, and by the more limited choices available to lay nurses. In 1973, two events altered the course of nursing unionization in Canada: the RNAO made a decision to support establishment of a separate, autonomous nursing union, and the Supreme Court of Canada made a decision, in 1974, to disallow certification of an SRNA supported staff nurses' unit as a collective bargaining agent on the grounds that SRNA was "management dominated." These events led to the creation of autonomous nursing unions in most provinces, separate from the provincial, professional nursing associations. While not all nurses agree with such strategies as strikes to resolve bargaining impasses, almost all support collective bargaining as an effective way to improve the quality of professional practice environments. Since registered nurses comprise the single largest category of Canadian health care providers, ensuring that they are adequately remunerated and satisfied with their work environments is pivotal to maintaining Canada's publicly funded and administered health care delivery system.

Notes

Introduction

1. The symbols of hospital and military nursing — caps, veils, uniforms, military medals, school pins, and rings — make up a large percentage of the artifact collection. Nurses' medical bags, syringe kits, lecture notes, and textbooks represent nursing practice. Memorabilia from the International Council of Nurses and the Canadian Nurses Association form the rest of the collection.

2. The portal www.civilization.ca/tresors/nursing/ncinto1e.html has specially-designed search and retrieval mechanisms. Over time, it is planned to add contextual information to the catalogue. A second phase will link selections from Library and Archives Canada material to the *Canadian Nursing History Collection Online* portal.

3. Kathryn McPherson, "Carving Out a Past: The Canadian Nurses Association War Memorial," *Histoire sociale/Social History* 29(58): 417–429 (November 1996); Dianne Dodd, "Nurses' Residences: Using the Built Environment as Evidence," *Nursing History Review* 9 (2001): 185–206.

4. John Murray Gibbon, and Mary S Mathewson, *Three Centuries of Canadian Nursing* (Toronto: The Macmillan Company, 1947).

5. Janet Ross Kerr, "A Historical Approach to the Evolution of University Nursing Education in Canada," in Janet Kerr, and Janetta MacPhail, eds., *Canadian Nursing: Issues and Perspectives* (Toronto: McGraw-Hill Ryerson, 1988); Sharon Richardson, "Transformation of the Canadian Association of University Schools of Nursing," *Western Journal of Nursing Research* 17 (1995): 416–34; Lee Stewart, *It's Up to You: Women at UBC in the Early Years* (Vancouver: UBC Press, 1990).

6. Edouard Desjardin, Suzanne Giroux, and Eileen E Flanagan, *Histoire de la profession infirmière au Québec* (Montreal: Association des infirmières de la province du Québec, 1970); André Petitat, *Les infirmières: De la vocation à la profession* (Montreal: Boréal, 1989); Marguerite Jean s.c.i.m., *Évolution des communauté religieuses de femmes au Canada de 1639 à nos jours* (Montreal: Fides, 1977).

7. G W L Nicolson, *Canada's Nursing Sisters* (Toronto: Samuel Stevenom Hockert Company, 1975).

8. Margaret Street, *Watch-Fires on the Mountain: The Life and Writings of Ethel Johns* (Toronto: University of Toronto Press, 1973); Marion Royce, *Eunice Dyke: Health Care Pioneer* (Toronto: Dundurn Press, 1983); Helen M Carpenter, *A Divine Discontent: Edith Kathleen Russell, Reforming Educator* (Toronto: Faculty of Nursing, University of Toronto, 1982); Marie-Claire Daveluy, *Jeanne Mance* (Montreal: Fides, 1962); Jean Coté, *Jeanne Mance, l'héroïque infirmière* (Outremont, QC: Quebecor, 1995); Natalie Rieger, *Jean Gunn, Nursing Leader* (Toronto: Fitzhenry & Whiteside, 1996); Diana Mansell, *Forging the Future: A History of Canadian Nursing* (Ann Arbor, MI: Thomas Press, 2003).

9. Judi Coburn, "'I See and Am Silent': A Short History of Nursing in Ontario," in Janice Acton, Penny Goldsmith, and Bonnie Shepard, eds., *Women at Work: Ontario, 1850–1930* (Toronto: Women's Educational Press, 1974), 127–63; Suzann Buckley, "Ladies or Midwives? Efforts to Reduce Infant and Maternal Mortality," in Linda Kealey, ed., *A Not Unreasonable Claim: Women and Reform in Canada, 1880s–1920s* (Toronto: The Women's Press, 1979), 131–49.

10. Michael Bliss, *Plague: A Story of Smallpox in Montreal* (Toronto: Harper Collins Publishers, 1991); Heather MacDougall, *Activists and Advocates: Toronto's Health Department, 1883–1983* (Toronto: Dundurn Press, 1990); Wendy Mitchinson, and Janice Dickin McGinnis, eds., *Essays in the History of Canadian Medicine* (Toronto: McClelland and Stewart, 1988).

11. Kathryn McPherson, *Bedside Matters: The Transformation of Canadian Nursing, 1900–1990* (Toronto: Oxford University Press, 1996); Cynthia Toman, "Crossing the Technological Line: Blood Transfusion and the Art and Science of Nursing, 1942–1990," (PhD diss., University of Ottawa, 1998); Kathryn McPherson, "Science and Technique: Nurses' Work in a Canadian Hospital, 1920–1939," in Dianne Dodd, and Deborah Gorham, eds., *Caring and Curing: Historical Perspectives on Women and Healing in Canada* (Ottawa: University of Ottawa Press, 1996), 71–101.

12. Coburn, "I See and Am Silent," 127–63; David Wagner, "The Proletarianization of Nursing in the United States, 1932–1946," *International Journal of Health Services* 10(2): 272 (1980); David Coburn, "The Development of Canadian Nursing: Professionalization and Proletarianization," *International Journal of Health Services* 18(3): 437–56 (1988); McPherson, *Bedside Matters*.

13. Linda White, "Who's in Charge Here? The General Hospital School of Nursing, St. John's, Newfoundland, 1903–30," *Canadian Bulletin of Medical History*, 11(1): 91–118 (1994); Meryn Stuart, "Shifting Professional Boundaries: Gender Conflict in Public Health, 1920–1925," in Dodd and Gorham, *Caring and Curing*.

14. Carlotta Hacker, *The Indomitable Lady Doctors* (Toronto and Vancouver: Clark, Irwin and Co., 1974); Veronica Strong-Boag, "Canada's Women Doctors: Feminism Constrained," in Kealey, *A Not Unreasonable Claim*, 109–29.

15. Mary Kinnear, *In Subordination: Professional Women 1870–1970* (Montreal and Kingston: McGill-Queen's University Press, 1995); Yolande Cohen, and Louise Bienvenue, "Emergence de l'identité professionnelle chez les infirmières québécoises, 1890–1927," *Canadian Bulletin of Medical History* 11(1): 119–51 (1994).

16. Veronica Strong-Boag, "Making a Difference: The History of Canada's Nurses," *Canadian Bulletin of Medical History* 8(2): 239 (1991).

17. Kathryn McPherson, and Meryn Stuart, "Writing Nursing History in Canada: Issues and Approaches," *Canadian Bulletin of Medical History* 11(1): 3–22 (1994).

18. François Rousseau, *La croix et le scalpel: Histoire des Augustines et de l'Hôtel-Dieu de Québec*, vols. I and II (Quebec: Éditions du Septentrion, 1989, 1994); Brigitte Violette, *Étude synthèse sur l'action des communautés religieuses de femmes dans le domaine de la santé publique au Québec (1639–1962)* (Quebec: Parks Canada, August 2001); The Clio Collective, *Quebec Women: A History*, trans. Roger Gannon, and Rosalind Gill (Toronto: The Women's Press, 1987); Micheline Dumont, *Les religieuses sont-elles féministes?* (Montreal: Bellarmin, 1995); Marta Danylewycz, *Taking the Veil: An Alternative to Marriage, Motherhood, and Spinsterhood in Quebec, 1840–1920* (Toronto: McClelland and Stewart, 1987).

19. Elizabeth Smyth, "Women Religious and Their Work of History in Canada, 1639–1978: A Starting Point for Analysis," *Historical Studies* (Canadian Catholic Historical Association) 64 (1998): 135–50; Dianne Dodd, and Brigitte Violette, "Women's Religious Congregations and Healthcare in Canada," paper presented at meeting of Parks Canada/Historic Sites and Monuments Board of Canada [HSMBC], July 2003, Ottawa, Submission Report #2003-36; Deborah Rink, *Spirited Women: A History of Catholic Sisters in British Columbia* (Vancouver: Sisters' Association Archdiocese of Vancouver, 2000).

20. Christina Bates, "Symbol of a Profession: One Hundred Years of Nurses' Caps," Canadian Nursing History Collection available online, Canadian Museum of Civilization, last updated 9 Sept. 2002, www.civilization.ca/hist/infirm/ininto1e.html; Kathryn McPherson "'The Case of the Kissing Nurse': Femininity, Sociability and Sexuality, 1920–1968," in McPherson, *Bedside Matters*.

Chapter 1

Lay Nursing from the New France Era to the End of the Nineteenth Century (1608–1891)

1. Marie-Françoise Collière is a French nurse and historian who has proposed a redefinition of nursing in a historical perspective, opposing the activities assigned to men and women in the health care field. Please refer to the suggested readings for some of her published works.

2. John Murray Gibbon, and Mary S Mathewson, *Three Centuries of Canadian Nursing* (Toronto: The Macmillan Co. of Canada Ltd., 1947), 3.

3. Étienne Michel Faillon, *Vie de Mlle Mance et histoire de l'Hôtel-Dieu de Villemarie dans l'île de Montréal, en Canada, Tome 1* (Villemarie: Soeurs de l'Hôtel-Dieu de Villemarie, 1854); Marie-Claire Daveluy, *Jeanne Mance. 1606–1673. Suivie d'un Essai généalogique sur les Mance et les De Mance, par M. Jacques Laurent* (Montreal and Paris: Fides, 1962); Dom Guy-Marie Oury, *Jeanne Mance et le rêve de M. de La Dauversière* (Chambray: C.L.D., 1983); Julie Noël, *L'œuvre de Jeanne Mance (1606–1673), co-fondatrice de Montréal, fondatrice de l'Hôtel-Dieu de Montréal et première infirmière laïque canadienne*, Historic Sites and Monuments Board of Canada, Agenda Paper 1998–16.

4. There are a number of works written about her, most notably Faillon, *Vie de Mlle Mance*; Rénald Lessard, "Les soins de santé au Canada aux XVIIième et XVIIIième siècles," in Normand Séguin, ed., *Atlas historique du Québec. L'institution médicale* (Sainte-Foy: Presses de l'Université Laval, Coll. Atlas historique du Québec, 1998), 3–36; Robert Lahaise, and Noël Vallerand, *La Nouvelle-France, 1524–1760* (Outremont: Lanctôt Éditeur, 1999), 62–3.

5. Marie Maupeou was a charitable widow who worked with St. Vincent de Paul; her book was *Recueil de recettes choisies, expérimentées et approuvées contre quantité de maux fort communs, tant internes qu'externes, invétérés et difficiles à guérir*. See Jeanne-Françoise Juchereau de Saint-Ignace and Marie Andrée Régnard Duplessis de Sainte-Hélène, *Les Annales de*

l'Hôtel-Dieu de Québec. 1636–1716, éditées dans leur texte original avec une introduction et des notes par dom Albert Jamet de l'Abbaye de Solesmes, (Quebec City: Hôtel-Dieu de Québec, 1939), 99.

6. Faillon, *Vie de Mlle Mance,* 42 (our translation). This detail is revealing, since it was not until 1653 that Étienne Bouchard agreed to act as the first surgeon at Villemarie on a five-year contract, and the first priest, Gabriel Souart, was allowed to practise medicine there "avec la permission du souverain Pontife" (with the permission of the sovereign pontiff). See Daveluy, *Jeanne Mance. 1606–1673,* 159, 160.

7. Daveluy, *Jeanne Mance. 1606–1673,* 251. It should be added that listed in the after-death inventory of Jeanne Mance, reproduced in its entirety in Daveluy (280–1), there is mention of a "a small cast-iron mortar and a pestle of the same material" and "a tin syringe, with its case" (our translation).

8. Faillon, *Vie de Mlle Mance,* 63 (our translation).

9. A term for medicinal herbs.

10. Quoted in Catherine Fortin-Morisset, "Jérémie, dit Lamontagne, Catherine (Aubuchon; Lepailleur de Laferté)," in *Dictionary of Canadian Biography, Vol. III: 1741–1770* (Toronto: University of Toronto Press, 1974), 314–5, available online: *Dictionary of Canadian Biography Online,* Library and Archives Canada, www.biographi.ca/EN/ShowBio.asp?BioId=35547. Fortin-Morisset also explains that, "In the 18th century French naturalists, supported by the intendants of New France, were trying to discover the medicinal and practical properties of the flora of Canada. Every year the intendants encouraged plant collecting and the dispatch of living or dried specimens to France on the king's vessels." See also Collectif Clio, "L'Ancien régime au feminine," *L'Histoire des femmes au Québec* (Montreal: Le Jour éditeur, 1992), 123; Lessard, "Soins de santé," 30.

11. Lessard, "Soins de santé." See also Jacques Bernier, *La médecine au Québec. Naissance et évolution d'une profession* (Quebec City: PUL, 1989), especially chapter 1, "Les premiers projets de réforme," 31–41.

12. Marianna O'Gallagher, *Grosse-Île: Gateway to Canada, 1832–1937* (Ste-Foy: Livres Carraig Books, 1984). The term "infirmière" was used in the French-language translation of this book; in the original documents reproduced in an appendix to the book, even those written in French used the title "nurse." See also Christine Chartré, *Le traitement des maladies contagieuses à la station de la Grosse-Île 1832–1927* (Parcs Canada, Patrimoine culturel et biens immmobiliers, Centre de services du Québec, 2001).

13. They were Ann McAuley, Cath O'Brien, M A Hum, Isabella Gillis, Ellen McCarthy, and Ellen Sullivan. See Christine Chartré, *Le traitement des maladies contagieuses à la station de la Grosse-Île 1832–1927.* See also O'Gallagher, *Grosse-Île,* 76; a photograph taken in 1909 shows seven nurses.

14. O'Gallagher, *Grosse-Île,* 113.

15. Chartré, *Traitement des maladies,* 74–5.

16. It should be noted that in addition to epidemics and economic crises, serious fires put some 20 000 people out on the streets in Quebec City in 1845 and destroyed 1500 dwellings in Montreal in 1866; see, on this subject, Collectif Clio, "Travailler sous un autre toit," in *L'Histoire des femmes au Québec,* chapter 7, 211–48.

17. One of them, Madame Olivier Berthelet, donated a house in which the Association planned to give "soup, clothing, and other items to the destitute." At the Association's general meeting it was also decided that home visits would be conducted to "ensure that those who needed it received their charity." Among the lay housekeepers, who, alone or with at most two maids and the charitable ladies, took care of orphans throughout these years, were Mrs J B Chalifoux, Miss Eulalie Petit, and the Misses Elmire and Delphine Morin. Marie-Claire Daveluy, *L'Orphelinat Catholique de Montréal* (Montreal: Le Devoir, 1919) (our translation).

18. In 1831, she opened a second, larger refuge, and then a third one in 1836. See Marguerite Jean, "Tavernier, Émilie (Gamelin)," *Dictionary of Canadian Biography, Vol. VIII: 1851–1860* (Toronto: University of Toronto Press, 1985), 863–5, available online: *Dictionary of Canadian Biography Online,* Library and Archives Canada, www.biographi.ca/EN/ShowBio.asp?BioId=38334.

19. France Gagnon, *L'Hospice Saint-Joseph de la Maternité de Québec, 1852–1876: prise en charge de la maternité hors-norme,* Cahier 70, Cahiers de recherche du GREMF, Groupe de recherche multidisciplinaire féministe (Quebec City, Université Laval, 1996), 47 (our translation).

20. I searched the Canadian censuses of 1861, 1871, 1881, and 1891 for Halifax, St. John, and Toronto, and the Toronto city directories from 1833 to 1891 for data on nurses and midwives. These records are available in the Toronto Reference Library.

21. Catherine Parr Trail, *I Bless You in My Heart: Selected Correspondence of Catherine Parr Trail,* eds. Carl Ballstadt, Elizabeth Hopkins, and Michael A Peterman (University of Toronto Press, 1996). See 102 and 51.

22. Elizabeth Jane Errington, *Wives and Mothers, School Mistresses and Scullery Maids: Working Women in Upper Canada 1790–1840* (Montreal and Kingston: McGill-Queen's University Press, 1995), 58.

23. Edith G Firth, ed., *The Town of York 1815–1834: Further Documents of Early Toronto* (University of Toronto Press, 1966), 227.

24. J T H Connors, "'Larger Fish to Catch Here Than Midwives': Midwifery and the Medical Profession in Nineteenth-Century Ontario" in Dianne Dodd, and Deborah Gorham, eds, *Caring and Curing: Historical Perspectives on Women and Healing in Canada* (Ottawa: University of Ottawa Press, 1994), 110.

25. Geoffrey Bilson, *A Darkened House: Cholera in Nineteenth Century Canada* (University of Toronto Press, 1980), 88.

26. W H Pearson, *Recollections and Records of Toronto of Old* (Toronto: William Briggs, 1914), 120. Pearson was talking of the 1840s.

27. Charlotte Gourlay Robinson, *Pioneer Profiles of New Brunswick Settlers* (Belleville, Ontario: Mika Publishing Company 1980), 42–9.

28. Isabella Beeton, *Beeton's Household Management* (London: Jonathan Cape Limited, 1968), a first edition facsimile. First published in bound edition in 1861.

29. S S Connell, "Case of Catalepsy," *Canadian Lancet* 4(7), 308–13 (March 1872).

30. Charles Kirk Clarke, *A History of the Toronto General Hospital* (Toronto: William Briggs, 1913), 82.

31. E C G[ordon], "Mrs Davis," *The Canadian Nurse* 1 (December 1905), 39.

32. It was such considerations that led to the conclusion that "the great foundations of Canadian communities that history has credited to the zeal and intellect of Bishop Bourget were in fact the appropriation of charities instituted by volunteer laywomen." Collectif Clio, "Travailler sous un autre toit," 233–4 (our translation).

33. Anne Summers, "The Mysterious Demise of Sarah Gamp: The Domiciliary Nurse and Her Detractors c. 1830–1860," *Victorian Studies* 32(3): 365–86 (1989).

Chapter 2

Canadian Midwifery: Blending Traditional and Modern Practices

Primary data for this report were gathered for the first author's doctoral and post-doctoral research on granny/traditional midwives and nurse-midwives in Newfoundland and Labrador and independent lay midwives in the 1970–1990s. Both authors conducted research on newly certified midwives in BC and the second author conducted interviews with Aboriginal elders, health professionals, and Aboriginal women during provincial midwifery legislation consultations.

1. J Fiske, "Carrier Women and the Politics of Mothering," in G Creese, and V Strong-Boag, eds. *British Columbia Reconsidered: Essays on Women* (Vancouver: Press Gang Publishers, 1992), 201.

2. F Boas, *Kwakiutl Ethnography*, Helen Codere, ed. (Chicago: University of Chicago Press, 1996), 61.

3. T Jeffries, "Sechelt Women and Self-Government," in G Creese and V Strong-Boag, eds. *British Columbia Reconsidered*, 91.

4. C Benoit, and D Carroll, "Aboriginal Midwifery in British Columbia: A Narrative Still Untold," *Western Geographic Series* 30 (1995): 221–46; Boas, *Kwakiutl Ethnography*.

5. James B Waldron, Ann Herring, T Kue Young, *Aboriginal Health In Canada: Historical, Cultural and Epidemiological Perspectives* (Toronto: University of Toronto Press, 1995).

6. J O'Neil, and P Kaufert, "The Politics of Obstetric Care: The Inuit Experience," in W Mitchinson, P Bourne, A Prentice, G Cuthbert Brandt, B Light, and N Black, eds., *Canadian Women: A Reader* (Toronto: Harcourt Brace,

1996); Quoted in Benoit and Carroll, "Aboriginal Midwifery in British Columbia," 240.

7. D Carroll, and C Benoit, "Aboriginal Midwifery in Canada: Merging Traditional Practices and Modern Science," in I Bourgeault, C Benoit, and R Davis-Floyd, eds., *Reconceiving Midwifery: Emerging Models of Care* (Kingston/Montreal: McGill-Queen's University Press, 2004): 263–86.

8. M Abbott, *The History of Medicine in the Province of Quebec* (Montreal: McGill University, 1931), 28.

9. S Buckley, "Ladies or Midwives? Efforts to Reduce Infant and Maternal Mortality," in Linda Kealey, ed., *A Not Unreasonable Claim: Women and Reform in Canada, 1880s–1920s* (Toronto: The Women's Press, 1979), 134.

10. Leslie C Biggs, "The Case of the Missing Midwives': A History of Midwifery in Ontario from 1795–1900," in Katherine Arnup, Andrée Lévesque, and Ruth Roach Pierson, eds., *Delivering Motherhood: Maternal Idealogies and Practices in the 19th and 20th Centuries* (London and new York: Routledge, 1990), 20–35.

11. N Langford, "Childbirth on the Canadian Prairies, 1880–1930," *Journal of Historical Sociology* 3 (1995): 278–302; Cited in L Rasmussen, C Savage, and A Wheeler, eds., *A Harvest Yet to Reap: A History of Prairie Women* (Toronto: The Women's Press, 1976), 78; E Silverman, *The Last Best West: Women on the Alberta Frontier, 1880-1930* (Montreal and London: Eden Press, 1984), 66; Personal communication with Karen Kobb, July 2003.

12. C Benoit, "Mothering in a Newfoundland Community: 1900–1940," in Arnup, Levesque, and Pierson, *Delivering Motherhood*, 185; Benoit, *Midwives in Passage*, 57; Benoit, "Midwives and Healers: The Newfoundland Experience," *Healthsharing* 5(1): 22–26, 23 (1983); Benoit, "Midwives and Healers," 24.

13. S Chard, "Tribute to Aunt Bertha: Bertha Anderson, Makkovik, 1872–1950," *Them Days Magazine* 4(1): 56–8 (1978).

14. Benoit, *Midwives in Passage*, 23, 49, 50.

15. Wendy Mitchinson, *Giving Birth in Canada*, 1900–1950 (Toronto: University of Toronto Press, 2002), 81; Benoit, field notes, Newfoundland, 1984.

16. K Kuusisto, "A Last Generation of Midwives": *Midwifery in 20th Century Nova Scotia, Canada* (Colchester, UK: University, Oral History Project, Social History Programme, 1997), 18, 19; J Mason, *A History of Midwifery in Canada*, Appendix 1. Task Force on the Implementation of Midwifery, Mary Eberts, Chairperson (Toronto: Ontario Government, 1987), 228.

17. Benoit, *Midwives in Passage*, 80, 81; Joyce Murphy, "Olive Bishop: Midwife-Nurse of Pass Island, South Coast of Newfoundland, Hermitage Bay," (Memorial University of Newfoundland Folklore and Language Archive (MUNFA), no. 75-285), 14–18.

18. Quoted in Benoit, *Midwives in Passage*, 3, 4.

19. Benoit, *Midwives in Passage*.

20. Cecilia Benoit, field notes (Labrador 1988–89).

21. Information provided to the authors on 1 March 2004 by Manitoba certified midwife, Kris Robinson, who worked with Lesley in Gjoa Haven in 1977–87.

22. Personal communication with Jo Lutley, July 2003; personal communication with Glad Reardon, 16 February 2004.

23. P Kaufert, and J O'Neil, "Analysis of a Dialogue on Risks in Childbirth: Clinicians, Epidemiologists, and Inuit Women," in S Lindenbaum and M Lock, eds., *Knowledge, Power & Practice* (Berkeley: University of California Press, 1993), 39, 40.

24. C Benoit, field notes (Newfoundland, 1984).

25. Bourgeault, Benoit, and Davis-Floyd, eds., *Reconceiving Midwifery.*

26. Cited in Hurlbert, "Midwifery in Canada: A Capsule in History," 31.

Chapter 3

The Trained Nurse: Private Duty and VON Home Nursing (Late 1800s to 1940s)

1. Barbara Keddy, Judy Glennis, Trudy Larsen, Pat Mallory, and Marg Storey, "The Personal Is Political: A Feminist Analysis of the Social Control of Rank and File Nurses in Canada in the 1920s and 1930s in Canada," *History of Nursing Society Journal* 4(3): 167–72 (1992/93).

2. Kathryn McPherson, *Bedside Matters: The Transformation of Canadian Nursing 1900–1990* (Ontario: Oxford University Press, 1996): 26, 51, 129.

3. Mary Kinnear, *In Subordination: Professional Women, 1870–1970* (Montreal and Kingston: McGill-Queen's University Press, 1995). Forty-five nurses, using the records of the Winnipeg General Hospital Alumnae Association responded to a questionnaire. See 108, 188–9, and footnote 45 on 212 (chapter 5); McPherson, *Bedside Matters.* McPherson interviewed a number of retired nurses in Manitoba; Barbara Keddy, "Private Duty Nursing Days of the 1920s and 1930s in Canada," *Canadian Woman Studies* 7(3): 99–101 (Fall 1986). Keddy interviewed 35 former nurses in Nova Scotia and her interviews are deposited in the Barbara Keddy Collection in the Public Archives of Nova Scotia.

4. Kathryn McPherson, *Bedside Matters*, 182.

5. Veronica Strong-Boag, *The New Day Recalled: Lives of Girls and Women in English Canada 1919–1939* (Toronto: Copp Clark Pitman Ltd., 1988), 65; McPherson, *Bedside Matters*, 57.

6. Jean Church, "New Trends in Private Duty," *Canadian Nurse* 33(9): 446–49 (September 1937).

7. George Weir, *Survey of Nursing Education in Canada* (Toronto, 1982), 89, as cited in Kinnear, *In Subordination*, 108.

8. McPherson, *Bedside Matters*, 95; Keddy, "Private Duty Nursing Days," 101; Susan Reverby, "Something Besides Waiting: The Politics of Private Duty Nursing Reform in the Depression," in Ellen Condliffe Langmann, ed., *Nursing History: New Perspectives, New Possibilities* (London: Teachers College, Columbia University, 1983), 133–56.

9. We are indebted to the RNABC History of Nursing for sending copies of the oral history tapes of Rebecca Bancroft, Surrey, British Columbia, who was interviewed by Audrey Stegan, 15 June 1987.

10. Sheila Penney, *A Century of Caring: The History of the Victorian Order of Nurses for Canada* (Victorian Order of Nurses, 1996). We are grateful to Ms Jennifer Stevens, Communications Manager, VON Ottawa, Canada, for her assistance and valuable information on the initiatives and changes within the VON that have kept this organization viable and held in such high regard throughout the country.

11. Keddy, "Private Duty Nursing Days," 101.

12. Mary Kinnear, *In Subordination;* Reverby, "Something Besides Waiting," in Langmann, *Nursing History: New Perspectives;* "Oral Histories of Nurses Who Worked in the 1920s and 1930s," Barbara Keddy Collection, Public Archives of Nova Scotia.

13. Keddy, "Oral Histories of Nurses."

14. Ibid.

15. Keddy, "Private Duty Nursing Days," 101.

16. Susan Reverby, *The Nursing Disorder: A Critical History of the Hospital–Nursing Relationship, 1860–1945* (PhD diss., Ann Arbor, MI, 1982), 197; Keddy, "Oral Histories of Nurses."

17. Keddy, "Oral Histories of Nurses."

18. Keddy, "Private Duty Nursing Days," 101.

19. Mabel McMullens, "Private Duty Nursing under Present Conditions," *The Canadian Nurse* 27(12): 643 (October 1931); Editorial, Department of Private Duty Nursing, "Functions and Standards in Private Duty," *The Canadian Nurse* 32(10): 463 (October 1936).

20. Jean Church, "New Trends in Private Duty," *The Canadian Nurse* 33 (September 1937): 446–449; Annual Report of Private Duty Section in BC for 1935–6, Vancouver, BC. With thanks to the RNABC for allowing access to this information.

21. George Weir, *Survey of Nursing Education;* McPherson, *Bedside Matters*, 135.

22. McPherson, *Bedside Matters*, 160.

Chapter 4

Healing the Body and Saving the Soul: Nursing Sisters and the First Catholic Hospitals in Quebec (1639–1880)

1. In 1960, out of 206 public hospitals in Quebec, 58 percent were the property of female religious communities, representing 66 percent of all hospital beds in the province. In addition, 25 percent of hospitals were owned by lay corporations and managed by a community, and nuns formed part of the staff. Danielle Juteau and Nicole Laurin, "La sécularisation et l'étatisation du secteur hospitalier au Québec de 1960 à 1966," in Robert Comeau, ed., *Jean Lesage et l'éveil d'une nation* (Montreal: Presses de l'Université du Québec, 1989), 156.

2. In Quebec, between 1639 and 1962, some 30 religious orders were associated with some mode of intervention in the health care field. Of this number, only two defined themselves as nursing orders: the Hospitallers of the Order of St. Augustine, called the Daughters of Mercy, and the Institute of the Religious Hospitallers of St. Joseph. Within these congregations there were choir sisters — the hospitallers — who provided care to the ill, and converse nuns — the domestics — who did manual labour to free up the hospitallers. This distinction endured until Vatican II (1965). To the two specifically designated nursing orders were added those whose activities in health care overlapped with charitable and/or educational enterprises, following the example of the Grey Nuns of Montreal, the Sisters of Providence, and the Sisters of Charity of Quebec City.

   See Claudette Lacelle, *L'apport social des communautés religieuses catholiques présentes au Canada avant 1940: une étude préparée à la demande de la Commission des lieux et monuments historiques du Canada dans le but d'identifier les communautés religieuses catholiques susceptibles de faire l'objet d'une commémoration en raison de leur contribution à l'histoire canadienne* (Environment Canada, National Parks Service, 1987, report on microfiche No. 425), 34–5; Brigitte Violette, *Étude synthèse sur l'action des congrégations religieuses de femmes dans le domaine de la santé au Québec (1639–1962), Rapport au Feuilleton préparé à l'intention de la Commission des lieux et monuments historiques du Canada* (Parks Canada, Centre de services du Québec, August 2001), Appendix 1.

3. This definition of the hospital flows largely from the omnipresence of clerics in the world of medicine in the Christian West, which explains why it took centuries of lay scientific discoveries before medicine officially left the sphere of monasteries and churches to become a scientific discipline and a lay domain. Hélène Laforce, *Histoire de la sage-femme dans la région de Québec* (Quebec City: Institut québécois de recherche sur la culture, "Prix Edmond-de-Nevers" coll., No. 4, 1985), 29.

4. See, notably, François Rousseau, *La croix et le scalpel: Histoire des Augustines et de l'Hôtel-Dieu de Québec, vol. 1, 1639–1892, and vol. 2, 1892–1989* (Quebec City: Éditions du Septentrion, 1989 and 1994); Denis Goulet, François Hudon, and Othmar Keel, *Histoire de l'hôpital Notre-Dame de Montréal, 1880–1980* (Montreal: VLB

éditeur, "Études québécoises" coll., 1993); Micheline D'Allaire, *L'Hôpital-Général de Québec, 1692–1764* (Montreal: Fides, 1971); Normand Perron, *Un siècle de vie hospitalière au Québec: Les Augustines et l'Hôtel-Dieu de Chicoutimi, 1884–1984* (Quebec City: Presses de l'Université du Québec, 1984); Johanne Daigle, "Devenir infirmière: le système d'apprentissage et la formation professionnelle à l'Hôtel-Dieu de Montréal, 1920 à 1970," (PhD diss., Department of History, Université du Québec à Montréal, 1990); François Guérard, *Histoire de la santé au Québec* (Montreal: Boréal, 1996).

5. Between 1639 and 1880, ten female religious orders and one male order were associated with the Catholic hospital network in Quebec.

6. Notre Dame Hospital was the first lay French-Canadian general hospital in Quebec. Goulet et al., *Histoire de l'hôpital Notre-Dame*, 46–7.

7. Jean Imbert quoted in Rousseau, *La croix et le scalpel*, vol. 1, 16 (our translation).

8. Matthew quoted in Rousseau, *La croix et le scalpel*, vol. 1, 16–7 (English translation: King James version).

9. Rénald Lessard, *Soins de santé au Canada: aux XVIIᵉ et XVIIIᵉ siècles* (Hull: Musée canadien des civilisations, 1989), 26 (our translation).

10. Goulet et al., *Histoire de l'hôpital Notre-Dame*, 12 (our translation).

11. Laforce, *Histoire de la sage-femme*, 28 (our translation).

12. In their turn, these two pioneer congregations transmitted their knowledge to newcomers to the hospital field. For example, before founding the Hôtel-Dieu de Trois-Rivières in 1697, the Ursulines learned about patient care and preparation of medications from the Augustine nuns of the Hôtel-Dieu de Québec. Before leaving for a mission in British Columbia, the Sisters of St. Anne went to the Hôtel-Dieu de Montréal, in 1858, to learn patient care from the Hospitallers of St. Joseph. See Rousseau, *La croix et le scalpel*, vol. 1, 105, and Deborah Rink, *Spirited Women: A History of Catholic Sisters in British Columbia* (Vancouver: Harbour Publishing, 2000), 26.

13. Daigle, *Devenir infirmière*, 132 (our translation).

14. Choir sister is a level in the hierarchy of a women's religious order and has nothing to do with musical skill; choir sisters were the rank above converse nuns and occupied the important posts in the community and the hospital (administrators, head nurses, pharmacists, etc.), whereas converse nuns were assigned to the menial tasks.

15. Quotation taken from the medical colloquium on the history of medicine in Canada, *Colloque sur les faits saillants de l'histoire de la médecine au Canada, tenu au Lac Beauport, le 7 octobre 1966* (Pointe-Claire, Quebec: Schering, 1966), 13 (our translation).

16. Since 1747, the Sisters of Charity (or Marguerite d'Youville's Grey Nuns), a community founded in the colony ten years earlier, had managed the Montreal General Hospital, replacing the Charron Brothers (or

Frères hospitaliers de la Croix et de Saint-Joseph), a male religious order founded in Canada in 1688, whose charities were collapsing under debt. The Grey Nuns were already providing home care to patients, and d'Youville had taken some ill people into her own home. In 1753, the letters patent issued by Louis XIV granted d'Youville the administration and ownership of the General Hospital. Denis Goulet and André Paradis, *Trois siècles d'histoire médicale au Québec: Chronologie des institutions et des pratiques au Québec (1639–1939)* (Montreal: VLB éditeur, "Études québécoises" coll., 1992), 62.

17. During the second half of the nineteenth century, discoveries by Pasteur and Lister led to major progress in microbiology and surgery. Anesthesia was developed in the 1830s; sterilization dates from the 1860s, and antiseptics from the 1870s. Lacelle, *L'apport social*, 26.

18. The College changed its name to the Professional Corporation of Physicians of Quebec in 1974, and in 1994 it became the Collège des médecins du Québec.

19. The faculty of medicine at Université Laval (1854) grew out of the Medical School of Quebec City (1845), the first francophone faculty. It was founded after McGill's faculty (1829), the first medical faculty in Quebec, which grew out of the Montreal Medical Institute (1823).

20. The affiliation between the faculty of medicine at Université Laval and the Hôtel-Dieu de Québec, in 1855, was not accepted right away; it seems that the Augustine nuns agreed only "to conform to the desires of their ecclesiastical superiors and avoid the physicians obtaining by force the consent they were demanding. In short, a solid, amiable arrangement in the guise of a trial basis seemed preferable and more likely to preserve their independence." Rousseau, *La croix et le scalpel*, vol. 1, 267 (our translation).

21. The training of hospitallers became an increasingly contentious issue; finally, in the early twentieth century, the physicians clearly indicated to the nuns that "their know-how acquired by mimicry and mastered by repetition would no longer suffice in adequate care of patients and that from now on their activities had to be based on book learning." Rousseau, *La croix et le scalpel*, vol. 2, 113 (our translation).

22. The Religious Hospitallers of St. Joseph turned away many requests from the Montreal School of Medicine and Surgery before agreeing, in 1850, "that visits to the medical wards could be made by each of the professors of the school, in turn, every three months for the space of one year" (our translation). As it had for been the Augustine nuns (see note 20 above), their bishop's intervention was decisive in the order's decision. Denis Goulet, *Histoire de la faculté de médecine de l'Université de Montréal, 1843–1993* (Montreal: VLB éditeur, "Études québécoises" coll., 1993), 24–32.

23. Guérard, *Histoire de la santé*, 27 (our translation).

24. Because the 1847 statute forced midwives practising in Quebec City, Montreal, and Trois-Rivières to pass an examination before two members of the College of Physicians and Surgeons of Lower Canada, the eight founders of the institute had taken practical training for 18 months before obtaining their certificates of competency on 12 July 1849. *Béatification et canonisation de la Servante de Dieu, Rosalie Cadron-Jetté, en religion Mère de la Nativité (1794–1864), fondatrice de l'Institut des Soeurs de Miséricorde de Montréal: positio sur les vertus et la renommée de sainteté*, vol. 1 (Rome: Congregation for the causes of saints, 1994) 165–7.

25. Ibid., 175 (our translation).

26. Dr Eugène-Hercule Trudel, house physician for the institution, had obtained, in October 1849, access to the Maternité Sainte-Pélagie for childbirth courses for the Montreal School of Medicine and Surgery. Goulet, *Histoire de la faculté*, 33.

27. To their three vows of poverty, chastity, and obedience was added a fourth one, that of "assisting in their labour fallen girls and women" and as a consequence to "form a corps of midwives." Avélina Paquin quoted in *Béatification*, 129 (our translation).

28. Ibid., 254 (our translation).

29. In this same letter, the superior related, "After a very painful childbirth in which the Doctor had been obliged to use forceps, two clerks behind the Doctor laughed and made fun of the patient and the labour. Permit me to remind you what occurred with Dr Gasquipy, who should, it seems to me, have known how to act during childbirths: in a single night he caused the death of two children and one girl, and the other girl after having suffered horribly almost died as well; the two children died without being baptised; he acted at all times in spite of the Sisters. Now for the girls, most of them say that if they had known they would be attended at childbirth by clerks, they never would have come here." Ibid., 254.

30. Quoted in Goulet et al., *Histoire de l'hôpital Notre-Dame*, 128–9. The works of Yolande Cohen tend to demonstrate that the Grey Nuns of Montreal, more than any other order, accentuated the professional aspect of their mission and were active parties in the hospital reform. See Yolande Cohen, "La contribution des Soeurs de la Charité à la modernisation de l'Hôpital Notre-Dame de Montréal," *Canadian Historical Review* 77(2): 185–220 (June 1996); Yolande Cohen, *Profession infirmière: Une histoire des soins dans les hôpitaux du Québec* (Montreal: Les Presses de l'Université de Montréal, 2000); Yolande Cohen, Jacinthe Pépin, Esther Lamontagne, and André Duquette, eds., *Les sciences infirmières: genèse d'une discipline. Histoire de la Faculté des sciences infirmières de l'Université de Montréal* (Montreal: Les Presses de l'Université de Montréal, 2002).

31. Rousseau, *La croix et le scalpel*, vol. 2, 94–5 (our translation).

32. Luciano Bozzini, Marc Renaud, Dominique Gaucher, and Jaime Llambias-Wolff, *Médecine et société: les années 80* (Laval, Éditions Saint-Martin, "Recherches et documents" coll., 1981), 16 (our translation). The authors of this collection offer a diversity of critical contributions

on issues around the relationship between health and society.

33. Hélène Laforce, "Les grandes étapes de l'élimination des sages-femmes au Québec du 17ᵉ au 20e siècle," in Francine Saillant and Michel O'Neill, eds., *Accoucher autrement: Repères historiques, sociaux et culturels de la grossesse et de l'accouchement au Québec* (Montreal: Éditions Saint-Martin, 1987), 177 (our translation).

Chapter 5

The Nightingale Influence and the Rise of the Modern Hospital

1. J M Gibbon, and Mary S Mathewson, *Three Centuries of Canadian Nursing* (Toronto: The Macmillan Company, 1947).

2. See for example the statistics listed in Appendix A of David Gagan and Rosemary Gagan's *For Patients of Moderate Means: A Social History of the Voluntary Public General Hospital in Canada, 1890–1950* (Montreal: McGill-Queen's University Press, 2002).

3. Dr Donald I MacLellan, *History of the Moncton Hospital: A Proud Past — a Healthy Future (1895–1995)* (Halifax: Nimbus Publishing, 1998), 2.

4. J T H Connor, *Doing Good: The Life of Toronto's General Hospital* (Toronto: University of Toronto Press, 2000), 5.

5. Gibbon, and Mathewson, *Three Centuries of Canadian Nursing*.

6. Vancouver Trades and Labor Council, Minutes, 23 June 1893, 392 (University of British Columbia Archives).

7. Charles Dickens, *The Life and Adventures of Martin Chuzzlewit*, (Boston, n.d.).

8. Cited in H E MacDermot, *History of the School of Nursing of the Montreal General Hospital* (Montreal, 1940), 7–8.

9. Ethel Johns, and Beatrice Fines, *The Winnipeg General Hospital and Health Sciences Centre School of Nursing 1887–1987* (Winnipeg: Alumnae Association Winnipeg General Hospital and Health Science Centre School of Nursing, 1988) (first published 1957), 1.

10. The most recent, and succinct, history of Nightingale's life and career can be found in Lynn McDonald, ed., *Florence Nightingale: An Introduction to Her Life and Family, vol. I of The Collected Works of Florence Nightingale* (Waterloo, ON: Wilfrid Laurier University Press, 2001).

11. For a detailed analysis of the Nightingale Fund and its role in the establishment of the St. Thomas's nursing school, see Monica E Baly, *Florence Nightingale and the Nursing Legacy* (London: Croom Helm, 1986).

12. Baly, *Florence Nightingale and the Nursing Legacy*.

13. Historian Carol Helmstadter has traced medical demands for skilled nursing — such as the efforts by young Joseph Lister, who in the 1850s established a fund for hiring a more skilled nurse in the surgery where he worked. Helmstadter, "The Passing of the Night Watch: Night Nursing Reform in the London Teaching Hospitals, 1856–90," *Canadian Bulletin of Medical History* 11(1): 23–69.

14. Carol Helmstadter, "Old Nurses and New: Nursing in the London Teaching Hospitals Before and After the Mid-Nineteenth-Century Reforms," *Nursing History Review* 1: 43–70; McDonald, *Florence Nightingale*, 41.

15. Bonnie Bulloch, and Vern L Bulloch, *The Emergence of Modern Nursing* (New York: Macmillan Company, 1964), 116.

16. Baly, *Florence Nightingale and the Nursing Legacy*, 138–41.

17. Baly, *Florence Nightingale and the Nursing Legacy*, 138–41; Judith Godden, "A 'Lamentable Failure'? The Founding of Nightingale Nursing in Australia, 1868–1884," *Australian Historical Studies* 32(117): 276–91 (2001).

18. Baly, *Florence Nightingale and the Nursing Legacy*, 144–7; Florence Nightingale's letters to Maria Machin, 1873–79, (McGill University Archives, MG 3046).

19. Victoria General Hospital, "Report of Commissioners Appointed to Enquire into Management," *Journal of the House of Assembly*, App. No. 15, 1896, Nova Scotia.

20. Linda White, "Who's in Charge Here? The General Hospital School of Nursing, St. John's Newfoundland, 1903–30," *Canadian Bulletin for the History of Medicine* 11(1): 91–118 (1994).

21. Vancouver General Hospital, Board of Directors, *Minutes*, Special Meeting, 10 April 1916.

22. Mary Poovey, *Uneven Developments: The Ideological Work of Gender in Mid-Victorian England* (Chicago: University of Chicago Press, 1988).

23. Florence Nightingale, *Notes on Nursing: What It Is, and What It Is Not* (Toronto: General Publishing Co., 1960). Publication information comes from the foreword to the 1946 edition by Virginia Dunbar, xviii.

24. This excerpt from "Santa Filomena" exemplifies Longfellow's contribution to the making of an icon:

> A lady with a lamp shall stand
> In the great history of the land,
> A noble type of good,
> Heroic womanhood.

25. See, for example, Elizabeth Marion Jamieson, and Mary Sewall, *Trends in Nursing History: Their Relationship to World Events* (Philadelphia: W B Saunders Company, 1940).

26. Gibbon, and Mathewson, *Three Centuries of Canadian Nursing*, 155.

27. Gagan, and Gagan in "Better, Brighter and Kinder Nurses," chapter 5 of *For Patients of Moderate Means*, make this point well.

28. The equivalent in 2004 dollars would not be much more than $100.

29. Kathryn McPherson, *Bedside Matters* (Toronto: Oxford University Press, 1996).

30. Kathryn McPherson, "Embodied Labour: The Occupational Health of Nurses, 1920–1940," paper presented to the Canadian Society for the History of Medicine, June 2003, Halifax, Nova Scotia.

31. McPherson, *Bedside Matters*, chapter 4.

32. Charles Rosenberg, *The Care of Strangers: The Rise of America's Hospital System* (New York: Johns Hopkins University Press, 1987), 221.

33. For more detailed information on the ethnic, racial, linguistic, and class composition of the nursing workforce, see McPherson, *Bedside Matters*, chapter 4.

34. On the recruitment of immigrant women into domestic service, see Marilyn Barber, "The Women Ontario Welcomed: Immigrant Domestics for Ontario Homes, 1870–1930," *Ontario History* 72(3): 148–72 (September 1980). On the place of black Canadian women in domestic service, see Agnes Calliste, "Canada's Immigration Policy and Domestics from the Caribbean," *Socialist Studies* 5 (1991): 143–7.

35. Kathryn McPherson, "The Case of the Kissing Nurse: Sexuality and Sociability in Canadian Nursing, 1920–1967," in K McPherson, C Morgan, and Nancy Forestell, eds., *Gendered Pasts: Historical Essays in Femininity and Masculinity in Canada* (Toronto: Oxford University Press, 1999).

36. Agnes Calliste, "Women of 'Exceptional Merit': Immigration of Caribbean Nurses to Canada," *Canadian Journal of Women and the Law* 6(1): 85–103 (1993); Karen Flynn, "Race, Class, and Gender: Black Nurses in Ontario, 1950–1980," (PhD diss., Department of Women's Studies, York University, 2002).

37. Aline Charles, "Women's Work in Eclipse: Nuns in Quebec Hospitals, 1940–1980," in G Feldberg, M Ladd-Taylor, A Li, and K McPherson, eds., *Women, Health and Nation: Canada and the United States since 1945* (Montreal: McGill-Queen's University Press, 2003).

Chapter 6

"Body Work," Medical Technology, and Hospital Nursing Practice

1. Anselm Strauss, Shizuko Fagerhaugh, Barbara Suczek, and Carol Wiener, *Social Organization of Medical Work* (Chicago: University of Chicago Press, 1985), ix. Strauss et al. described "body work" primarily as work on patients' malfunctioning bodies, acknowledging but neglecting the concept of working with one's own body. See also Cynthia Toman, "Blood Work: Canadian Nursing and Blood Transfusion, 1942–1990," *Nursing History Review* 9 (2001): 51–78 and Kathryn McPherson, *Bedside Matters: The Transformation of Canadian Nursing, 1900–1990* (Toronto: Oxford University Press, 1996), 74.

2. See Kathryn McPherson, "Science and Technique: Nurses' Work in a Canadian Hospital, 1920–1939," in Dianne Dodd, and Deborah Gorham, eds., *Caring and Curing: Historical Perspectives on Women and Healing in Canada* (Ottawa: University of Ottawa Press, 1994), 71–101, 75–7; and Bertha Harmer, *Textbook of the Principles and Practice of Nursing* (New York: The Macmillan Company, 1923).

3. Gertrude Armstrong Fawcett, audio-taped interview with author, 16 March 1999, at Ottawa.

4. Isabel Hampton Robb, *Nursing: Its Principles and Practice for Hospital and Private Use* (Toronto: J F Hartz, 1914), 151, 160–2.

5. Chris Dooley, "'They Gave Their Care, but We Gave Loving Care': Defining and Defending Boundaries of Skill and Craft in the Nursing Service of a Manitoba Mental Hospital during the Great Depression," *Canadian Bulletin of Medical History* 21(2): in press (2004); and Veryl M Tipliski, "Parting at the Crossroads: The Development of Education for Psychiatric Nursing in Three Canadian Provinces, 1909–1955," *Canadian Bulletin of Medical History* 21(2): in press (2004).

6. Standardized techniques were specific procedures with step-by-step instructions for performing tasks. They developed during the early 1900s, partially in relation to Taylorism or the Scientific Management movement, which focused primarily on efficiency or the "one best way of doing things" to get the most work out of labourers for the least amount of time and energy. Schools of nursing developed huge procedure books detailing every possible routine to follow for a range of tasks from making any one of approximately 15 to 20 kinds of beds, to dissolving morphine tablets for injection, to preparing the body after death, and much more. These standardized techniques were designed for safety — to prevent students from injuring patients and to prevent patients from picking up hospital infections (during the period before antibiotics were available to fight infections, these could literally be deadly). Standardized techniques were also designed to exploit free student labour and to extract meticulous obedience to supervisors.

7. Jean Milligan, audio-taped interview with author, 29 October 1997, at Ottawa.

8. See the *Rules for Nurses: The Lady Stanley Institute Training School of the County of Carleton General Protestant Hospital* (Ottawa: Crain Printers, n.d.), 6; and McPherson, "Science and Technique," 78–9.

9. Barbara Logan Tunis, *In Caps and Gowns: The Story of the School for Graduate Nurses, McGill University, 1920–1964* (Montreal: McGill University Press, 1966), 38; and Harmer, *Textbook of the Principles and Practice of Nursing*.

10. Hampton Robb, *Nursing: Its Principles and Practice*, 288.

11. Bertha Harmer, and Virginia Henderson, *Principles and Practice of Nursing*, 4th ed. (New York: The Macmillan Company, 1939), 598–617.

12. George M Weir, *Survey of Nursing Education in Canada* (Toronto: University of Toronto Press, 1932), 498, 15; Dorothy M (Grainger) Anderson, in E A Landells, ed., *The Military Nurses of Canada: Recollections of Canadian Military Nurses*, vol. 1 (White Rock, BC: Co-Publishing, 1995), 411.

13. Minutes, General Medical Board of the Ottawa Civic Hospital, 26 November 1954, MG 38, City of Ottawa Archives [hereafter as COA].

14. Hospital Annual Report [hereafter as HAR], Ottawa Civic Hospital Archives [hereafter as OCHA], 1944, 23–4.

15. Cynthia Toman, "Crossing the Technological Line: Blood Transfusion and the Art and Science of Nursing, 1942–1990," (MScN thesis, University of Ottawa, 1998).

16. Patricia Crossley, audio-taped interview with author, 26 January 1998, at Ottawa.

17. Minutes, General Medical Board, 28 September 1951, MG 38, COA; Minutes, Faculty Organization Folder, 15 January 1947, box 6, COA; Nursing Policy Book, 15 February 1954; "Blood Pressure," Nursing Procedure Book, July 1954, OCHA.

18. Esther Lucile Brown, "Nursing for the Future: A Report Prepared for the National Nursing Council," (n.p., 1948), 81, OCHA.

19. H W Henderson, "Delegation of Special Procedures: The Current Situation," address to the Ontario Hospital Association, 1 December 1981, College of Nurses of Ontario [hereafter as CNO].

20. Henderson, "Delegation of Special Procedures," 3; Helen G McArthur, "A College of Nurses for Ontario," *Canadian Nurse* 56(6): 515–8 (1960); and Helen K Mussallem, "Professional Nurses' Associations," in Alice J Baumgart, and Jenniece Larsen, eds., *Canadian Nursing Faces the Future*, 2nd ed., (Toronto: Mosby Year Book, 1992), 495–517.

21. Elizabeth Fenton, retired chief technologist of the OCH Blood Bank from 1943–1985, personal communication with author, 22 May 1998.

22. "Judicial Inquiry, vol. I–III," COA, MG 38, vol. 36. Judge Macdougall's decision is found in "Civic Hospital," Minutes of the City Council, 2 August 1949, 673, COA. See also, Minutes, Medical Advisory Board, 8 April 1952, MG 38, box 17, COA.

23. H E MacDermot, *History of the School of Nursing of the Montreal General Hospital* (Montreal: The Alumnae Association, 1940, re-issued 1961), 77.

24. Donna Zschoche, and L E Brown, "Intensive Care Nursing: Specialism, Junior Doctoring, or Just Nursing?" *American Journal of Nursing* (November, 1969): 2373.

25. Margarete Sandelowski, "'Making the Best of Things': Technology in American Nursing, 1870–1940," *Nursing History Review* 5(1997): 4; and Margarete Sandelowski, *Devices and Desires: Gender, Technology, and American Nursing* (Chapel Hill, NC: The University of North Carolina Press, 2000).

26. Kathy Slattery, audio-taped interview with author, 10 February 1998, at Ottawa.

27. Audio-taped interviews of Pat Doucett, Connie Buckley, and Gwen Hefferman with the author and Evelyn Kerr during the spring of 1995, at Ottawa.

28. Doucett interview; and Wilbert Keon, audio-taped interview with Evelyn Kerr and the author on 14 March 1995, at Ottawa.

29. Titled as "Nov 10/70 1130 AM," this poem was found in an unpublished, personal collection called "Poems from the Bards," in the possession of Pat Doucett, Ottawa, Ontario.

30. Rosemary Prince Coombs, "Active-Care Hospital Nurse Expands Her Role," *Canadian Nurse* 66(10): 23–27 (October 1970); and Rosemary Prince Coombs, "Creating a Therapeutic Environment," *Canadian Nurse* 61(11): 889–95 (November 1965).

31. Wendy McKnight Nicklin, audio-taped interview with author, 21 April 1998, at Ottawa.

Chapter 7

Public Health Nursing

1. This story is recounted in Monica M Green, *Through the Years with Public Health Nursing: A History of Public Health Nursing in the Provincial Government Jurisdiction British Columbia* (Ottawa, ON: Canadian Public Health Association, 1984), 101–7.

2. Amy V Wilson, *No Man Stands Alone* (London: Hodder & Stoughton, Ltd., 1965), 3.

3. Green, *Through the Years with Public Health Nursing*, 104.

4. University-based post-diploma programs in public health were established in 1919 in five Canadian universities with financial support from the Canadian Red Cross and /or the Rockefeller Foundation. Prior to 1919, and for a short period thereafter, the Victorian Order of Nurses for Canada operated Training Centres for graduates of diploma nursing programs in several major Canadian cities. See Diana J Mansell, *Forging the Future: A History of Nursing in Canada* (Ann Arbor, MI: Thomas Press, 2004); Kathryn McPherson, *Bedside Matters: The Transformation of Canadian Nursing, 1900–1990* (Toronto, ON: Oxford University Press, 1996); Sheila Penney, *A Century of Caring: The History of the Victorian Order of Nurses for Canada* (Ottawa, ON: VON Canada, 1996).

5. Wilson, *No Man Stands Alone*.

6. Bessie J Banfill, *Pioneer Nurse* (Toronto, ON: Ryerson Press, 1967), 9.

7. Margaret Scott Nursing Mission, *Annual Report for 1908* (Winnipeg, MB, 1908).

8. Kate Brightly Colley, *While Rivers Flow: Stories of Early Alberta* (Saskatoon, SK: Prairie Books, 1970); Gertrude LeRoy Miller, *Mustard Plasters and Handcars: Through the Eyes of a Red Cross Outpost Nurse* (Toronto, ON: Natural Heritage/Natural History Inc., 2000); Joyce Nevitt, *White Caps and Black Bands: Nursing in Newfoundland to 1934* (St. John's, NL: Jefferson Press, 1978).

9. Olive Matthews, "Child Welfare," *The Canadian Nurse* 16(1): 16 (1920).

10. Green, *Through the Years with Public Health Nursing*, 18.

11. Douglas O Baldwin, *She Answered Every Call: The Life of Public Health Nurse Mona Gordon Wilson (1894–1981)* (Charlottetown, PE: Indigo Press, 1997); Banfill, *Pioneer Nurse*; Colley, *While Rivers Flow*; Mary E Hope, *Lamp on the Snow* (London: Angus & Robertson, 1955); Miller, *Mustard Plasters and Handcars.*

12. Geoffrey Bilson, *A Darkened House: Cholera in Nineteenth-Century Canada* (Toronto, ON: University of Toronto Press, 1980); R D Defries, ed., *The Development of Public Health in Canada* (Ottawa, ON: Canadian Public Health Association, 1940).

13. Helen MacMurchy, "New Field for Nurses," *The Canadian Nurse*, 3(9): 487 (1907).

14. These incidents are documented in Heather MacDougall, *Activists and Advocates: Toronto's Health Department 1883–1993* (Toronto, ON: Dundurn Press, 1990), 128.

15. The two national anti-tuberculosis societies were the National Sanatorium Association, founded in 1896, and the Canadian Association for the Prevention of Consumption and Other Forms of Tuberculosis, founded in 1901. See MacDougall, *Activists & Advocates*; Katherine McCuaig, *The Weariness, the Fever, and the Fret: The Campaign against Tuberculosis in Canada 1900–1950* (Montreal, QC: McGill-Queen's University Press, 1999).

16. City of Winnipeg Health Department, Annual Report for the Year Ending December 1914 (Winnipeg, MB, 1915).

17. Montreal's Tuberculosis League hired a nurse from the VON in 1907 to provide similar services in that city. In 1909, tuberculosis nursing was established in Winnipeg and Colchester County by the local anti-tuberculosis societies. Vancouver's anti-tuberculosis society hired its first full-time nurse in 1914. R D Defries, ed., *The Federal and Provincial Health Services in Canada: A Volume Commemorating the Fiftieth Year of the Canadian Public Health Association and of the Canadian Journal of Public Health 1910–1959* (Ottawa, ON: Canadian Public Health Association, 1959); John Murray Gibbon, *The Victorian Order of Nurses for Canada: 50th Anniversary 1897–1947* (Montreal, QC: Southam Press, 1947); M L Meiklejohn, "Anti-tuberculosis Work in Canada," *The Canadian Nurse* 3(11): 581–5 (1907); Marion Royce, *Eunice Dyke, Health Care Pioneer: From Pioneer Public Health Nurse to Advocate for the Aged* (Toronto, ON: Dundurn Press, 1983); Glennis Zilm, and Ethel Warbinek, "Early Tuberculosis Nursing in British Columbia," *The Canadian Journal of Nursing Research* 27(3): 65–82 (1995). Christina Mitchell wrote a very informative article about her work in *The Canadian Nurse*. See Christina A Mitchell, "Chronic Tuberculosis," *The Canadian Nurse* 3(2): 54–6 (1907).

18. Two Canadian medical historians have examined the history of tuberculosis in Canadian society during this era. Although these monographs provide a detailed description of Canada's efforts to control and eradicate tuberculosis, neither source provides much discussion of the role that public health nurses played in this campaign. See McCuaig, *The Weariness, the Fever, and the Fret*; George Jasper Wherrett, *The Miracle of the Empty Beds: A History of Tuberculosis in Canada* (Toronto, ON: University of Toronto Press, 1977).

19. City of Winnipeg Health Department, *Annual Report for the Year Ending December 1908* (Winnipeg, MB, 1909); Defries, ed., *The Development of Public Health in Canada*; MacDougall, *Activists & Advocates*; Mona Gleason, "Race, Class and Health: School Medical Inspection and 'Healthy' Children in British Columbia, 1890–1930," *Canadian Bulletin of Medical History* 19(1): 95–112 (2002); Neil Sutherland, *Children in English-Canadian Society* (Waterloo, ON: Wilfrid Laurier Press, 2000).

20. All of these experiences are recounted in Gleason, "Race, Class and Health."

21. City of Winnipeg Health Department, *Annual Report for the Year Ending December 1910* (Winnipeg, MB, 1911); City of Winnipeg Health Department, *Annual Report for the Year Ending December 1914* (Winnipeg, MB, 1915); Gibbon, *The Victorian Order of Nurses for Canada*; MacDougall, *Activists & Advocates*; Royce, *Eunice Dyke, Health Care Pioneer.*

22. Denyse Baillargeon, "Gouttes de lait et soif de pouvoir: Les dessous de la luttel contre la moralité infantile à Montreal, 1910–1935," *Canadian Bulletin of Medical History* 15(1): 27–57 (1980).

23. Margaret Scott Nursing Mission, *Annual Report for 1909* (Winnipeg, MB, 1909).

24. Eunice Dyke, cited in Royce, *Eunice Dyke, Health Care Pioneer*, 49.

25. Defries, ed., *The Federal and Provincial Health Services in Canada*; John F Hutchinson, *Champions of Charity: War and the Rise of the Red Cross* (Boulder, CO: Westview Press, 1996); Susan E Riddell, "Curing Society's Ills: Public Health Nurses and Public Health in Rural British Columbia, 1916–1946 (MA thesis, Simon Fraser University, 1991); Meryn E Stuart, "Let Not the People Perish for Lack of Knowledge: Public Health Nursing and the Ontario Rural Child Welfare Project, 1916–1930" (PhD diss., University of Pennsylvania, 1987).

26. Douglas Baldwin, "Interconnecting the Personal and Public: Support Networks of Mona Wilson," *Journal of Nursing Research* 23(3): 26 (1995).

27. Meryn Stuart, "'Half a Loaf is Better than No Bread': Public Health Nurses and Physicians in Ontario, 1920–1925," *Nursing Research* 41(1): 21 (1992).

28. Ethel Johns, "Ideals of Public Health Nursing," *The Canadian Nurse* 14(3): 910 (1918).

29. This story and further discussion about the sometimes difficult working relationship between public health nurses and physicians in Northern Ontario appears in Stuart, "'Half a Loaf is Better than No Bread,'" 21–7. See also Meryn Stuart, "Ideology and Experience: Public Health Nursing and the Ontario Rural Child Welfare Project, 1920–1925," *Canadian Bulletin of Medical History* 6 (1989): 111–31.

30. Wilson, *No Man Stands Alone*, 23.

31. The exact nature of the public health nurses' practice varies from one province and community to another. Two recent textbooks describe in considerable detail the range of roles and programs provided by public health nurses in Canada. See Lynette Leesburg Stamler and Lucie Yui, *Canadian Community Health Nursing* (Don Mills, ON: Pearson Education Canada, 2005); Miriam J Stewart, *Community Nursing: Promoting Canadians' Health*, 2d ed. (Toronto, ON: W B Saunders, 2000).

32. For an in-depth analysis of the global impact of reduced support for public health and communicable disease control systems during the last quarter of the twentieth century see Laurie Garrett, *The Coming Plague: Newly Emerging Diseases in a World Out of Balance* (New York: Penguin Books, 1994); and Laurie Garrett, *Betrayal of Trust: The Collapse of Global Public Health* (New York: Hyperion Books, 2000).

Chapter 8

Religious Nursing Orders of Canada: A Presence on All Western Frontiers

1. A "large" hospital is defined as one having more than 200 beds. John Murray Gibbon, and Mary S Matthewson, *Three Centuries of Canadian Nursing* (Toronto: The Macmillan Company, 1947), 484–91.

2. Jean-François Cardin, Claude Couture, and Gratien Allaire, *Histoire du Canada: Espace et différences* (Quebec: Les Presses de l'Université Laval, 1996), 33.

3. Estelle Mitchell, *Les Soeurs Grises de Montréal à la Rivière-Rouge, 1844–1984* (Montreal: Éditions du Méridien, 1987), 9–21.

4. Archives des Soeurs Grises de Montréal (at Montreal) (hereafter ASGM), Lettres de Saint-Albert, 1858–1877. Letter of Sister Emery in Lac Sainte Anne to Mother Deschamps at Montreal, 13 April 1860, 35. The original in French: "Ici, il faut être de tous les métiers. Il y a quelques jours j'ai montré à un pauvre homme à vanner de l'orge. C'était un peu extraordinaire de voir une Soeur Grise à un tel ouvrage...."

5. ASGM, Lettres de Saint-Albert, 1858–1877. Letter of Sister Emery in Saint-Albert to Mother Slocombe at Montreal, 6 January 1871, 247–53.

6. Deborah Rink, *Spirited Women: A History of Catholic Sisters in British Columbia* (Vancouver: Harbour Publishing, 2000), 6–27.

7. Margaret Cantwell, and Mary George Edmond, in *North to Share: The Sisters of Saint Ann in Alaska and the Yukon Territory* (Victoria: Sisters of Saint Ann, 1983), 91, give the following description of this fundraising event: A week-long Christmas bazaar was organized by a club, the 60 Ladies, to help pay off more of the hospital debts. A promotional folio, The Paystreak, appeared a few times to inform people of the bazaar, the types of debts, and the amount to be paid off. Dawson people came in crowds to the bazaar. Sister Mary Jules of the Sacred Heart, who had joined Sister Pauline as hospital cook, roasted turkeys for the "restaurant." Sister Pauline made candies; other sisters offered paper flowers dipped in wax. Sister Joseph adorned a handkerchief with Brussels lace. There was great rivalry among the booths, all adding excitement and colour to the bazaar. At the end, the president of the 60 Ladies presented the sisters with $12 000.

8. Cantwell, and George Edmond, *North to Share*, 79–106; Frances Backhouse, *Women of the Klondike* (Vancouver: Whitecap Books, 1995), 113–52.

9. John Murray Gibbon, and Mary S Matthewson, *Three Centuries of Canadian Nursing* (Toronto: The Macmillan Company, 1947), 484–91.

10. Claudia Helen Popowich, *To Serve Is to Love: The Canadian Sisters Servants of Mary Immaculate* (Toronto: University of Toronto Press, 1971), 2–17.

11. Ibid., Howard Palmer, and Tamara Palmer, *Alberta: A New History* (Edmonton: Hurtig Publishers, 1990).

12. Popowich, *To Serve Is to Love*, 46.

13. Ibid., 2–121.

14. For comparable examples from Quebec, see Normand Perron, *Un siècle de vie hospitalière au Québec: Les Augustines de l'Hôtel-Dieu de Chicoutimi, 1884–1994* (Chicoutimi: Presses de l'Université du Québec, 1984) and Yolande Cohen, *Profession infirmière, une histoire des soins dans les hôpitaux du Québec* (Montreal: Les Presses de l'Université de Montréal, 2000).

15. Pauline Paul, "A History of the Edmonton General Hospital 1895–1970: 'Be Faithful to the Duties of Your Calling'" (PhD diss., University of Alberta, Edmonton, 1994).

16. More details of this conflict can be found in: Archives des Soeurs Grises de Montréal (at Edmonton) (hereafter ASGME), Newspaper file, *Edmonton Bulletin*, 30 March 1899; ASGME, Newspaper file, *Edmonton Bulletin*, 10 April 1899; ASGME, EGH, Chroniques, 17 June 1897.

17. Pauline Paul, and Janet Ross Kerr, "A Philosophy of Care: The Grey Nuns of Montreal," in Bob Hesketh, and Frances Swyripa, eds., *Edmonton: The Life of a City* (Edmonton: NeWest Press, 1995).

18. Cohen, *Profession infirmière.*

19. Thérèse Castonguay, SGM, *A Mission of Caring, Catholic Health Association of Alberta: A Chronicle of the First Fifty Years* (Edmonton: Catholic Health Association of Alberta, 1991).

20. Paul, "A History of the Edmonton General Hospital 1895–1970."

21. Dr Édouard Desjardins, Suzanne Giroux, and Eileen C Flanagan, "Les écoles supérieures d'infirmières," in *Histoire de la profession infirmière au Québec* (Montreal: L'Association des infirmières et infirmiers de la province de Québec, 1970), chapter 18, 120–32.

22. Paul, and Ross Kerr, "A Philosophy of Care."

23. Cantwell, and George Edmond, *North to Share*, 99.

24. ASGME, EGH, Chroniques, 1915 to 1928, 24 June 1928.

25. ASGME, EGH, Chroniques, 1933 to 1960. A record number of 11 sisters went to the 1936 annual meeting, which celebrated the tenth birthday of l'Association Canadienne française de l'Alberta.

Chapter 9

Outpost Nursing in Canada

1. Letters from Maude Weaver to her mother and to her sister, Gwen, 21 July and 24 July (likely 1933). Originals held by Beth Boegh and Margaret Boone, daughters of Maude Weaver Boone. Our thanks to them both for permission to use this excerpt from her letters.

2. Relatively little has yet been written on this phenomenon in relation to nurses in Canada. See Cathy Leigh James, "Gender, Class and Ethnicity in the Organization of Neighbourhood and Nation: The Role of Toronto's Settlement Houses in the Formation of the Canadian State, 1902–1914," (PhD diss., OISE, University of Toronto, 1997). Some American authors have begun to explore the connection between women's health and social welfare work and the emergence of the social welfare state: Linda Gordon, *Pitied but Not Entitled: Single Mothers and the History of Welfare, 1890–1935* (New York: The Free Press, 1994); Molly Ladd-Taylor, *Mother-Work: Child Welfare, and the State, 1890–1930* (Urbana: University of Illinois Press, 1994); "Introduction," Seth Koven, and Sonya Michel, eds., *Mothers of a New World: Maternalist Politics and the Origins of Welfare States* (London: Routledge, 1993).

3. These included Vernon, Revelstoke, Kaslo, Barkerville, and Rock Bay in British Columbia; Red Deer, Indian Head, and Yorkton in Saskatchewan; Dauphin and Swan River in Manitoba; Copper Cliff, North Bay, Thessalon, New Liskeard, and Fort William in Ontario; and Pictou in Nova Scotia.

4. Sheila Penney, *A Century of Caring: The History of the Victorian Order of Nurses for Canada* (Ottawa: VON Canada, 1996), 15.

5. Meryn Stuart, "Shifting Professional Boundaries: Gender Conflict in Public Health, 1920–1925," in Dianne Dodd, and Deborah Gorham, eds., *Caring and Curing: Historical Perspectives on Women and Healing in Canada* (Ottawa: University of Ottawa Press, 1994), 49–70; Cynthia Comacchio, "'The Infant Soldier': The Great War and the Medical Campaign for Child Welfare," *Canadian Bulletin of Medical History*, 5(2): 99–119 (Winter 1988); Desmond Morton, and Glenn Wright, *Winning the Second Battle: Canadian Veterans and the Return to Civilian Life 1915–1930* (Toronto: University of Toronto Press, 1987).

6. Dianne Dodd, "Helen MacMurchy: Popular Midwifery and Maternity Services for Canadian Pioneer Women," in Dodd and Gorham, *Caring and Curing*, 135–61.

7. Monica Green, *Through the Years with Public Health Nursing* (Ottawa: Canadian Public Health Association, 1984).

8. A knitting circle is a group of women who organize to have knitting done by volunteers. They then sell the products and use the proceeds to support some cause.

9. Edgar House, *The Way Out: The Story of NONIA, 1920–1990* (St. John's Creative Publishers, 1990); Joyce Nevitt, *White Caps and Black Bands: Nursing in Newfoundland to 1934* (St. John's: Jefferson Press, 1978).

10. Sharon Richardson, "Frontier Health Care: Alberta's District and Municipal Nursing Services, 1919 to 1976," *Alberta History* 46 (1998): 5–8; also Richardson, "Political Women, Professional Nurses, and the Creation of Alberta's District Nursing Service, 1919–1925," *Nursing History Review* 6 (1998): 25–50.

11. Jayne Elliott, "Keep the Red Cross Flag Flying: The Red Cross Outposts in Ontario, 1922–1984," (PhD diss., Queen's University, 2004).

12. Nicole Rousseau, and Johanne Daigle, "Medical Service to Settlers: The Gestation and Establishment of a Nursing Service in Quebec, 1932–1943," *Nursing History Review* 8 (2000): 95–116; Johanne Daigle, and Nicole Rousseau, "Le service médical aux colons. Gestation et implantation d'un service infirmier au Québec (1932–1943)," *Revue d'histoire de l'Amérique française* 52(1): 47–72 (1998); Daigle, Rousseau, Francine, and Saillant, "Des traces sur la neige. La contribution des infirmières au développement des régions isolées du Québec au XXième siècle," *Recherches féministes* 6(1): 93–103 (1993).

13. Rousseau, and Daigle, "Medical Service to Settlers."

14. Judith Zelmanovits, "'Midwives Preferred': Maternity Care in Outpost Nursing Stations in Northern Canada, 1945–1988," in Georgina Feldberg, Molly Ladd-Taylor, Alison Li, and Kathryn McPherson, eds., *Women, Health and Nation: Canada and the United States since 1945* (Montreal and Kingston: McGill-Queen's University), 164.

15. Conlin Sterritt worked as an outpost nurse in the Peace River District from 1920 to 1932. Irene Stewart, *These Were Our Yesterdays: A History of District Nursing in Alberta* (Altona, MN: D W Friesen and Sons, 1979), 21.

16. Gertrude LeRoy Miller, *Mustard Plasters and Handcars*, 11.

17. Stewart, *These Were Our Yesterdays*, 20–32.

18. Zelmanovits, "Midwives Preferred," 165, 161; Letter from Louise de Kiriline to her mother, 24 June 1928, Louise de Kiriline Lawrence Papers. Trans. Jayne Elliott. NA, MG31, J18, Vol. 12, File 2-2.

19. Stewart, *These Were Our Yesterdays*, 138.

20. Letter to Dianne Dodd from Mrs Annie Lane, Salvage, dated 11 May 1998. Mrs Lane, who remembers at least eight nurses serving her community, began knitting at the age of 13 or 14 and continued well into her seventies.

21. Interview, Margaret Maclachlan with Jayne Elliott, Cornwall, ON, 10 February 2000.

22. Zelmanovits, "Midwives Preferred," 173.

23. Ibid., 177–8.

Chapter 10

Caregiving on the Front: The Experience of Canadian Military Nurses during World War I

1. To learn more about the life and work of Florence Nightingale, see F B Smith, *Florence Nightingale: Reputation and Power* (London: Croom Helm, 1982), and Vern L Bullough, Bonnie Bullough, and Marietta P Stanton, *Florence Nightingale and Her Era: A Collection of New Scholarship* (New York: Garland, 1990).

2. Few works have been devoted solely to the history of military nurses in Canada. John Gibbon and Mary Matthewson devote a chapter to the subject in their study *Three Centuries of Canadian Nursing* (Toronto: The Macmillan Company, 1974 [1947]). The studies of G W L Nicholson, *Seventy Years of Service* (Ottawa: Borealis Press, 1977) and *Canada's Nursing Sisters* (Toronto: Samuel Stevens, Hakkert & Co., 1975), on the medical services in the Canadian Armed Forces, are more explicit. For an excellent bibliography and recent review of the historiography of military nurses in Canada, see the introduction and bibliography in Susan Mann, *The War Diary of Clare Gass 1915–1918* (Montreal: McGill-Queen's University Press, 2000).

3. Nicholson, *Canada's Nursing Sisters*, 27.

4. Ibid., 33–4.

5. Ibid., 44.

6. Ibid., 44–5.

7. Statistics compiled from figures drawn from *Department of Trade and Commerce (Census and Statistics Office) Fifth Census of Canada*, 1911 (Ottawa: L Taché Printer, 1912).

8. This information was extracted from 25 interviews conducted with military nurses of the Canadian Expeditionary Force from 1977 to 1979 by Margaret Allemang, as part of the *Canadian Nursing Sisters of World War I Oral History Program* (Toronto: University of Toronto, Faculty of Nursing, 1977–79).

9. Nicholson, Canada's *Nursing Sisters*, 52.

10. Ibid., 46.

11. Ibid., 73.

12. Marion Wylie, *Canadian Nursing Sisters of World War I Oral History Program*. Interview conducted by Margaret Allemang, Toronto, Faculty of Nursing, University of Toronto, 1979, 22.

Chapter 11

"Ready, Aye Ready": Canadian Military Nurses as an Expandable and Expendable Workforce (1920–2000)

1. Jean S Wilson, "Notes from the National Office," *The Canadian Nurse* 35(8) (August 1939).

2. Mary M Bower White, audio-taped interview with author at Surrey, BC, on 20 October 2001.

3. Lee Anne Quinn, as quoted by Michelle Gagné in "Airevac Nurses in War Zones," *The Canadian Nurse* 92(2): 34 (February 1996).

4. Elizabeth B Pense Neil, audio-taped interview with Norma Fieldhouse at Kingston, Ontario, in March 1987, Oral History Collection, Margaret M Allemang Centre for the History of Nursing.

5. Elizabeth Smellie, "A Message from the Matron-in-Chief," *The Canadian Nurse* 36(9): 622–3 (September 1940).

6. Jessie Morrison, "Address to Royal Alexandra Hospital Nurses Alumnae, Edmonton, 9 December 1974," 87.4, 91.30, and 92.10, Alberta Association of Registered Nurses Museum and Archives.

7. Dorothy Surgenor Maddock, audio-taped interview with author at Ottawa, Ontario, on 26 June 2001.

8. Helen M Ross O'Brien in E A Landells, ed., *The Military Nurses of Canada: Recollections of Canadian Military Nurses* [hereafter Military Nurses of Canada], vol. 1 (White Rock, BC: Co-Publishing, 1995 and 1999), 159.

9. Ethel Johns, "This Heritage of Freedom," *The Canadian Nurse* 36(7): 403 (July 1940).

10. Gaëtane LaBonté Kerr, audio-taped interview with Lisa Weintraub at Montreal, Quebec, on 11 April 1985, Concordia Oral History Project, ISN 167796, National Archives of Canada [hereafter NA]; Gaëtane LaBonté Kerr, in Landells, *Military Nurses of Canada*, vol. 1: 338; and Lisa Bannister, producer, *Equal to the Challenge: An Anthology of Women's Experiences during World War II* (Ottawa: Department of National Defence, 2001): xiii–xv.

11. Edna O Waugh Beattie in Landells, *Military Nurses of Canada*, vol. 1: 78; Joan M Gore Spring in Landells, *Military Nurses of Canada*, vol. 1: 408; Marion Rhae Nichols Stewart in Landells, *Military Nurses of Canada*, vol. 1: 409; and Margaret H Middleton Counter in Landells, *Military Nurses of Canada*, vol. 1: 82.

12. George M Weir, *Survey of Nursing Education in Canada*, 498 and 15.

13. Elizabeth Smellie, "Minutes of the Matron's Conference," Ottawa, 27–29 May 1943, "Correspondence and Minutes of Meetings regarding Nursing Sisters, July 43/October 45," 147.73 C 132009 (D2) and "Appointment Statistics," 000.8 (D93), National Department of Defence, Directorate of History and Heritage.

14. Evelyn Pepper, in Landells, *Military Nurses of Canada*, vol. 1: 45–6; and Evelyn A. Pepper, Gaëtan (LaBonté) Kerr, Harriet J T Sloan, and Margaret D McLean, "'Over There' in World War II," *The Canadian Nurse* 62(11): 32 (November 1966).

15. Jean Ellen Wheeler Keays, audio-taped interview with Sheila Zerr at White Rock, BC, on 16 August 1994, Registered Nurses Association of British Columbia Library.

16. Frances Oakes, audio-taped interview with author at Guelph, Ontario on 15 May 2001; W R Feasby, ed., *Official History of the Canadian Medical Services*, vol. 1: *Organization and Campaigns* (Ottawa: Queen's Printer, 1956): 439.

17. Surgenor Maddock interview.

18. Marian McEwen, in Landells, *Military Nurses of Canada*, vol. 3: 251–2.

19. Constance Betty Nicolson Brown, audio-taped interview with the author at Ottawa, Ontario on 3 June 2001.

20. Doris Carter, *Never Leave Your Head Uncovered: A Canadian Nursing Sister in World War Two* (Waterdown, ON: Potlatch Publications, 1999): 12; White interview; and Kathleen (Rowntree) Bowman, in Landells, *Military Nurses of Canada*, vol. 1: 79.

21. T S Wilson, "Resuscitation in Battle Casualties," *Journal of the Canadian Medical Services* 2(5): 520 (1945).

22. F Mills, "A Letter from a Field Surgical Unit C.M.F. (Overseas)," *Journal of the Canadian Medical Services* 1(3): 187 (March 1944); Feasby, *Official History of the Canadian Medical Services*, vol. 1: 189.

23. Agnes J Macleod, "With a RCAMC Casualty Clearing Station," *The Canadian Nurse* 37(2): 95–6 (February 1941).

24. Jean Dorgan in Landells, *Military Nurses of Canada*, vol. 1: 128.

25. "Tells of Death of Winnipeg Nursing Sister," news clipping, Winnipeg General Hospital Nurses Alumnae Archives; "Last Post," *The Canadian Nurse* 38(12): 938–939 (December 1942); Marjorie (Cowan) Horton, in Landells, *Military Nurses of Canada*, vol. 1: 554–5.

26. Cynthia Toman, "'Officers and Ladies': Canadian Nursing Sisters, Women's Work, and the Second World War," (PhD diss., Department of History, University of Ottawa, 2003).

27. Tritt Aspler interview.

28. Cox Walker interview.

29. This information comes from 1145 Second World War Nursing Sisters' personnel files held by Library and Archives Canada. The data was generated from a routine document filled out by Department of Veterans Affairs counsellors when demobilizing armed forces personnel. The questions asked about plans related to veterans' entitlements for education, small business and land grants, resettlement needs, etc. This research was originally done while preparing my doctoral thesis. (See note 26 above.)

30. Roe Dewart interview.

31. Helen K Mussallem, audio-taped interview with author at Ottawa, Ontario, on 24 September 2001; Marion Lindeburgh, "Postwar Planning Committee," *The Canadian Nurse* 42(9): 791–2 (September 1946); and Barbara Logan Tunis, *In Caps and Gowns: The Story of the School for Graduate Nurses, McGill University, 1920–1964* (Montreal: McGill University Press), 19.

Chapter 12

Enough but Not Too Much: Nursing Education in English Language Canada (1874–2000)

1. Brian Abel-Smith, *A History of the Nursing Profession* (London: Heinemann, 1960), 73.

2. Theresa Christy, *Cornerstone for Nursing Education: A History of the Division of Nursing Education of Teachers College, Columbia University, 1899–1947* (New York: Teachers College Press), 36.

3. John M Gibbon, and Mary S Mathewson, *Three Centuries of Canadian Nursing* (Toronto: The Macmillan Company, 1946), 145.

4. Rondalyn Kirkwood, "The Development of University Nursing Education in Canada, 1920–1975: Two Case Studies," (PhD diss., University of Toronto, 1988), 276–7.

5. Kathryn McPherson, *Bedside Matters*, 10.

6. Blanche Duncanson, "The Development of Nursing at the Diploma Level" in Mary Quale Innis, ed., *Education in a Changing Society* (Toronto: University of Toronto Press, 1970), 109–29.

7. Rae Chittick, interview with Rondalyn Kirkwood, Vancouver, 12 August 1983, taped transcript.

8. Pauline Paul, "Nursing Education Becomes Synonymous with Nursing Service: The Development of Training Schools" in Janet Ross-Kerr, ed., *Prepared to Care: Nurses and Nursing in Alberta* (Edmonton: University of Alberta Press, 1998), 129–53.

9. Glennis Zilm, and Ethel Warbinek, *Legacy: History of Nursing Education at the University of British Columbia, 1919–1994* (Vancouver: University of British Columbia Press, 1994), 76–7.

10. George Weir, *The Survey of Nursing*, 379, 383.

11. Helen K Mussallem, *Spotlight on Nursing Education: The Report of the Pilot Project for the Evaluation of School of Nursing in Canada* (Ottawa: Canadian Nurses Association, 1960).

12. Helen Carpenter, *A Divine Discontent: Edith Kathleen Russell: Reforming Educator* (Toronto: University of Toronto School of Nursing, 1982), 15.

13. R B Ferguson, "Operating a Nurse Training School: The Financial Picture," *The Canadian Hospital* (27) (January 1951): 37–9.

14. A R Lord, *Report of the Evaluation of the Metropolitan School of Nursing, Windsor Ontario* (Ottawa: Canadian Nurses Association, 1952), 53.

15. C G Costello, and T Castonguay, *The Evaluation of a Two-Year Experimental Nursing Program, Regina Grey Nuns Hospital* (Regina: Grey Nuns Hospital, 1969).

16. Moyra Allen, and Marie Reidy, *Learning to Nurse: The First Five Years of the Ryerson Nursing Program* (Toronto: Registered Nurses Association of Ontario, 1971).

17. Margaret Allemang, "Nursing Education in the United States and Canada: 1873–1950," (PhD diss., University of Washington, 1974), 248.

18. Ethel Johns, "The University in Relation to Nursing Education," *Modern Hospital* 15(2): 1–5 (August 1920).

19. M Adelaide Nutting to Isabel Stewart, 16 July 1919, "History of Nursing Archives [microfilm]" (Ann Arbor Michigan: University Microfilms International), quoted in G L Dickson, "The Unintended Consequences of a Male Professional Ideology for the Development of Nursing Education," *Advances in Nursing Science*, 15(3): 67–83 (1993).

20. Robin Harris, *A History of Higher Education in Canada, 1664–1960* (Toronto: University of Toronto Press, 1976), 412.

21. Stephen Leacock, "We Are Teaching Women All Wrong," *Colliers* 68 (31 December 1921): 15, quoted in Margaret Gillett, *We Walked Very Warily: A History of Women at McGill* (Montreal: Eden Press Women's Publications, 1981), 15.

22. Elizabeth Logan, interview with Lynn Kirkwood, December 1987, Wolfville, Nova Scotia.

23. Edith Kathleen Russell, "The Canadian Nurse and Canadian Nursing," *The Canadian Nurse* 24(12): 627–30, 628 (December 1928).

24. Kirkwood, 127.

Chapter 13

Professionalism and Canadian Nursing

1. "Dorothy Macham: The Driving Force of Women's College," *Globe and Mail*, 24 August 2002, F7.

2. Diana Mansell, *Forging the Future: A History of Canadian Nursing* (Michigan: Thomas Press, 2003), 8.

3. Yolande Cohen, Jacinthe Pepin, Esther Lamontagne, and André Duquette, *Les sciences infirmières: genèse d'une discipline. Histoire de la Faculté des sciences infirmières de l'Université de Montréal* (Montreal: University of Montreal Press, 2002), 22–8.

4. Margaret Levi, "Functional Redundancy and the Process of Professionalization: The Case of Nurses in the United States," *Journal of Health Politics, Politics and Law* 5(2): 334, 343 (Summer 1980).

5. Shirley Marie Stinson, "Deprofessionalization in Nursing?" (EdD diss., Columbia University, 1969); David Wagner, "The Proletarianization of Nursing in the United States, 1932–1946," *International Journal of Health Services* 10(2): 272 (1980).

6. Cynthia Toman, "Trained Brains Are Better Than Trained Muscles: Scientific Management and Canadian Nurses, 1910–1919," *Nursing History Review* 11 (2003): 93.

7. Mary Kinnear, *In Subordination: Professional Women 1870–1970* (Montreal and Kingston: McGill-Queen's University Press, 1995), 7.

8. Margaret M Street, "Canadian Nursing in Perspective: Past, Present and Future," Keynote Address, Fiftieth Anniversary of the University of Alberta Hospital and the University of Alberta School of Nursing, 15 November 1974, University of Alberta, Edmonton.

9. Mary Agnes Snively, "The Toronto General Hospital Training School for Nurses," *The Canadian Nurse* 1(1): 6–8 (March 1905).

10. Dorothy Riddell (colleague of Alice Munn), videotaped interview with Diana Mansell in 1988.

11. Yolande Cohen, *Profession infirmière: Une histoire des soins dans les hôpitaux du Québec* (University of Montreal Press, 2000), 88.

12. Kathryn McPherson, *Bedside Matters*, 6–12.

13. Sioban Nelson, *Say Little, Do Much: Nurses, Nuns and Hospitals in the Nineteenth Century* (Philadelphia: University of Pennsylvania Press, 2001).

14. Terence Fay, *A History of Canadian Catholics: Gallicanism, Romanism, and Canadianism* (McGill-Queen's University Press, 2002), 147.

15. Cohen, *Profession infirmière*, 93–102.

16. Brigitte Violette, *Étude synthèse sur l'action des congrégations religieuses de femmes dans le domaine de la santé au Québec* (1639–1962), Historic Sites and Monuments Board of Canada/Parks Canada Report, August 2001.

17. Claudette Lacelle, *L'apport social des communautés religieuses catholiques présentes au Canada avant 1940: une étude préparée à la demande de la Commission des lieux et monuments historiques du Canada dans le but d'identifier les communautés religieuses catholiques susceptibles de faire l'objet d'une commémoration en raison de leur contribution à l'histoire canadienne*, Environment Canada, Parks Canada, Microfiche # 425, 1987, 37.

18. Esther Lamontagne, and Yolande Cohen, "Les Soeurs Grises à l'Université de Montréal, 1923–1947: De la gestion hospitalière à l'enseignement supérieur en nursing," *Historical Studies in Education* 15(2): 289, 291–2 (2003).

19. Cohen, et al., *Les sciences infirmières*.

20. Authored by Sister Denise Lefebvre, Adèle Levasseur, Germaine Dessureau, and Flore Bellemare.

21. Lamontagne, and Cohen, "Les Soeurs Grises à l'Université de Montréal," 273–97.

22. Yolande Cohen, and Éric Vaillancourt, "L'identité professionnelle des infirmières canadiennes-françaises à travers leurs revues (1924–1956)," *Revue d'histoire de l'Amérique française* 50(4): 537–70 (printemps 1997).

23. Edouard Desjardin, Eileen Flanagan, and Suzanne Giroux, *Heritage: History of the Nursing Profession in Quebec from the Augustinians and Jeanne Mance to Medicare* (Quebec: Association des infirmières et infirmiers de la province du Québec, 1971), 115; George Weir, as quoted in Desjardin, et al., *Heritage*, 85; Violette, *Étude synthèse*, 164.

24. Johanne Daigle, "L'éveil syndical des 'religieuses laïques': l'émergence et l'évolution de l'Alliance des infirmières de Montréal, 1946–66," in Marie Lavigne, and Yolande Pinard, eds., *Travailleuses et féministes: Les femmes dans la société québécoise* (Montreal: Boréal Express, 1983), 119; Yolande Cohen, and Michèle Dagenais, "Le Metier d'infirmière: Savoir feminine et reconnaissance professionelle," *Revue d'histoire de l'Amérique française* 41(2): 155–77 (1987).

25. Cohen, et al., *Les sciences infirmières*, 131–5 (Alice Girard quote, our translation).

Chapter 14

Unionization of Canadian Nursing

1. Annie F Lawrie, "A Plea for the General Duty Nurse," *The Canadian Nurse* 38(6): 409 (June 1942).

2. Kathleen W Ellis, "Breezes Blow Through the West," *The Canadian Nurse* 39 (January 1943): 23.

3. Helen A Saunders, "Facing the Facts," *The Canadian Nurse* 42 (March 1946): 215.

4. Alice Baumgart, and Mary Wheeler, "The Nursing Work Force in Canada," in Alice Baumgart, and Jenniece Larsen, eds., *Canadian Nursing Faces the Future*, 2d ed. (St. Louis: Mosby Year Book, 1992), 49.

5. Mark Bray, and Jacques Rouillard, "Union Structure and Strategy in Australia and Canada," *Labour/Le Travail* 38 and *Labour History* 71 (1996), 218.

6. Sharon Richardson, "'Lively Combat': Kathleen Ellis and the Canadian Nurses' Association's Lobby during the Second World War," *Canadian Bulletin of Medical History* 17 (2000), 209–27.

7. Isabel LeBourdais, "Collective Bargaining — RNAO," *The Canadian Nurse* 61 (July 1965): 529–30.

8. Esther Beith, "Report of the Labour Relations Committee," *The Canadian Nurse* 42 (September 1946): 693–5.

9. M E K, "Should We?" *The Canadian Nurse* 42 (November 1946): 935.

10. Evelyn E Hood, "Collective Bargaining," *The Canadian Nurse* 50 (December 1954): 968–9; Evelyn E Hood, "Economic Security in British Columbia," *American Journal of Nursing* 56 (1956): 583–5; Evelyn E Hood, "Province-wide Bargaining for Nurses," *The Canadian Nurse* 57 (November 1961): 1064–5; Glenna Rowsell, "Ups and Downs of Economic Progress," *The Canadian Nurse* 63(11): 26–9 (November 1967).

11. Kathryn McPherson, *Bedside Matters*, 22.

12. Phyllis M Jensen, "The Changing Role of Nurses' Unions," in Baumgart, and Larsen, *Canadian Nursing Faces the Future*, 560.

13. Rowsell, "Ups and Downs of Economic Progress," 27–9; Jensen, "The Changing Role of Nurses' Unions," 561–3.

14. Bray, and Rouillard, "Union Structure and Strategy in Australia and Canada," 220–1.

15. Raelene Frances, Linda Kealey, and Joan Sangster, "Women and Wage Labour in Australia and Canada, 1880–1980," *Labour/Le Travail* 38 (Fall 1996) and *Labour History* 71 (November 1996): 87.

16. Bray, and Rouillard, "Union Structure and Strategy in Australia and Canada," 221.

17. Baumgart, and Wheeler, "The Nursing Work Force in Canada," 51–2.

18. "RNAO Supports Central Union to Replace Bargaining Units," *The Canadian Nurse* 69 (July 1973): 8; "Ontario Nurses' Association Formed for Province-Wide Bargaining," *The Canadian Nurse* 70 (March 1974): 11–2; "Labour Relations Board Approves Central Union for Ontario Nurses," *The Canadian Nurse* 70 (March 1974): 8.

19. "SRNA Ends All Involvement in Collective Bargaining after Supreme Court Ruling," *The Canadian Nurse* 69 (December 1973): 12 and 14; "SUN Negotiates First Contract, Saskatchewan Salaries Now Competitive," *The Canadian Nurse* 70 (July 1974): 6.

20. Jensen, "The Changing Role of Nurses' Unions," 564–6.

21. Kathleen Connors, "100 000 New Members Later, Canada's Nurse Leader to Retire," Canadian Federation of Nurses' Unions Press Release, March 2002, Ottawa, ON.

22. Marjorie McIntyre, and Carol McDonald, "Unionization: Collective Bargaining in Nursing," in Marjorie McIntyre, and Elizabeth Thomlinson, eds., *Realities of Canadian Nursing: Professional, Practice and Power Issues* (Philadelphia: Lippincott, Williams & Wilkins, 2003), 324.

23. Desmond Morton, "Government Union Workers: A Review Article," *Labour/Le Travail* 35 (Spring 1995): 300.

24. Bray, and Rouillard, "Union Structure and Strategy in Australia and Canada," 222.

25. Judith Hibberd, "Strikes by Nurses," in Baumgart and Larsen, *Canadian Nursing Faces the Future*, 583–5.

26. McIntyre, and McDonald, "Unionization: Collective Bargaining in Nursing," 328–9; Janet C Ross-Kerr, "Emergence of Nursing Unions as a Social Force in

Canada," in Janet C Ross-Kerr, and Marilynn J Wood, eds., *Canadian Nursing: Issues and Perspectives*, 4th ed. (Toronto: Mosby, 2003), 299.

27. Hibberd, "Strikes by Nurses," 586, 589.

28. Janet C Ross-Kerr, *Prepared to Care: Nurses and Nursing in Alberta* (Edmonton: University of Alberta Press, 1998), 284–5.

Selected Readings

Allard, Geneviève. "Des anges blanc sur le front : l'expérience de guerre des infirmières militaires canadiennes pendant la Première Guerre mondiale." *Bulletin d'histoire politique* 8(2–3): 119–33 (Winter 2000).

Allen, Moyra, and Marie Reidy. *Learning to Nurse: The First Five Years of the Ryerson Nursing Program.* Toronto, ON: Registered Nurses Association of Ontario, 1971.

Baillargeon, Denyse. "Gouttes de lait et soif de pouvoir : les dessous de la lutte contre la moralité infantile à Montréal, 1910–1935." *Canadian Bulletin of Medical History* 15(1): 27–57 (1980).

Baldwin, Douglas O. *She Answered Every Call: The Life of Public Health Nurse Mona Gordon Wilson (1894–1981).* Charlottetown, PEI: Indigo, 1997.

Banfill, Bessie J. *Pioneer Nurse.* Toronto, ON: Ryerson, 1967.

Baumgart, Alice J, and Rondalyn Kirkwood. "Social Reform vs Educational Reform: University Nursing Education in Canada, 1919–1960." *Journal of Advanced Nursing* 15 (1990): 510–6.

Baumgart, Alice J, and Jenniece Larsen. *Canadian Nursing Faces the Future.* Toronto, ON: Mosby, 1992.

Beaton, Marilyn, and Jeanette Walsh. *From the Voices of Nurses: An Oral History of Newfoundland Nurses who Graduated Prior to 1950.* St. John's, NL: Jesperson, 2004.

Benoit, C. *Midwives in Passage: The Modernisation of Maternity Care.* St John's, NL: Memorial University, Institute of Social and Economic Research, 1991.

Boschma, Geertje. *Faculty of Nursing on the Move: University of Calgary, 1969–2004.* Calgary, AB: University of Calgary Press, 2004.

Bourgeault, Ivy Lynn, Cecilia Benoit, and Robbie Davis-Floyd, eds. *Reconceiving Midwifery: Emerging Models of Care.* Kingston, ON and Montreal, QC: McGill-Queen's University, 2004.

Bramadat, Ina J, and Karen Chalmers. "Nursing Education in Canada: Historical 'Progress'— Contemporary Issues." *Journal of Advanced Nursing* 14 (1989): 719–26.

Bramadat, Ina J, and Marion I Saydak. "Nursing on the Canadian Prairies, 1900–1930: Effects of Immigration." *Nursing History Review* 1 (1993): 105–18.

Calliste, Agnes. "Antiracism Organizing and Resistance in Nursing: African Canadian Women." *Canadian Review of Sociology and Anthropology* 33(3): 361–90 (August 1996).

———— "Women of 'Exceptional Merit': Immigration of Caribbean Nurses to Canada." *Canadian Journal of Women and the Law* 6(1): 85–103 (1993).

Cantwell, Margaret, and Mary George Edmond. *North to Share, The Sisters of Saint Ann in Alaska and the Yukon Territory.* Victoria, BC: Sisters of Saint Ann, 1983.

Care, Dean, David Gregory, John English, and Peri Venkatesh. "A Struggle for Equality: Resistance to Commissioning of Male Nurses in the Canadian Military, 1952–1967." *Canadian Journal of Nursing Research* 28(1): 103–17 (1996).

Carpenter, Helen. A Divine *Discontent: Edith Kathleen Russell, Reforming Educator.* Toronto, ON: University of Toronto School of Nursing, 1982.

Carter, Doris V. *Never Leave Your Head Uncovered: A Canadian Nursing Sister in World War Two.* Waterdown, ON: Potlatch, 1999.

Castonguay, Thérèse, SGM. *A Mission of Caring, Catholic Health Association of Alberta: A Chronicle of the First Fifty Years.* Edmonton, AB: Catholic Health Association of Alberta, 1991.

Chartré, Christine. *Le traitement des maladies contagieuses à la station de la Grosse-Île, 1832–1927.* Quebec, QC: Parks Canada, 2001.

Clint, Mabel. *Our Bit. Memories of War Service by a Canadian Nursing Sister.* Montreal, QC: Alumnae Association of the Royal Victoria Hospital, 1934.

Coburn, Judy. "I See and I am Silent: A Short History of Nursing in Ontario." In Linda Kealey, ed., *Women and Work: 1950–1930.* Toronto, ON: Canadian Women's Educational Press, 1974.

Cohen, Yolande. "La contribution des Soeurs de la Charité à la modernisation de l'Hôpital Notre-Dame de Montréal," *Canadian Historical Review* 77(2): 185–220 (June 1996).

———. *Profession, infirmière : une histoire des soins dans les hôpitaux du Québec.* Montreal, QC: Université de Montréal, 2000.

Cohen, Yolande, and Louise Bienvenue. "Émergence de l'identité professionelle chez les infirmières québécoises, 1890–1927." *Canadian Bulletin of Medical History* 11 (1994): 119–51.

Cohen, Yolande, and Michèle Dagenais. "Le métier d'infirmière : savoir féminin et reconnaissance professionelle." *Revue d'histoire de l'Amérique française* 41(2): 155–77 (1987).

Cohen, Yolande, Jacinthe Pépin, Esther Lamontagne, and André Duquette. *Les sciences infirmières : genèse d'une discipline; Histoire de la Faculté des sciences infirmières de l'Université de Montréal.* Montreal, QC: Université de Montréal, 2002.

Connor, J T H. *Doing Good: The Life of Toronto's General Hospital.* Toronto, ON: University of Toronto, 2000.

Daigle, Johanne. "Devenir infirmière : les modalités d'expression d'une culture soignante au XXᵉ siècle." *Recherche féministe* 4(1): 67–86 (1991).

———. "L'éveil syndical des 'religieuses laïques' : l'émergence et l'évolution de l'Alliance des infirmières de Montréal, 1946–1966." In Marie Lavigne and Yolande Pinard, eds., *Travailleuses et féministes : Les femmes dans la société québécoise.* Montreal, QC: Boréal Express, 1983.

Daigle, Johanne, and Nicole Rousseau. "Medical Service to Settlers: The Gestation and Establishment of a Nursing Service in Quebec, 1932–1943." *Nursing History Review* 8 (2000): 95–116.

D'Allaire, Micheline. *Les communautés religieuses de Montréal, Tome I. Les communautés religieuses et l'assistance sociale à Montréal, 1659–1900.* Montreal, QC: Éditions du Méridien, 1997.

Daveluy, Marie-Claire. *Jeanne Mance, 1606–1673.* Montreal, QC and Paris: Fides, 1962.

Desjardin, Edouard, Eileen Flanagan, and Suzanne Giroux. *Heritage: History of the Nursing Profession in Quebec from the Augustinians and Jeanne Mance to Medicare.* Quebec, QC: The Association of Nurses of the Province of Quebec, 1971; and *Histoire de la profession infirmière au Québec.* Montreal, QC: L'Association des infirmières et infirmiers de la province du Québec, 1970.

Dodd, Dianne, and Deborah Gorham. *Caring and Curing: Historical Perspectives on Women and Healing in Canada.* Ottawa, ON: University of Ottawa, 1994.

Drees, Laurie Meijer, and Lesley McBain. "Nursing and Native People in Northern Saskatchewan, 1930s–1950s." *Canadian Bulletin of Medical History* 18(1): 2001.

Feldbert, Georgina, Molly Ladd-Taylor, Alison Li, and Kathryn McPherson, eds. *Women, Health and Nation: Canada and the United States since 1945.* Montreal, QC: McGill-Queen's University, 2003.

Gagan, David, and Rosemary Gagan. F*or Patients of Moderate Means: A Social History of the Voluntary Public General Hospital in Canada, 1890–1950.* Montreal, QC: McGill-Queen's University, 2002.

Gagnon, France. *L'Hospice Saint-Joseph de la Maternité de Québec, 1852–1876.* Cahier 70, Cahiers de recherche du GREMF, Groupe de recherche multidisciplinaire féministe. Quebec, QC: Université Laval, 1996.

Gagnon, Hervé. *Soigner le corps et l'âme : les hospitalières de Saint-Joseph et l'Hôtel-Dieu de Montréal, XVIIᵉ–XXᵉ siècles.* Sherbrooke, QC: Productions GGC, 2002.

Gibbon, John M, and Mary S Mathewson. *Three Centuries of Canadian Nursing.* Toronto, ON: The Macmillan Company, 1946.

Gleason, Mona. "Race, Class and Health: School Medical Inspection and 'Healthy' Children in British Columbia, 1890–1930." *Canadian Bulletin of Medical History* 19(1): 95–112, 2002.

Goulet, Denis, François Hudon, and Othmar Keel. *Histoire de l'hôpital Notre-Dame de Montréal 1880–1980.* Montreal, QC: VLB éditeur,1992.

Green, H Gordon. *Don't Have Your Baby in the Dory: A Biography of Myra Bennett.* Montreal, QC: Harvest House, 1974.

Green, Monica M. *Through the Years with Public Health Nursing: A History of Public Health Nursing in the Provincial Government Jurisdiction British Columbia.* Ottawa, ON: Canadian Public Health Association, 1984.

House, Edgar. *The Way Out; The Story of NONIA, 1920–1990.* St. John's NL: Creative Publishers, 1990.

Jean, Marguerite. *Évolution des communautés religieuses de femmes au Canada de 1639 à nos jours.* Montreal, QC: Fides, 1977.

Keddy, Barbara. "Private Duty Nursing in the 1920s and 1930s in Canada." *Canadian Woman Studies* 7(3): 99–101 (Fall 1986).

Kinnear, Mary. *In Subordination: Professional Women 1870–1970.* Kingston, ON and Montreal, QC: McGill-Queen's University, 1995.

Kirkwood, Rondalyn. "Blending Vigorous Leadership and Womanly Virtues: Edith Kathleen Russell at the University of Toronto, 1920–1952." *Canadian Bulletin of Medical History* 11 (1994): 175–205.

Lacelle, Claudette. *L'apport social des communautés religieuses catholiques présentes au Canada avant 1940.* Ottawa, ON: Parks Canada Report No. 425, 1987.

Laforce, Hélène. *Histoire de la sage-femme dans la région de Québec.* Quebec, QC: Institut québécois de recherche sur la culture, 1985.

Lamontagne, Esther, and Yolande Cohen. "Les Soeurs Grises à l'Université de Montréal, 1923–1947 : de la gestion hospitalière à l'enseignement supérieur en nursing." *Historical Studies in Education* 15(2): 273–97 (2003).

Landells, E A, ed. *The Military Nurses of Canada: Recollections of Canadian Military Nurses.* Vols. 1–3. White Rock, BC: Co-Publishing, 1995–99.

Laurin, Nicole, Danielle Juteau, and Lorraine Duchesne. *À la recherche d'un monde oublié. Les communautés religieuses de femmes au Québec de 1900 à 1970.* Montreal, QC: Le Jour, 1991.

MacDougall, Heather. *Activists and Advocates: Toronto's Health Department 1883–1993.* Toronto, ON: Dundurn Press, 1990.

MacQueen, Joyce M. "Who the Dickens Brought Sarah Gamp to Canada?" *Canadian Journal of Nursing Research* 21(2): 27–37 (Summer 1989).

Mann, Susan. *The War Diary of Clare Gass, 1915–1918.* Montreal, QC: McGill-Queen's University, 2000.

Mansell, Diana J. *Forging the Future: A History of Nursing in Canada.* Ann Arbor, MI: Thomas Press, 2003.

McDonald, Lynn, ed. Florence Nightingale: *An Introduction to her Life, Work, Family and Domestic Arrangements.* Vol. 1. The Collected Works of Florence Nightingale. Waterloo, ON: Wilfred Laurier University, 2001.

McPherson, Kathryn. *Bedside Matters: The Transformation of Canadian Nursing 1900–1990.* Toronto, ON: Oxford University, 1996.

McPherson, Kathryn, and Meryn Stuart. "Writing Nursing History in Canada: Issues and Approaches." *Canadian Bulletin of Medical History* 11 (1994): 3–22.

Miller, Gertrude LeRoy. *Mustard Plasters and Handcars: Through the Eyes of a Red Cross Outpost Nurse.* Toronto, ON: Natural Heritage Books, 2000.

Mitchell, Estelle. *Les Soeurs Grises de Montréal à la Rivière-Rouge, 1844–1984.* Montreal, QC: Éditions du Méridien, 1987.

Mitchinson, Wendy. *Giving Birth in Canada, 1900–1950.* Toronto, ON: University of Toronto, 2002.

Mussallem, Helen. "Spotlight on Nursing Education: The Report of the Pilot Project for the Evaluation of Schools of Nursing in Canada." Ottawa, ON: Canadian Nurses Association, 1960.

Nelson, Sioban. *Say Little, Do Much: Nurses, Nuns and Hospitals in the Nineteenth Century.* Philadephia, PA: University of Pennsylvania, 2001.

Nevitt, Joyce. *White Caps and Black Bands: Nursing in Newfoundland to 1934.* St. John's NL: Jefferson Press, 1978.

Nicholson, G W L. *Canada's Nursing Sisters.* Toronto, ON: Samuel Stevens, Hakkert, 1975.

———. *Seventy Years of Service.* Ottawa, ON: Borealis Press, 1977.

O'Neil, J, and P Kaufert. (1996) "The Politics of Obstetric Care: The Inuit Experience." In W Mitchinson, P Bourne, A Prentice, G Cuthbert Brandt, B Light, and N Black, eds., *Canadian Women: A Reader.* Toronto, ON: Harcourt Brace, 1996: 416–429.

Paul, Pauline. "The Contribution of the Grey Nuns to the Development of Nursing in Canada: Historical Issues." *Canadian Bulletin of Medical History* 11 (1994): 207–17.

Paul, Pauline, and Janet Ross-Kerr. "A Philosophy of Care: The Grey Nuns of Montreal." In Bob Hesketh and Frances Swyripa, eds., *Edmonton: The Life of a City.* Edmonton, AB: NeWest Press, 1995.

Paulson, E, G Zilm, and E Warbinek. "Profile of a Leader: Pioneer Government Advisor Laura Holland, RN, RRC, CBE, LLD (1883–1956)." *Canadian Journal of Nursing Research* 13(3): 36–9 (2000).

Pearson, Anne. *The Royal Jubilee Hospital School of Nursing 1891–1982.* Victoria, BC: Royal Jubilee Hospital Nurses Alumnae Association, 1985.

Penney, Sheila. *A Century of Caring: The History of the Victorian Order of Nurses for Canada.* Ottawa, ON: VON Canada, 1996.

Perron, Normand. *Un siècle de vie hospitalière au Québec : Les Augustines de l'Hôtel-Dieu de Chicoutimi, 1884–1994.* Quebec, QC: Université du Québec, 1984.

Petitat, André. *Les infirmières : de la vocation à la profession.* Montreal, QC: Boréal Express, 1989.

Popowich, Claudia Helen. *To Serve is to Love; The Canadian Sisters Servants of Mary Immaculate.* Toronto, ON: University of Toronto, 1971.

Richardson, Sharon. "Alberta's Provincial Travelling Clinic, 1924–42. Canadian Bulletin of Medical History 9(1): 245–63 (2002).

———. "Frontier Health Care: Alberta's District and Municipal Nursing Services, 1919 to 1976." *Alberta History* 46(1): 5–8 (Winter 1998).

———. "Political Women, Professional Nurses, and the Creation of Alberta's District Nursing Services, 1919–1976." *Nursing History Review* 6 (1998): 25–50.

Rink, Deborah. *Spirited Women, A History of Catholic Sisters in British Columbia.* Vancouver, BC: Harbour Publishing, 2000.

Ross-Kerr, Janet. *Prepared to Care: Nurses and Nursing in Alberta, 1859–1996.* Edmonton, AB: University of Alberta, 1998.

Ross-Kerr, Janet, and Jannette MacPhail, eds. *Canadian Nursing: Issues and Perspectives.* Toronto, ON: McGraw-Hill Ryerson, 1988.

Rousseau, François. *La croix et le scalpel. Histoire des Augustines et de l'Hôtel-Dieu de Québec I : 1639–1892;* and *La croix et le scalpel. Histoire des Augustines et de l'Hôtel-Dieu de Québec II : 1892–1989.* Quebec, QC: Éditions du Septentrion, 1989 and 1994.

Royce, Marion. Eunice Dyke: *Health Care Pioneer; From Pioneer Public Health Nurse to Advocate for the Aged.* Toronto, ON: Dundurn Press, 1983.

Scott, J Karen, and Joan E Kieser, eds. *Northern Nurses: True Nursing Adventures from Canada's North.* Oakville, ON: Kokum Publications, 2002.

Stewart, Irene. *These Were Our Yesterdays: A History of District Nursing in Alberta.* Altona, MB: D W Friesen and Sons, 1979.

Street, Margaret M. *Watch-Fires on the Mountains: The Life and Writings of Ethel Johns.* Toronto, ON: University of Toronto, 1973.

Strong-Boag, Veronica. "Making a Difference: The History of Canada's Nurses." *Canadian Bulletin of Medical History* 8(2): 231–48 (1991).

Stuart, Meryn. "Half a Loaf is Better than No Bread: Public Health Nurses and Physicians in Ontario, 1920–1925." *Canadian Journal of Nursing Research* 41(1): 21–27 (1992).

———. "Ideology and Experience: Public Health Nursing and the Ontario Rural Child Welfare Project, 1920–1925." *Canadian Bulletin of Medical History* 6 (1989): 111–31.

———. "War and Peace: Professional Identities and Nurses' Training, 1914–1930." In Elizabeth Smyth, Sandra Acker, Paula Bourne, and Alison Prentice, eds., *Challenging Professions: Historical and Contemporary Perspectives on Women's Professional Work.* Toronto, ON: University of Toronto, 1999: 171–93.

Stuart, Meryn, and Cynthia Toman, eds. *Canadian Bulletin of Medical History*, Special Issue on Nursing 21(2): 2004.

Toman, Cynthia. "Blood Work: Canadian Nursing and Blood Transfusion, 1942–1990." *Nursing History Review* 9 (2001): 51–78.

———. "'An Officer and a Lady': The Shaping of Military Nurses, 1939–1945." In Andrea Martinez and Meryn Stuart, eds., *Out of the Ivory Tower: Taking Feminist Research to the Community.* Toronto, ON: Sumach Publications, 2003: 89–115.

———. "'Trained brains are better than trained muscles': Scientific Management and Canadian Nursing, 1910–1939." *Nursing History Review* 11 (2003): 89–108.

Twohig, Peter. *Challenge and Change: A History of Dalhousie School of Nursing, 1948–1989.* Halifax, NS: Fenwood Publishing, 1998.

Violette, Brigitte. *Étude synthèse sur l'action des communauté religieuses de femmes dans le domaine de la santé au Québec (1639–1962).* Historic Sites and Monuments Board of Canada Report. Ottawa, ON: Parks Canada, August, 2001.

White, Mary M. *Hello War, Goodbye Sanity.* Surrey, BC: Mary M White, 1992.

Zilm, Glennis, and Ethel Warbinek. "Early Tuberculosis Nursing in British Columbia." *Canadian Journal of Nursing Research* 27(3): 65–82 (1995).

———. *Legacy: History of Nursing Education at the University of British Columbia 1919–1994.* Vancouver, BC: University of British Columbia School of Nursing, 1994.

Contributors

Geneviève Allard holds an MA (History) from Université Laval and currently works at Library and Archives Canada. She was, for a time, one of the archivists responsible for governmental military records. She is now managing projects to make cultural resources available on the Internet. Her research interests include military and medical history, with a specialized focus on military medicine, military nursing, and mental illness in the First World War. Her publications include "Des anges blanc sur le front: L'expérience de guerre des infirmières militaires Canadiennes pendant la Première Guerre mondiale" in *Bulletin d'histoire politique* (2000).

Christina Bates is the curator for Ontario history at the Canadian Museum of Civilization and is the author of *Out of Old Ontario Kitchens*. Specializing in social history and women's history, she has published in journals such as *Material History Review, Dress* (Costume Society of America) and *Muse* (Canadian Museums Association), and has contributed to books such as *Framing Our Past: Canadian Women's History in the Twentieth Century* and *Fashion: A Canadian Perspective*. She is chair of the Canadian Nursing History Collection Committee, and curator of the "A Caring Profession" exhibition on the history of Canadian nursing.

Cecilia Benoit completed her PhD at the University of Toronto and is currently a professor in the Department of Sociology at the University of Victoria. She has published journal articles and book chapters on mothering in Canada and a number of other high-income countries, comparative health and welfare systems, midwives' caring work in cross-national perspective, and Aboriginal midwifery in BC and other areas of Canada. She is author of *Midwives in Passage* (1991) and *Women, Work and Social Rights* (2000), and co-editor of *Birth By Design* (2001) and *Reconceiving Midwifery* (2004). Cecilia is a core partner of one of the five national Centres of Women's Health, NNEWH (located at York University).

Dena Carroll holds BA Sociology and MBA degrees from the University of Victoria. She has been involved with Aboriginal women's health, urban Aboriginal health centres, and health policy issues in British Columbia for over a decade. Dena is a member of the Chippewa of Nawash Band in Cape Croker, Ontario, and has published work relating to Aboriginal midwifery in BC and other areas of Canada, health care regionalization, and maternal health care. Dena is a community partner with one of the five national Centres of Women's Health, NNEWH (located at York University) and also serves on NNEWH's Research, Network and Training Committee.

Dianne Dodd (PhD Carleton) is an historian for Parks Canada, National Historic Sites and Coordinator of the Women's History Initiative. She has published in the areas of contraception, domestic technology, public health and nursing, and is co-editor, with Deborah Gorham, of *Caring and Curing: Historical Perspectives on Women and Healing in Canada*.

Jayne Elliott, a former nurse, recently received a PhD in the Department of History at Queen's University. Her interest in the history of rural medicine and nursing in Canada provides the focus for her dissertation and the article "Blurring the Boundaries of Space: Shaping Nursing Lives at the Red Cross Outposts in Ontario, 1922–1945" (*Canadian Bulletin of Medical History*, 2004).

Barbara Keddy, PhD, RN, is a co-founder of the Canadian Association for the History of Nursing and Professor of Nursing, Women's Studies, and Sociology at Dalhousie University. Dr Keddy teaches qualitative research methodologies, philosophical and methodological issues in knowledge and research, and the sociology of women and aging. Her current research interests include women and fibromyalgia, mid-life black women's health, and women and menopause.

Lynn Kirkwood, BN, PhD, was an associate professor in the Faculty of Nursing at Queen's University from 1974 to 2000 and is now retired. Her doctoral dissertation was an historical comparison of the development of two university schools of nursing and she has published in nursing and women's history journals as well as written two monographs related to nursing education.

Diana Mansell, RN, PhD, University of Calgary, currently has an adjunct appointment with the Faculty of Nursing, University of Calgary. She has been active in nursing for more than 35 years and is a past president of the Canadian Association for the History of Nursing. She is author of *Forging the Future: A History of Nursing in Canada* (2003).

Marion McKay holds a bachelor and a master's degree in Nursing from the University of Manitoba, and an MA (History) from the University of Manitoba/University of Winnipeg. She has recently received her PhD in the History Department at the University of Manitoba. She has held an SSHRC Doctoral Fellowship in support of her research on the early years of public health in Winnipeg. Prior to joining the Faculty of Nursing at the University of Manitoba, she worked for several years as a public health nurse.

Kathryn McPherson teaches history at York University and is chair of York's School of Women's Studies. She is author of *Bedside Matters: The Transformation of Canadian Nursing, 1900–1990* and has co-edited several volumes of essays, including *Gendered Pasts: Historical Essays in Femininity* and *Masculinity in Canada and Women, Health and Nation: Canada and the United States since 1945*.

Pauline Paul is Associate Professor, Faculty of Nursing, University of Alberta, and is author of numerous publications on the history of nursing, including "The Contribution of the Grey Nuns to the Development of Nursing in Canada: Historiographical Issues" in the *Canadian Bulletin of Medical History* (1994).

Sharon Richardson, RN, PhD, is an associate professor in the Faculty of Nursing, University of Alberta, in the areas of Canadian nursing and Canadian health care history, trends, and issues. She has published extensively on the history of Canadian nursing and health care. In over 35 years of professional nursing experience in direct care, administration, and teaching, in locales as varied as southern Ontario, the High Arctic, central Alberta, and interior British Columbia, Sharon has personally experienced many of the changes in the Canadian nursing labour force, including unionization. Most recently, she was president of the Alberta Association of Registered Nurses.

Nicole Rousseau, BA, BSc Santé (Nursing), MN, PhD (Nursing) is retired following a career as a professor at the Faculté des sciences infirmières, Université Laval. Her publications include articles co-authored with historian Johanne Daigle on the origins and evolution of the Quebec Medical Service to Settlers.

Cynthia Toman, RN, PhD is Assistant Professor at the University of Ottawa School of Nursing, guest curator for the military nursing module in the "A Caring Profession" exhibition on the history of Canadian nursing at the Canadian Museum of Civilization, and consultant to the Canadian War Museum on military nursing. Her doctoral dissertation is titled: "'Officers and Ladies': Canadian Nursing Sisters, Women's Work and the Second World War." She has published numerous articles on nursing history related to practice, gender, and medical technology in addition to military nursing.

Brigitte Violette holds a PhD (History) from l'Université de Montréal and now works as an historian with Parks Canada. For Parks Canada she has conducted an in-depth study of female religious communities in the health sector in Quebec and researched the settlement of the Gaspé Peninsula. She has also written historical notes for a number of commemorative plaques for the Historic Sites and Monuments Board of Canada. Her publications include "Entre l'émigration de la misère et l'eldorado mythique: genèse d'une petite-bourgeoisie franco-américaine (Fall River, 1870–1920)," in *Les parcours de l'histoire: Hommage à Yves Roby* (2002).

Judith Young, BScN, MScN, MA, now retired following a career as a pediatric nurse and teacher, was a founding member of the Canadian Association for the History of Nursing (1986). She has published historical articles focusing on the early years of the Hospital for Sick Children, Toronto, and on the care of hospitalized children between 1875 and 1975, and also co-authored *A Guide to Nursing Historical Materials in Ontario* (1994). She recently received an MA in History from York University.